10^{α}

9585

ALCOHOL

and

YOUR HEALTH

Louise Bailey Burgess

CHARLES

Charles Publishing
Los Angeles

Published in the United States by
Charles Publishing Company, Inc.
8350 Santa Monica Boulevard
Los Angeles, California 90069
and simultaneously in Canada by
Copp-Clark, Toronto, Ontario

Library of Congress Catalog Card Number 72-83315
ISBN Number 0-912880-01-5

First Edition September 1973
Manufactured in the United States of America

DEDICATION

*To my college-age grandchildren,
Sarah and Molly and Jerry, all non-users
of alcohol, whose abundant good health, keen
creative minds and strong moral character
are a constant source of joy and pride
to their parents and me.*

TABLE OF CONTENTS

FOREWORD

Alcohol and Your Health brings needed attention to the serious problems that can result from consumption of alcoholic beverages. We see the problems created by the drinking driver. The waste in the lives of our people, both old and young, that results from usage of this addicting drug is demonstrated. Various programs to combat the destructive nature of alcohol consumption among different segments of our society are examined. In general, this work is an account of the real cost to our society that results from usage of alcoholic beverages. It looks at the economic, physical, and mental waste created by America's most misused drug. The information presented by Mrs. Burgess in this volume should be more widely understood. The battle against the use and/or misuse of alcohol could then be won.

It was evident to me long before I came to the Congress that a comprehensive national program to help states and communities deal with problems related to alcohol consumption was among the nation's most urgent needs. As a City Judge in Salt Lake City one of my jurisdictions was the criminal court, the court before which anyone charged with drunkenness was brought for sentencing. During those years, alcoholism, from a legal standpoint, was treated like any other anti-social behavior problem. Although many of us realized then that it was an illness, we had no machinery for treating it. All we could do was sentence anyone picked up on a charge of drunkenness to a jail sentence—or, as an alternative, hand down a "floater" sentence which meant the defendant had to get out of town within twenty-four hours. This usually meant the problem was passed on to another court in another city where the same pattern would be followed.

It was a heartbreaking, baffling experience, a losing game every day of the week. The same drunks came before me day after day. I would give them a sentence that was long enough for them to "dry out." But they would be back again in a few days. Competent professional treatment was needed, but there was no way to provide it.

Thus, I know from personal experience as a judge, and from my general experience with the alcohol addicted—an experience that everyone inevitably has—what a towering medical and social problem this addiction represents to our society. It is a problem unequaled in its impact on life today. Its effects are so devastating, and so intermingled with our other problems, that it is impossible to estimate the total cost caused by its wide incidence.

When I came to the Senate I resolved that as soon as I could I would begin to work on legislation which, hopefully, would give the states and communities the help they needed to meet this tragic health-social problem. This has been one of my major fields of endeavor. In 1965, I introduced the Senate's first bill to bring the resources of the Federal government to bear on the problems resulting from alcohol consumption. When Senator Harold Hughes, a reformed alcoholic, came to the Senate, I readily deferred to his leadership and joined him and Senator Javits in developing a much broader bill, S. 3835, which the Senate passed on August 10, 1970.

Thus the Comprehensive Alcohol Abuse, Alcoholism Prevention, Treatment and Rehabilitation Act of 1970—Public Law 91—616—became Federal law on December 31, 1970.* As a result of this legislation, the future is brighter for millions of American families tragically affected by alcoholism.

—Frank E. Moss
United States Senator

*Public Law 91-616 is reproduced in full, beginning on page 203.

PREFACE

Despite the U.S. Department of Health, Education, and Welfare's *Special Report to the U.S. Congress on Alcohol & Health* in December of 1971, which defined use of beverage alcohol as the nation's No. 1 drug problem, the majority of our people still think of it as a beverage rather than a drug and unthinkingly accept the use of alcoholic beverages as part of our way of life.

Alcohol beverage consumption is at an all-time high. One in five adults knows some family member who drinks too much. Statistically one in 14 adults will become addicted. Physicians agree there is no way to tell in advance who may be susceptible, who will become addicted.

I have three grandchildren. I want them—I want every man, woman and child—to know the entire truth about the use of beverage alcohol: that it can all too often damage and destroy health, happiness and life itself.

My faith is in youth. They want a better world, a better future. Knowing the facts, many young people will no longer be ignorantly, innocently trapped. With no cure for alcoholism, with "recovery" dependent upon never taking another drink—absolutely forever—how many young people may well ask themselves, "Why start?"

It has been irrefutably established that moderation does not work because alcohol is an addictive drug. Though addiction may have progressed beyond one's own will power to control it, there is, in addition to many help agencies, a Power in the Universe greater than self. Acknowledgment of this is an all-important tenent for many who seek rehabilitation and recovery as, for instance, in Alcoholics Anonymous.

When Arnold Toynbee was asked by what this age would be remembered, he dared to believe "a better life possible for all people. We have it in our hands to give to history some new and unexpected turn."

I wrote this book because I believe we have history in our hands and that, given the facts, we will give it a new and important turn.

Louise Bailey Burgess
San Diego, California
September, 1973

1

ALCOHOL: ITS PROPERTIES AND EFFECTS

". . . the drug alcohol, will mire millions of Americans in a state of dependency, and maim or kill millions of others."

—Merlin D. DuVal, M.D.
U.S. Assistant Secretary for Health and Scientific Affairs

1

alcohol, n. 1. Also called ethyl alcohol, grain alcohol, ethanol, fermentation alcohol, spirits of wine, Cologne spirit. a colorless, limpid, volatile, flammable, water-miscible liquid C_2H_5OH, having an etherlike odor and pungent, burning taste, the intoxicating principle of fermented liquors, produced by yeast fermentation of certain carbohydrates, as grains, molasses, starch, or sugar, or obtained synthetically by hydration of ethylene or as a by-product of certain hydrocarbon syntheses: used chiefly as a solvent in the extraction of specific substances, in beverages, medicines, organic synthesis, lotions, tonics, colognes, rubbing compounds, as an automobile radiator antifreeze, and as a rocket fuel. 2. any intoxicating liquor containing this spirit. 3. *Chem.* any of a class of chemical compounds having the general formula ROH, where R represents an alkyl group and −OH a hydroxyl group, as in methyl alcohol, CH_3OH, or ethyl alcohol, C_2H_5OH. [<NL<ML<Ar *al-kuhul* the powered antimony, the distillate]

Only a portion of this definition is applicable to the terms of reference within this volume. We are not concerned with the use of cologne, antifreeze, or rocket fuel; we *are* deeply concerned with definition 2: "any intoxicating liquor containing this spirit."

THE ALCOHOLIC SCOREBOARD

36,000,000 Americans harmed directly or indirectly because of alcoholism or problem drinking.	**$21,700,000,000** latest annual expenditure by Americans for alcoholic beverages according to the Distilled Spirits Institute.
9,000,000 alcoholics or problem drinkers.	**$15 BILLION** annual economic drain because of alcoholism-in lost work time, health and welfare costs, property damage etc.
200,000 new cases of alcoholism each year.	**15%** (approximate) of the 400,000 patients in state mental hospitals are under treatment for the problem of alcoholism.
28,400 of the 50,000 killed in traffic accidents each year had alcohol in their blood at the time of the accident.	**OVER HALF** the states report alcoholism the most frequent diagnosis for first admissions to state hospitals.
500,000 disabling injuries are suffered in crashes involving problem drinkers.	**1/3** of all suicides are alcohol-related. **1/2** of all homicides are alcohol-related.
34,800 or more than half of the 60,000 nonhighway accidental deaths are alcohol involved.	**STEADY INCREASE** in the number of alcoholics admitted to state hospitals.
11,000 death certificates annually list alcoholism or alcoholic psychoses as cause.	**10-12 YEAR DECREASE** in life expectancy of every alcoholic.
2,000,000 (approximate) arrests each year for public drunkenness = 40% of all non-traffic arrests.	**IMPOSSIBLE** to estimate human suffering related to alcoholism, from broken homes, deserted families and problems of children of alcoholic parents.

The statistics used in *The Alcoholic Scoreboard* with one exception are based on material in a statement by Vernon E. Wilson, M.D. before the Senate Subcommittee on Alcoholism and Narcotics, March 8, 1971. Dr. Wilson is the Administrator of the Health Services and Mental Health Administration, U.S. Department of Health, Education and Welfare.

4

The Properties of Beverage Alcohol

The most widely consumed alcoholic beverages are beer, wine, and distilled spirits.

Beer is made of cereal grains fermented into a broth; wine is produced by the natural fermentation of grapes or other fruits; hard liquor (spirits) is produced through distillation. The process of distillation utilizes the difference in boiling point between alcohol and water. Alcohol, made from a variety of agricultural products, primarily barley, oats, and potatoes, boils at a lower temperature than water. When the solution of alcohol in water is boiled, a mixture or distillate containing about 95 percent alcohol results. The vapor condenses when drawn through a coil submerged in cold water, giving a liquid that has a very high alcoholic content.

Beer usually contains about 4 percent alcohol. Dinner wines, like beaujolais or chablis, are 10 to 12 percent alcohol. Dessert wines such as sherries contain more alcohol, somewhere between 17 and 20 percent. Distilled beverages, commonly called "hard liquor," range from 40 to 50 percent alcohol. A can of beer, a glass of wine and a cocktail or highball each contains approximately the same amount of alcohol.

The "proof" of a given alcoholic beverage is determined by doubling the percentage factor of pure alcohol it contains. The proof of a beverage containing 40 percent pure alcohol is obtained by multiplying the amount of pure alcohol by 2. Thus, a 40-percent alcoholic beverage is 80 proof. Some alcoholic beverages, including wine and beer, list the percentage rather than the proof. A wine of 14 percent is 28 proof; beer of 4 percent is 8 proof.

Obviously, this two-way standard of measuring and advertising alcoholic content can be confusing to the consumer. A 20-percent wine may be thought to contain only one-fourth the alcoholic content of an 80-proof whiskey; whereas, in fact, the wine contains one-half as much alcohol as the whiskey.

In answer to the question "Are beer and wine less harmful than distilled liquor?" Dr. Lindsay R. Curtis, in *Quiz Book—Funda-*

---

*The annual $21-plus billion expenditure for alcoholic beverages shown in The Alcoholic Scoreboard has been updated in The Second Report of the National Commission on Marihuana and Drug Abuse, issued March 1973, to $24 billion.

mental Facts Concerning Beverage Alcohol, says: "This claim is often made, but overlooks the way in which these beverages are consumed by the average drinker. Beer, with an alcoholic content of but 4 percent sounds much weaker than whiskey, with 40 to 50 percent of alcohol, but the quantities imbibed are very different. The steady beer or wine drinker may be consuming as much alcohol as the man who drinks whiskey. The ethyl alcohol in all these beverages is the same alcohol and has the same effect on the drinker." As Thomas Edison said, "Putting alcohol into the body is like putting sand in a motor."

How Alcohol Affects Us

Nearly all the foods we ingest must be digested and changed before the human system accepts them for use. Alcohol, however, almost immediately enters into the bloodstream in the same form in which imbibed. It then moves through the liver to the many parts of the body, including the brain. Alcohol is absorbed into the bloodstream so quickly that moments after it is swallowed it can be found in all tissues, organs, and secretions of the body.

It takes three hours for three one-ounce drinks of distilled spirits (hard liquor) to be cleared out of the body of a healthy 160-pound person. The body starts to do this clearing out through a process of 10 percent elimination and 90 percent oxidation. Oxidation is accomplished chiefly in the liver, where the alcohol is changed into acetaldehyde, a flammable, poisonous material, then to acetate (the acid of vinegar), and finally into water and carbon dioxide.

Alcohol supplies calories but no minerals, no proteins, no vitamins. Alcohol has no nutritional value.

A low level of alcohol in the blood, as would result from taking one drink an hour, has a mild tranquilizing effect since alcohol is a central nervous system depressant. Yet at first it may seem to stimulate. The brain consists of many layers, and alcohol's initial effects are exerted upon the upper parts of the brain where self-control patterns are stored. After a drink or two or three, depending upon the individual, a lack of self-control generally occurs, along with loss of inhibitions and, generally, greater volubility. If drinking continues, however, the alcohol frequently causes a switch to aggressive behavior and severe depression as well as other asocial behavior patterns.

6

Additional, continued imbibing can depress brain activity to a point where memory as well as muscular coordination and balance will be disturbed. Beyond this state, further drinking may have serious consequences. Severe nervous or mental disorders can result from heavy drinking over a period of many years. And, if the alcohol anesthetizes the deepest levels of the brain, coma or death may occur. Alcohol is the most common cause of convulsions. Recent research has shown that alcohol destroys irreplaceable brain cells. Like various other drugs, alcohol frequently produces withdrawal symptoms at the time its intake is discontinued.

Government Concern

At the 1971 American Medical Association in Atlantic City, New Jersey, Dr. Robert B. Forney of Indianapolis said of alcohol: "If it were just coming on the market now, it would be available only by prescription."

Dr. Roger O. Egeberg, Assistant Secretary for Health and Scientific Affairs, U.S. Department of Health, Education, and Welfare, in an address sponsored by the National Institute of Mental Health in Washington, D.C. in the summer of 1970, defined the alcohol problem as the "Number One health problem in this country." Dr. Egeberg called for an all-out research effort that would take precedence even over studies on narcotics and other illicit drugs.

Dr. Merlin K. DuVal, Assistant Secretary for Health and Scientific Affairs, U.S. Department of Health, Education, and Welfare (HEW) in '71, stated in that department's *First Special Report to the U.S. Congress on Alcohol & Health*,* that ". . . the drug alcohol, will mire millions of Americans in a state of dependency, and maim or kill millions of others."

This concern by government about the hazards of alcohol to the American consumer should, it is hoped, result in some protective measures—measures similar to those regarding other commodities considered deleterious and/or dangerous to public health. Every package of cigarettes, for instance, carries the warning that smoking is dangerous; dietetic soft drinks are differentiated from non-dietetic; the use of cyclamates and DDT are now viewed as

---

*This Report is published in full at the back of this book.

harmful. It remains an imponderable, therefore, that alcoholic beverages are not labeled as being a drug and "dangerous to your health."

It would seem that the National Institute on Alcohol Abuse and Alcoholism (NIAAA), established to carry out HEW's policies regarding alcohol and the public's health under Public Law 91—616, and the Surgeon General might well consider the labeling of alcohol-beverage containers as having a high priority.

2

ALCOHOLISM

"If alcoholism were a communicable disease, a national emergency would be declared."

—Dr. William C. Menninger

2

What Is An Alcoholic?

The World Health Organization states that "Alcoholics are those excessive drinkers whose dependence upon alcohol has attained such a degree that it shows a noticeable mental disturbance or an interference with their bodily or mental health, their interpersonal relations, and their smooth social and economic functioning; or who show the prodromal signs of such developments." This, of course, is but one of many varying descriptions of the alcoholic.

Dr. William C. Menninger once said: "If alcoholism were a communicable disease, a national emergency would be declared."

The word "disease" is frequently and generally used to denote the alcoholic's condition. If alcoholism is a disease, then it most certainly is a noncommunicable, after-the-fact one. For these reasons, the word "addiction" is replacing the word "disease" as the more accurate description of the physio-psychological state of alcoholism. The "diseases" that result from alcoholism are the results rather than the causes of the addiction. NIAAA has pointed out that "Alcoholism would be impossible without alcohol."

11

"Our concept of alcoholism as a disease is that, contrary to many other diseases, alcoholism is self-induced," stated Dr. C. Anthony D'Alonzo, medical director of E.I. du Pont de Nemours & Company, testifying in late 1969, before the Senate Subcommittee on Alcoholism and Narcotics, at Mt. Sinai Hospital in New York. "We must assume that one who cannot drink does not have to, or at least should not . . . thus, the disease is preventable."

According to Dr. D'Alonzo, "The alcoholic individual has been variously described as infantile, recessive, neurotic, selfish, irresponsible, and possessed of excessive momism. He has been accused of being a derelict and of lacking in moral substance. He has been linked to various and sundry psychiatric disorders, syndromes, and patterns. It has been our experience that the alcoholic, when sober, is just like the sober nonalcoholic. He is the person working or living next to you. When he is sober and not drinking at all, he is generally indistinguishable by personality, appearance, mannerism, or character from the other people . . . When he is drinking, however, he is apprehensive, anxious, jittery, perspiring, suspicious, easily swayed, and weak."

There is no scientific data to predetermine which drinking person will become addicted. As Dr. Curtis puts it, "A rotten bridge would be safe to cross *if* the timbers would not give way while you were crossing. The number of people who have not been able to continue to take alcoholic liquors moderately is large enough to make alcoholism one of the three leading social evils. Taking frequently such a habit-forming drug . . . is as unsafe as trusting one's weight to a rotten bridge which is known to be liable to go down under one."

Warning Signals

Alcoholism is a complex, progressive disorder; it creeps up on its victims and grows more virulent year by year. If not treated it ends, with few exceptions, in permanent mental damage, physical incapacity or early death. The chronic alcoholic has a physical and psychological dependence (addiction) on the drug alcohol. He can't stop drinking once he's started, even though alcohol is destroying his life.

Though there are warning signals, alcoholism happens without the drinker's conscious knowledge. Contrary to popular belief, the alcoholic is not found in great numbers on skid row; he is found among all strata of society. He may reside in an urban complex or suburban or rural community. He is not restricted to any particular nationality or race (although there seems to be less incidence of alcoholism among the Jewish and Italian people, and extremely high incidence among American Indians). There is no evidence that alcoholics consume any required amount of alcohol to support their habit. Authorities have concluded that the alcoholic is identified not by *how much* he drinks, but by *when* he drinks, *how* he drinks, *why* he drinks, and the ultimate effect of his drinking upon his personality.

Alcoholic addiction begins with social drinking. Insidiously, the drinking becomes more frequent. Then the drinker begins to find excuses for imbibing at times other than social occasions and readily makes excuses to himself for doing so, frequently blaming everyday problems. As anxieties and guilt increase, he may develop into a lone drinker, often "sneaking" an extra drink, becoming increasingly bitter toward his family, society, and his friends. He does his best to hide his condition from others and begins to worry about not being able to obtain alcohol. Finally, "blackouts" can occur; he finds it difficult to recall past and recent events. Much of what happened the evening previous, for instance, is hazy, or he remembers nothing of it at all, beginning with the point of "blackout." The alcoholic blackout does not mean a loss of consciousness, or even the individual's slumping into a chair or sofa in an apparent or actual physical eclipse. He will seem to others merely to have imbibed too much—far too much, perhaps—but he will be ambulatory and maintain a conversation, even tell or listen to a joke or two with laughter.

The next day he will be able to remember nothing of what he said or what was said to him; he will have suffered a "lost" hour, or two hours, or perhaps an entire weekend if on a binge. This is the man or woman who, the morning after, cannot recall driving home or where the car was left parked. In panic, he'll hurry outdoors to search for the car. Locating it finally, he'll return indoors, the panic easing but still there. A drink, he tells himself, will help settle him. And he has a stiff jolt to wash away the dismay, and the inner shame and embarrassment. The jolt will "settle" him, for awhile; then as the vicious cycle begins repeating itself he will need another, and another.

He is in serious trouble. He must have help.

However, helping him is generally not easy. As pointed out by Cecil Carle in one of his newspaper series which appeared in Southern California's *Valley News* "Treating the alcoholic is like the recipe for rabbit stew: first you must catch the rabbit. All recovered alcoholics know how true this is. Rarely has an alcoholic readily admitted that he is suffering from this killer disease until he is in deep trouble and the way out is torturous or impossible."

The Woman Alcoholic

This is as true of women problem drinkers and alcoholics as of men. The vast majority of women alcoholics tend to hide their drinking; they're generally expert at covering up the signs of their addiction. They usually are harder to reach and to help than men with alcohol-related problems. This is a major problem, since today it is believed that there are almost as many female as male alcoholics.

Part of the problem with alcoholism among women is the staunch double standard about drinking, even in these permissive times. Society will frequently tolerate a man who cannot hold his liquor (all too often it is incorrectly looked upon as being "amusing" or "manly"). But there is scorn for the woman who drinks too much in public. As a result, the female does her best to hide and deny her indulgences until it can no longer remain hidden.

But no double standard exists in the warning symptoms. The woman drinker often displays the same danger signs as the male. As a rule, warnings occur earlier than in the man headed toward alcoholism. Thus, if she will take heed in time, she may be able to stop drinking.

The High-Income Alcoholic

The upper-class alcoholic generally drinks for the same reasons as those in the lower socioeconomic groups—a sense of in-

14

adequacy, dependency problems, anxiety, depression, loneliness, rage, repressed sexuality, and fear of advancing age.

There are a number of private hospitals where those who can afford expensive treatment are given the utmost privacy while fighting to rid themselves of alcohol addiction. One of these is the Silver Hill Foundation in New Canaan, Connecticut. It is a beautiful, wooded country clublike area of 60 acres which includes a golf course, tennis courts, gymnasium, and indoor swimming pool. Every "guest" has a private room at Silver Hill where, says research director Dr. John S. Tamerin, "abstinence is [considered] the beginning, not the end of treatment."

By this, of course, Dr. Tamerin, formerly a research associate at the National Center for Prevention and Control of Alcoholism, means that, like a hard-drug addict, the alcohol addict is never actually cured; his only "cure," once he has gained the will to abstain, is to remain abstinent. One drink following detoxification and regained control and he'll be "hooked" again.

Medical director of this private psychiatric hospital, Dr. Charles P. Neumann, claims that 50 percent of those treated have been able to remain free of alcohol during the past 7 years. Differences in wealth and position, Dr. Neumann says, play no major role in the making of an alcoholic.

One case history from Silver Hill files is that of a corporate executive who in his fifties developed feelings of anxiety and concern associated with advancing age. Divorce and remarriage didn't work. During these years he attempted to offset his deeper feelings with alcohol. Because of his executive status, he was able to conceal his excessive drinking for a number of years. When he was fifty-nine, however, management, aware of his condition and the consequent cost and embarrassment to the firm, told him he must do something about it or retire. He is presently striving to do something about it and regain his former prestige. But this man will have a difficult time making it back to his executive suite since, like many alcoholics who have waited too long to seek help, he shows evidence of organic mental deterioration.

The case of this particular man is not rare, especially among the affluent who are in trouble with alcohol. As three physicians in a paper presented to the Academy of Psychosomatic Medicine observed: "It is possible that because of their high intelligence and

15

verbal glibness, these people [high income] can successfully deny and conceal the impact of their drinking.

"It is precisely the hazard of wealth and power and the fact that these individuals can take care of themselves so well, that their illness can be concealed until the individual patient may in certain instances no longer be amenable to treatment."

The Raleigh Hills Treatment Centers, located on the west coast, comprise another of the private systems available to those experiencing problems due to excessive use of alcohol. The hospitalization segment of their program is normally ten to twelve days, though longer periods are recommended whenever necessary. Facilities are situated at Redwood City and Newport Beach, California; Portland, Oregon; and Spokane, Washington. Raleigh Hills states that a major factor contributing to its 49 percent recovery ratio is a thorough follow-up during the year after the patient's hospitalization.

The Pain of Alcoholism

That all alcoholics lead a painful existence, which they strive to hide from the world, is attested to by the book, *Marty Mann Answers Your Questions about Drinking and Alcoholism* [Holt, Rinehart and Winston]: "Alcoholism hurts in every department of your life. Physically, the alcoholic always feels sick . . . very sick . . . except, of course, when he's had enough drinks not to feel anything. Mentally, the suffering is acute, because you can't stay high or drunk all the time, and at sober moments . . . especially about three o'clock in the morning . . . you know exactly what's happening to you, you see your life going down the drain, and you don't know why or what to do about it. Emotionally, it hurts terribly, since you are losing all you value and love, you are hurting those who love you, and you seem powerless to do anything about it. Socially, your life is a shambles, your friends begin to disappear, no one wants to come to see you, and they no longer invite you out. So far as your career is concerned, it's appalling, because your ability to function is gradually dwindling: whatever you do, you can no longer do it well. And financially it's a disaster . . . Ask any alcoholic whether his alcoholism was painful, and I think he will agree with me."

The alcoholic is generally a desocialized person. He doesn't belong; he probably has ostracized himself from the primary social group to which he should belong. He is alienated, living in two worlds. He very often is a sociable person; he likes to be with others, wishes to be the life of the party. But he can't do it without alcohol. Alcohol helps him feel as if he "belongs" and, in time, all too often forces him to withdraw. He becomes aware of others not wanting to be in his company, so he also moves away from them. By the time he has recognized that his drinking is beyond control, he usually has exhausted the patience of most of his friends as well as the members of his family. He is alone.

The Doctor and the Alcoholic

Many physicians are reluctant to accept alcoholic patients. "They're just too much trouble," one doctor said. "There's no way to control them. They get loaded and call you all hours of the night. They bug you. They won't follow orders. In short, they're the world's worst patients."

The medical director of the Alcohol and Drug Dependence Clinic of the Tennessee Psychiatric Hospital in Memphis, Dr. David H. Knott, states that one out of every seven persons who goes to a physician has a drinking problem, and that the patient cloaks the truth with a symptom for another illness. The physician often does not try to ferret out the true problem. "We're not talking about the skid row bum," Dr. Knott said, addressing an audience of about 200 doctors and health workers at a California seminar. "Rather, we're talking about the chronic drinker who denies that he has a problem and whose physician is unable or unwilling to confront him with it." Dr. Knott went on to say that there was no intent to indict physicians. "We're just trying to educate them. We want to increase their suspicions that there might be something below the surface of the patient's problems . . . "

There are, of course, a number of doctors who have dedicated themselves to helping the alcohol addicted. One of these is Dr. Ruth Fox of New York City, who began treating alcoholics thirty years ago. Dr. Fox says that she finds it necessary to devote two hours to the first appointment with a patient, the initial 45 minutes usually spent extracting an admission that there is a drinking problem.

When she started in this special practice, Dr. Fox states that the

17

average age of her patients was 45 years, whereas today it is 30 to 31. This can be a hopeful rather than a pessimistic sign. A patient of 30 presumably has not ingested as much alcohol as one 15 years older, presumably has more resiliency, and thus if he or she can get "clean" and stay "clean"—that is, remain abstinent—has an excellent chance for a normal, happy and successful life.

This is not to mean that the man or woman of 45 has less chance of attaining and maintaining lifetime sobriety. Virtually every medical authority in the field of alcoholism can cite numerous examples of "cured" alcoholics whose ages range from the teens through the eighties. Nonetheless, it remains a fact that with the passing of each year, the tolerance of man's body, and brain, for alcohol irrevocably decreases.

Most alcoholics are, at the least, difficult patients. But when the doctor takes his oath he vows to attend the difficult. In New York City today, 60 percent of the physicians do not treat alcohol addiction, and the other 40 percent admit that only 1 percent of their practice involves the treatment of alcoholics. Little wonder, then, that alcoholism has until very recently been recognized as "the illness that goes untreated" and "the cause conservatively of 86,000 deaths annually in this country."

States one authority: ". . . there is almost no education in our medical schools about alcoholism . . . The nature of alcoholism and the emotions associated with it."

In short, doctors' drinking habits as a group may distort their attitudes toward their patients with alcohol-related problems, and lead to under-diagnosis.

One doctor who is committed to working with alcoholics says of his collegues: ". . . this is not a job for the inexperienced—it is one of the toughest assignments in the world. Many have no faculty to do it . . . No good doctor, be he a general practitioner or an industrial physician, can fail to appreciate . . . the so-called hidden aspects of drinking, a staggering problem not yet adequately explored . . . .

"How then can any physician say that he is not interested in the problem of alcoholism? The problem of alcoholism is the problem of people, and the problems of people are in the province of the physician."

While alcoholism is indeed a problem of people, those hurt most

18

by the problem are the very young, who must so often remain under a roof where one or both parents are alcoholics. Texas District judges, for example, have estimated that over 60 percent of dependent children are the result of either parent, or both, using alcohol extensively. Judge Mildred Lilley, Los Angeles Marital Relations Court, has stated that "75% to 95% of marriages separated by divorce have alcohol as a part."

A Pilot Help Program

The alcoholic needs help. Will he seek help? Will he accept it? Who can help him?

Help *is* available. There are more deeply-concerned, dedicated people who want to help the alcoholic than he realizes. Here is what one relatively small help-agency accomplished, as reported at the hearings before the Special Subcommittee on Alcoholism and Narcotics, May 1970, by Daniel L. Howe, director, Alcoholism Information Center, Helena, Montana:

> When we first began our program* in Helena, we found amongst the general populace a very sick and apathetic attitude toward the alcoholic and his or her well-being, a very immature concept of alcoholics. In surveys we took we recognized that the people were stating that there is a problem and they felt that something should be done about it but their personal actions did not follow their beliefs.
>
> Hospitals that we dealt with saw the need for emergency care, but they always found excuses why they themselves could not establish treatment facilities.
>
> Law enforcement agencies, courts and prisons in the State, and in the county and on the city level, stated that alcoholism was causing more than 75 percent of their workload, but in our efforts to establish programs for them in the beginning, they were hesitant to change their present mode of dealing with the problem drinker.
>
> High school administrators stated 90 percent of their students were drinking, but they were at a stalemate as to what to do.
>
> Churches and civic organizations bemoaned the severity of the problems, but refused to speak about it from their pulpits and to the local press.
>
> The welfare departments and social agencies claimed that their case-

---

*A miniature test-pilot program based on theories included within bill S. 3835, which became Public Law 91–616.

loads were more and more the result of alcoholism, but only voiced a loud lament as a solution.

On the city and county level, the officials mumbled in confusion.

It was in this state of affairs that we found the community, and in which we began our pilot program.

. . . but after our beginning, after a relatively short period of time, 6 months, there is now enthusiasm, there is now a concern among all those agencies which I formerly mentioned showed such apathy, showed such ignorance.

This has come through the dedication of my staff, and I think it probably has come from the fact that we are a pilot program and do have the auspices and do have the concern of the Federal Government behind us.

When we first introduced ourselves to State official or local social agencies dealing with the problem, they would ask us if we were AA [Alcoholics Anonymous], as if it were a bad word. We told them no, that we supported it, but that our main backing was that we were a pilot project for the Health, Education, and Welfare Department. The minute we made that statement there were open ears. There was acceptance of our presence, and there was an immediate concern.

I believe there is a copout of the adult generation to place an exaggerated emphasis on the problem of drugs so as to avoid the real issue, alcoholism. I am not trying to minimize the problems drugs create, but to say that the problem of drugs is going to become an increasing problem in the United States and therefore we ought to look at that instead of alcoholism is naive, because alcoholism is growing at a rate far faster than that of drugs.

Where to Go for Help

Here is a suggested list of places to go for help.*

A superior in charge at work.

The nearest National Council on Alcohol (NCA) office.

Alcoholics Anonymous (AA).

A teacher or professor at school.

A clergyman.

A social worker.

Salvation Army.

Veterans Administration.

---

*A detailed, state-by-state listing of help agencies is to be found in the Appendices, beginning on page 179.

A doctor.

A hospital (though many hospitals still insist on treating problem drinkers and alcoholics under a mental-patient label. Presently it is estimated that approximately one of every three of the 1.5 million patients in state mental hospitals, for instance, are under treatment for alcoholism).

The above are not placed in order of preference. The troubled person should talk first with whomever he would feel most comfortable. The wife or husband of a person in trouble with alcohol should *not* attempt to "cure," for despite well-meant intentions more harm than good can result. If there is no AA, NCA or other agency nearby, write or phone the closest United States Department of Health, Education, and Welfare (HEW) office for information as to the nearest available help.

Anyone in trouble with alcohol should seek help, and *quickly*, for sudden death is the alcoholic's most constant drinking partner. Twenty-four percent of alcoholic deaths are violent—by fire, poisoning, suicide, accidents, and falls; 33 percent of sudden and unexpected deaths among young adults are attributable to alcoholism; alcoholics have a nearly 45 percent greater chance of dying in automobile accidents than nonalcoholics.

Alcoholics Anonymous

AA was founded in 1935 by a stockbroker and a surgeon, both hopeless alcoholics. Describing themselves as "a fellowship of men and women who share their experience, strength, and hope with each other," they not only helped themselves but set out to share their recovery experience freely with anyone who may have an alcohol-related problem.

The organization is concerned solely with the personal recovery and continued sobriety of its members. AA itself engages in no research, no medical or psychiatric treatment, although members often individually participate in such activities.

The first of the 12 steps in the AA program states: "We admitted we were powerless over alcohol—that our lives had become unmanageable." After acknowledging the need of a Power greater than self, the person who remains with the program relies on the aid of other alcoholics. The twelfth step calls for his helping others, not only for their sake but also for his own continued

21

sobriety. All of this occurs in a fellowship in which the alcoholic is unconditionally accepted as a peer.

Those who have entered and remained in the Alcoholics Anonymous program have found it has replaced, at least in part, their previous social activities. As a group, AA members seek to live without a drink from day-to-day, each member knowing the others stand ready to help in any emergency. To the person who is trying to change his lifestyle, readjustment is made less lonely through group meetings as well as by parties in the homes of AA members.

Offshoot organizations of AA have been effective in helping family members of the alcoholic. Al-Anon, an organization for spouses, relatives, and friends of alcoholics, is available whether or not the alcoholic is in AA. Al-Ateen, which shall be discussed further in chapter 4, is a parallel organization for teenage children of an alcoholic parent; Al-Atots is for still younger children.

Despite its proven worth, so complex is alcoholism that only an estimated 700,000 out of 9 million alcoholics—a mere 14 percent who so desperately need help—have found their way to, and remained with, the AA program.

Deterrents

Synthetic tranquilizers are being used to help acute cases of alcoholism. Other therapeutic aids, such as control of fluid and electrolyte balance, permit most patients who have recovered from delirium, hallucinations and tremors to start additional treatment.

With the more acute stages of intoxication passed, the alcoholic is not "cured." He must begin a long-range program of special treatment, which, of course, involves his not drinking. The most widely used and best known of the so-called deterrent agents to the consumption of alcohol beverages are Antabuse—frequently referred to as "the four-day insurance policy"—or Temposil. A patient regularly taking either of these compounds, with the slightest intake of alcohol suffers a pounding headache, flushing, nausea, and other severely unpleasant symptoms. That person can become very ill and death may occur in rare instances.

Such deterrents are, obviously, merely a temporary means to help the alcoholic not drink. Often the alcoholic patient is put into some program of psychotherapy. He has to be prepared

22

psychologically to accept the fact that the rest of his life must be spent without alcohol.

(See chart, pages 26-27, for the stages that lead to alcohol addiction and recovery.)

The recovering alcoholic who finds professional psychotherapy beyond his financial means should locate the nearest public health clinic. Many industries arrange for aid to their alcoholic employees. Also, many clergymen have increasingly interested themselves in this problem and can be of help in rendering advice and counsel. And there is Alcoholics Anonymous, which has chapters in most communities and will help lead the troubled drinker to a psychotherapy facility as an adjunct to AA aid.

The only hope for the permanent "curing" of an alcoholic is abstinence. In the past, attempts to control alcoholism have been punitive. The offender was thrown into jail or a mental institution. Today, attitudes are changing. As one leading authority in the field of alcoholism has declared:

"We must remove drunkenness as a socially accepted form of behavior. Every time we laugh at a performer or at anyone who is drunk, we are socially sanctioning drunken behavior, approving of someone who has gotten sick with a drug."

Teaching Programs

To render aid to the alcoholic there also are emerging agencies—some governmental, some privately sponsored—devoted to converting nonprofessional people into trained counselors to alcoholics and problem drinkers. The South Oaks Foundation, a recently formed nonprofit research group, sponsors a counselor training program at the South Oaks Hospital in Amityville, New York. This program, which supplies direly needed specialists to work as counselors who will also help to treat and rehabilitate the alcohol addicted, is among the first of its kind in the nation.

Those who enroll in the 40-week course become involved in lectures, field trips, introduction to treatment, and on-the-job casework. Upon completion of the course, the counselors are prepared to treat alcoholics in private industry, labor organizations, health clinics, and guidance centers. Among those now attending the South Oaks training program are a few former alcoholics, a priest, a doctor, and a bartender, all whose work have introduced

A CHART OF ALCOHOL

ENLIGHTENED AND INTERESTING WAY OF
LIFE OPENS UP WITH ROAD AHEAD TO
HIGHER LEVELS THAN EVER BEFORE

GROUP THERAPY AND
MUTUAL HELP CONTINUE

INCREASING TOLERANCE

RATIONALIZATIONS RECOGNIZED

CONTENTMENT IN SOBRIETY

CARE OF PERSONAL APPEARANCE

CONFIDENCE OF EMPLOYERS

FIRST STEPS TOWARDS
ECONOMIC STABILITY

INCREASE OF EMOTIONAL CONTROL

APPRECIATION OF REAL VALUES

FACTS FACED WITH COURAGE

RE-BIRTH OF IDEALS

NEW CIRCLE OF STABLE FRIENDS

NEW INTERESTS DEVELOP

FAMILY AND FRIENDS
APPRECIATE EFFORTS

ADJUSTMENT TO FAMILY NEEDS

NATURAL REST AND SLEEP

REALISTIC THINKING

DESIRE TO ESCAPE GOES

REGULAR NOURISHMENT
TAKEN

RETURN OF SELF ESTEEM

DIMINISHING FEARS
OF THE UNKNOWN
FUTURE

APPRECIATION OF POSSIBILITIES
OF NEW WAY OF LIFE

START OF GROUP THERAPY

ONSET OF NEW HOPE

PHYSICAL OVERHAUL BY DOCTOR

SPIRITUAL NEEDS EXAMINED

RIGHT THINKING BEGINS

ASSISTED IN MAKING
PERSONAL STOCKTAKING

MEETS FORMER ADDICTS NORMAL AND HAPPY

STOPS TAKING ALCOHOL

TOLD ADDICTION CAN BE ARRESTED

LEARNS
ALCOHOLISM
IS AN ILLNESS

HONEST DESIRE FOR HELP

REHABILITATION

Reprinted from
THE BRITISH
JOURNAL OF
ADDICTION
Vol. 54, No. 2

Chart can be obtained from National Council on Alcoholism

ADDICTION AND RECOVERY

them to the severe difficulties of the alcoholic and the problem drinker.

At one of the early program meetings Dr. Maxwell Weisman, psychiatrist and director of the Division of Alcoholism Control of the Maryland Department of Health, asked for a raise of hands from those people who drank. Approximately a dozen responded and Dr. Weisman said, "One of you is now or surely will be an alcoholic. Which one is it?"

When laughter rippled throughout the audience of 35 persons, the doctor stated, "Why the laughter? If I said, 'One of you surely will have, say, cancer,' would you laugh? Of course not. Even here in this group, why is there this flippant attitude toward alcoholism?"

There Can Be Cause for Optimism

As stated on page 82 of the December 1971 HEW *First Special Report on Alcohol & Health* (printed in full at the back of this book), alcoholism is chronic and often recurring, and "has multiple causations including genetic, biological, psychological, and sociological factors. These factors are found in different combinations and with different relative importance in each alcoholic person. To be successful, treatment must take these various issues into account. The body and its chemistry must be considered. So also must the love, hate, and fear that reside in the unconscious level of our minds—between spouses, among children and parents, within social groups and, ultimately, in the broad spectrum of society as it encourages or prevents alcoholicm.

"Alcoholism is a complicated disorder, but it can be treated successfully. Any technique used indiscriminately will be much less successful. When the proper treatment modalities are utilized for the unique needs of the particular patient, however, we indeed have cause for optimism."

ARE YOU AN ALCOHOLIC?

To answer this question ask yourself the following questions and answer them as honestly as you can.

	Yes	No
1 Do you lose time from work due to drinking?	☐	☐
2 Is drinking making your home life unhappy?	☐	☐
3 Do you drink because you are shy with other people?	☐	☐
4 Is drinking affecting your reputation?	☐	☐
5 Have you ever felt remorse after drinking?	☐	☐
6 Have you gotten into financial difficulties as a result of drinking?	☐	☐
7 Do you turn to lower companions and an inferior environment when drinking?	☐	☐
8 Does your drinking make you careless of your family's welfare?	☐	☐
9 Has your ambition decreased since drinking?	☐	☐
10 Do you crave a drink at a definite time daily?	☐	☐
11 Do you want a drink the next morning?	☐	☐
12 Does drinking cause you to have difficulty in sleeping?	☐	☐
13 Has your efficiency decreased since drinking?	☐	☐
14 Is drinking jeopardizing your job or business?	☐	☐
15 Do you drink to escape from worries or trouble?	☐	☐
16 Do you drink alone?	☐	☐
17 Have you ever had a complete loss of memory as a result of drinking?	☐	☐
18 Has your physician ever treated you for drinking?	☐	☐
19 Do you drink to build up your self-confidence?	☐	☐
20 Have you ever been to a hospital or institution on account of drinking?	☐	☐

If you have answered YES to any one of the questions, there is a definite warning that **you may be alcoholic.**

If you have answered YES to any two, the chances are that you **are an alcoholic.**

If you have answered YES to **three or more, you are definitely an alcoholic.**

(The above Test Questions are used by Johns Hopkins University Hospital, Baltimore, Md., in deciding whether or not a patient is alcoholic.)

27

3

THE DRINKING
DRIVER

*". . . It is the drinking driver who is
the menace, the one who thinks himself
keener, stronger and quicker when he is
duller, weaker and slower."*

—Dr. George B. Cutten
Past President of Colgate University

3

Alcohol Impairs Driving Skill

Approximately 45,000 Americans were killed in combat during the many years of war in Vietnam. Within any recent two-year span of this same period, over 50,000 were killed on U.S. streets and highways as the result of alcohol-related accidents. In 1970, 500,000 disabling injuries were suffered in automobile crashes involving problem drinkers. In data collected from 7,000 blood-alcohol determinations of dead drivers and pedestrians, California's Traffic Safety Foundation learned that 82 percent had a percentage level of 0.10 [one-tenth of one percent] or higher of alcohol in their blood. [In that state, up to 0.10 is the legal allowable percentage of alcohol in the blood. See page 38 for the legally acceptable percentage in all states.]

The drinking driver cannot accurately gauge how much or how little alcohol in his own bloodstream is "safe." According to Dr. George B. Cutten, past president of Colgate University, "Alcohol interferes with the performance of skilled movements, while the victim judges himself to be more skilled. It weakens his muscular powers while he considers himself stronger. It slows his reaction time, but he is sure he is speedier . . . He will soon run into a telegraph pole or precipitate himself into a ditch and eliminate himself from traffic. It is the drinking driver who is the menace, the one who thinks himself keener, stronger and quicker, when he is duller, weaker and slower.

"The reaction time—the time which elapses between sensory stimulus, such as seeing another car, and when we move our arms to steer the car—is about one-fifth of a second," states Cutten. "Alcohol slows this so that alcoholized reaction time may be two, three, four, or even more fifths of a second. At 60 m.p.h. a car travels 18 feet in one-fifth of a second. So instead of 18 feet, the car may travel 36, 54, or 72 feet before the driver takes any action, and usually that means trouble."

One drink slows a person's reflexes. After many years of experimentation, Dr. Francis G. Benedict, director of the Carnegie Nutrition Laboratory, said: "We have found that the consumption of even a small quantity of wine retards eye action to a point where it is unsafe for a person who had drunk wine to drive an automobile."

Levels as low as 0.05 percent alcohol in the blood may seriously impair the driving skills of certain persons; as the level increases to 0.10 percent (five to six ounces of alcohol), the American Medical Association states that "the degree of intoxication is such that the driving skills of everyone are dangerously altered."

The individual who likes to believe he drives *better* with a few drinks in him isn't likely to pay any attention whatever to blood levels and critical zones.

If you are reading this swiftly, perhaps too swiftly, then let John C. Rogers, writing in *Parade* magazine, give you pause as he quotes Willard Y. Howell, a director in the Department of Transportation, on the fact that over 20,000 highway deaths in the United States last year involved individuals considered problem drinkers: "That comes to 385 deaths a week. But do you hear any public outcry about that shocking figure? If a 747 jet crashed every week killing 385 persons, we would demand a grounding of that aircraft."

The drinking driver involved in a nonfatal accident, if it is a first offense, generally receives a fine or a warning, or both. If it is a second or third offense, the driver's license is usually suspended for a given period of time; the judge might insist upon a jail sentence being served as well.

Merely suspending a license, many authorities have discovered, fails as a deterrent. In a west-coast state, for instance, a recent study revealed that 68 percent of drivers whose licenses were revoked continued driving. In this same state, out of a group of 1,000 drivers who killed someone under the influence of liquor, only 25 percent received felony convictions for drunk driving, and less than 5 percent went to jail.

The Department of Transportation (DOT), which labels the drunk driver as the No. 1 highway killer, estimates that of the drivers whose licenses have been suspended or revoked for repeated drunk driving offenses, 80 percent continue to drive.

Once behind the wheels of their vehicles, heavy drinkers and alcoholics obviously become a dire city-street and highway threat. DOT estimates that though these drivers represent but a small fraction—about 7 percent—of those involved in accidents, they are responsible for approximately two out of three of all alcohol-related traffic deaths. The other third is caused by the "social" and "moderate" drinker.

That something can be done to decrease both fatal and nonfatal accidents by drinking drivers was proved in an experiment conducted by a lone Chicago jurist, Cook County Traffic Court Judge Raymond Berg. Judge Berg decided that during the final two weeks of December 1970—the Christmas holiday—all those convicted of a drunk-driving charge would be sentenced not only to loss of license for one year but also to a mandatory minimum seven days in jail. The results: Fatalities in Chicago decreased 65 percent during that period as compared with the same period of previous years. Injuries decreased 50 percent. There was an 80 percent drop in automobile crashes in which drunkenness played a part.

Who is the Alcoholic Driver?

Drinking drivers have been found to be as unlike in their driving skills and experiences as they are in imbibing tolerances and attitudes. "If you drink, don't drive" is a well-meant admonition. It is also one that realists know is not generally observed in our society.

Though two out of three fatal accidents are caused by the 7 percent mentioned above, social drinkers, comprising the great majority of imbibers, make up a large proportion of those involved in alcohol-related auto accidents. A Midwest study of 250 defendants convicted of DWI (driving while intoxicated) showed that 20 percent were problem drinkers or alcoholics while 80 percent were of the social or occasional-imbiber group.

This study was supervised by Dr. Edward J. Kelleher, director of the Chicago Circuit Court's psychiatric institute; and included also Dr. Arthur L. Conrad, director of the Circuit Court's traffic safety and education division, and Traffic Court Judge Berg. Examinations of the drivers were conducted by the professional staff of the psychiatric institute, consisting of psychiatrists, psychiatric social workers, clinical psychologists, and a brainwave technician.

"Upon examining and analyzing these defendants, as well as a group of nondefendants," the study reported, "it was further disclosed that the existence of a deplorable but prevalent attitude among the driving public exists . . . the attitude that the DWI laws are made for chronic alcoholics, not for the occasional or social drinker. Regrettably, we believe this attitude is being unwittingly encouraged by the current emphasis placed almost exclusively on the alcoholic driver."

Department of Transportation Program

DOT has recently established a seven-year, four-pronged program in an attempt to stem the tide of highway deaths related to the drinking driver. Jerome A. Holiber, Chief, Technical Office of Alcohol Countermeasures Programs Division, states: "The Office of Alcohol Countermeasures has been charged by the Department of Transportation with developing an effort to combat the tremendous toll of death and injury caused on our highways by drunk drivers. The thrust of our program occurs in four areas: a national public education campaign; research and development programs; Federal matching fund support for State and community alcohol safety programs; and Alcohol Safety Action Projects (ASAPs)."

Thirty-five ASAPs are underway in states and communities throughout the country. These multifaceted programs focus on law enforcement, traffic courts, special driver counseling, and public education in order to establish systematic ways of approaching the problem.

The Tampa, Florida, ASAP uses a new kind of questionnaire-interview to help distinguish between drinking drivers and drunken drivers. As part of the Los Angeles County ASAP program, television cameras have been installed in the dashboards of a number of patrol cars to apprehend drinking drivers who attempt to elude lawmen. Other DOT-funded ASAP cities also are initiating new, original measures to differentiate between the habitual drinking driver and the social drinking driver. Arrests have increased in most cities having ASAP programs.

The skeptics, pointing to the ever mounting toll of alcohol-related highway accidents and mortalities, contend that such programs have not succeeded, and cannot succeed, and insist that sterner measures be employed.

One director of an ASAP project was challenged: "And if that [rehabilitation] does not work?"

"Then," the director replied, "this country is faced with a continuing, serious problem it may never solve."

Legal Definitions of the Alcoholic Driver

The inconsistent regulations of the various states as to what percentage of alcohol in the blood constitutes a presumptively unsafe level contributes to a large degree to the nation's, and the individual citizen's, confusion about drinking and driving—a confusion substantially responsible for the shockingly high accident rate on our streets and highways.

The terms "Implied Consent" and "Presumptive Limit" add to the confusion for many drivers, though neither is difficult to understand. Implied Consent is the law which states that if you drive on a public street and are arrested, you have "implied" that

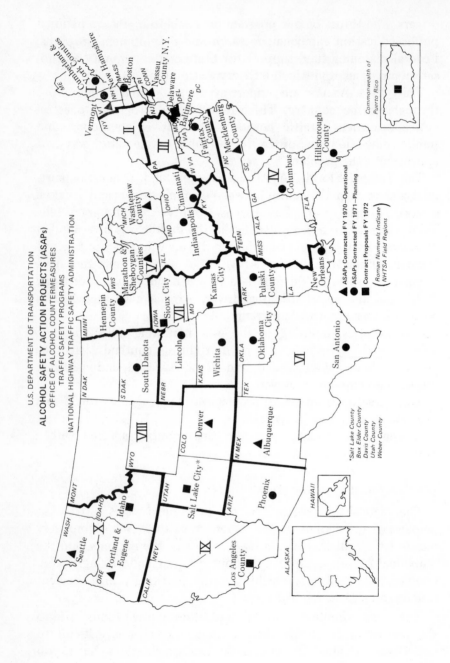

U.S. DEPARTMENT OF TRANSPORTATION

ALCOHOL SAFETY ACTION PROJECTS (ASAPs)

OFFICE OF ALCOHOL COUNTERMEASURES

TRAFFIC SAFETY PROGRAMS

NATIONAL HIGHWAY TRAFFIC SAFETY ADMINISTRATION

▲ ASAPs Contracted FY 1970—Operational

● ASAPs Contracted FY 1971—Planning

■ Contract Proposals FY 1972

(Roman Numerals Indicate
  NHTSA Field Regions)

*Salt Lake County
 Box Elder County
 Davis County
 Utah County
 Weber County

Commonwealth of
Puerto Rico

36

you have given your "consent" to a chemical test for alcohol. Refusal to submit or failure to complete the test can result in the loss of your driver's license for a stipulated period of time. The arrested person generally has a choice of blood, breath, or urine tests. He does *not* have the right to consult with an attorney or doctor before deciding which test he'll take. He does *not* have the right to an attorney or doctor while taking the test.

In Denver, Colorado, the police put a person arrested for drunk driving directly on TV. At the station house, the suspect is requested to take a sobriety test—Implied Consent. Refusal means automatic loss of his driver's license. With agreement, a television camera is switched on. The suspect answers a few questions, is told to touch his nose with his finger, walk a straight line, and so forth. Aware that his actions are being recorded, he strives to make the best showing possible. Later, when his case is heard in court, the "performance" is played back for judge and jury on a TV monitor. No matter how circumspect and sober the suspect may now appear, the film, together with the BAC (Blood Alcohol Concentration) report, constitutes irrefutable evidence of his condition when arrested.

The Presumptive Limit law explains the meaning of the alcohol chemical test. In California, for instance, below 0.05 percent a defendant is "presumed" to be sober (although he may not be). Between 0.05 and 0.09 percent, no presumption is made either way. With a blood-alcohol level of 0.10 percent or higher, a driver is presumed "under the influence of alcohol."

[The state-by-state variance of legally-acceptable percentage of alcohol in the blood is shown on the next two pages.]

Safer Percentage Levels

If we would hope to save some (hopefully many) of those half-million persons who are disabled and also offset to a substantial degree the over 25,000 killed each year due to alcohol-related traffic accidents, then a safer level than 0.10 percent would seem to be between 0.05 and 0.07 percent of alcohol in the blood, depending upon the individual's weight and chemistry.

There is a relation between alcohol concentration in the body and a drinker's weight, quantity of food in the stomach, amount of liquor consumed, time over which consumed, and time since

37

State	Year "Chemical Test" Law Enacted	Presumptive Level	Year "Implied Consent" Law Enacted
Alabama	1969	0.10%	1969
Alaska	1969	0.10%	1969
Arizona	1947	0.10%	1969
Arkansas	1957	0.10%	1969
California	1969	0.10%	1966
Colorado	1957	0.10% (ID-.05%)	1967
Connecticut	1964	0.10%	1964
Delaware	1954	0.10%	1969
Florida	1967	0.10%	1967
Georgia	1968	0.10%	1968
Hawaii	1961	0.15%	1967
Idaho	1952	0.08%	1955
Illinois	1957	0.10%	1971
Indiana	1939	0.10%	1969
Iowa	1963	0.10% (*)	1964
Kansas	1954	0.10%	1955
Kentucky	1968	0.10%	1968
Louisiana	1968	0.10%	1968
Maine	1947	0.10%	1969
Maryland	1959	0.15% (ID-.10%)	1969
Massachusetts	1960	0.15%	1967
Michigan	1960	0.15% (ID-.10%)	1967
Minnesota	1967	0.10%	1961
Mississippi	1971	0.15%	1971
Missouri	1964	0.15%	1965
Montana	1957	0.10%	1971
Nebraska	1949	0.10%	1959
Nevada	1958	0.10%	1969
New Hampshire	1949	0.15%	1965
New Jersey	1950	0.15% (ID-.10%)	1966

State	Year "Chemical Test" Law Enacted	Presumptive Level	Year "Implied Consent" Law Enacted
New Mexico	1969	0.10%	1969
New York	1941	0.12% (ID-.08%)	1953
North Carolina	1962	0.10%	1966 (**)
North Dakota	1960	0.10%	1959
Ohio	1967	0.10%	1967
Oklahoma	1967	0.15%	1967
Oregon	1949	0.10%	1965
Pennsylvania	1968	0.10%	1968
Rhode Island	1966	0.10%	1966
South Carolina	1949	0.10%	1969
South Dakota	1959	0.15%	1959
Tennessee	1953	0.10%	1969
Texas	1971	0.10%	1969 (**)
Utah	1967	0.08%	1957
Vermont	1964	0.10%	1958
Virginia	1956	0.15% (ID-.10%)	1962
Washington	1968	0.10%	1968
West Virginia	1968	0.10%	1968
Wisconsin	1947	0.15%	1970
Wyoming	1955	0.15%	1971
District of Columbia	1968	0.15%	has none

(*) Provides that the presumption arises when the blood-alcohol level is more than the specified percentage.

(**) Does not provide for revocation or suspension under refusal.

(ID) State also has a lesser offense of "driving while impaired" with lower presumptive levels and separate penalties.

Above statistics are from the National Safety Council's TRAFFIC SAFETY MONOGRAPH No. 2, "Testing the Drinking Driver."

the last drink. If eight ounces of 80 to 90 proof liquor were ingested in an hour to an hour-and-one-half by a person of 150 pounds, the alcohol level in the blood would be around 0.15 percent. This person would be bordering on heavy intoxication. It would take ten hours for complete elimination of the alcohol in the blood. With 0.15 percent in the blood, a person is a minimum of five hours removed from driving safely.

Says Horace E. Campbell, M.D., chairman, Automotive Safety Committee, Colorado State Medical Society: "If the object is to prevent motor car crashes, then the legal limit [of alcohol in the blood] will eventually have to be brought to that level at which most people do not demonstrate impaired driving ability; i.e., at least to the level of 0.05%, a point which the realistic Norwegians accepted almost 40 years ago."

Indiana University's Department of Police Administration states that blood-alcohol levels over 0.04 percent are definitely associated with increased accident involvement, adding that when the level reaches 0.06 percent, the probability of causing an accident is twice that of the no-alcohol level; at 0.10 percent, the probability is six times greater; and at 0.15 percent it is 25 times greater.

In Ohio, 25 percent of the 15- to 19-year-old drivers killed in accidents had alcohol levels of more than 0.10 percent. In Wisconsin, for drinking drivers in the same age group, the percentage was doubled when blood-alcohol proved to be in excess of 0.10 percent.

Experiments Show Effects of Alcohol on Driving

In Canada, an interesting and informative experiment relative to the percentage of alcohol in the blood was conducted with eight skilled professional racing drivers acting as the "guinea pigs." On a test course, a comparison of their changes in driving judgement, attitude and skill was made during a series of four "dry" runs (without alcohol) and four "wet" runs (with alcohol), with blood-alcohol levels from 0.04 to 0.15 percent. A Canadian research team, headed by H. Ward Smith, Ph.D., director of the Centre of Forensic Sciences, reported:

"The most notable finding appeared to be a failure to sense the attitude or position of the car. This showed especially on curves

THE AVERAGE EFFECTS OF ALCOHOL

1·2 **BOTTLES OF BEER or COCKTAILS** • FLUSHING OF THE SKIN • INHIBITIONS BEGIN TO RECEDE • HEART SPEEDS UP • GAIETY	BLOOD-ALCOHOL LEVEL **4** ────── 100's of 1%
3·4 **BOTTLES OF BEER or COCKTAILS** • JUDGMENT IS SLOWER • GIDDINESS • COORDINATION IS A BIT OFF . . .	BLOOD-ALCOHOL LEVEL **6** ────── 100's of 1%
5·6 BOTTLES OF BEER or COCKTAILS • VISION A BIT BLURRED • SPEECH A LITTLE FUZZY • REACTION TIME SLOWED	BLOOD-ALCOHOL LEVEL **10** ────── 100's of 1%
6·8 **BOTTLES OF BEER or COCKTAILS** • STAGGERING • SEEING DOUBLE • LOSS OF BALANCE	BLOOD-ALCOHOL LEVEL **16** ────── 100's of 1%
15·20 **BOTTLES OF BEER or COCKTAILS** • SKIN IS CLAMMY • PUPILS ARE DILATED UNCONSCIOUSNESS	BLOOD-ALCOHOL LEVEL **40** ────── 100's of 1%
20·25 **BOTTLES OF BEER or COCKTAILS** • ALCOHOLIC POISONING=DEATH	**50** ALCOHOL LEVEL ────── 100's of 1%

The American Business Men's Research Foundation

41

and is connected with the deep muscle sense which is the balancing mechanism of the body. Since there was a reduction in this feeling, the driver reacted to visual clues which only come after something has happened. His driving response was therefore late and usually exaggerated. This gave a choppy, weaving, jerky action to the car. The drivers said that things were happening too fast and they seemed to be driving behind the car rather than ahead of it. This is notable because racing drivers need to plan far ahead of the car and are quite accustomed to doing this. In this study, changes in driving ability were shown in all drivers at levels between 0.04% and 0.08%. At higher levels up to 0.15%, the results were even more prominent in terms of impairment in driving ability."

A demonstration at Ontario Motor Speedway, Ontario, California, supervised by law enforcement officers and Dr. Slade Hulbert, a UCLA research psychologist, showed impaired driving performance with blood-alcohol levels well below the 0.10 maximum set by state law. Dr. Hulbert's studies indicated that "alcohol can impair driving skills although the driver may be unaware of it—until the crash," reported Harry Nelson, Los Angeles *Times* medical writer. Participating in the demonstration sponsored by the Los Angeles County Medical Association were Bob Bondurant, a professional race-driver instructor; George Follmer, winner of the Riverside Grand Prix; Bob Earl, one of Bondurant's co-instructors, and several others, including a woman driver. Nelson described the demonstration:

> Bondurant devised a precision driving course which the subjects were asked to drive in as fast a time as possible while knocking over as few roadmarkers as possible. They did the course while sober and then repeated it under the influence of alcohol.
>
> In every case performance deteriorated after drinking.
>
> "I was surprised. I thought I was doing a good job," Bondurant said. His driving score dropped from 1:30 while sober to 2:18 when "drunk," although legally he was not drunk because his blood-alcohol level was 0.08.
>
> The score denotes the time required to run the course after penalties made for cones knocked over and other factors.
>
> Each of the subjects drank from 2 to 10 ounces of vodka or scotch over a time period of about 45 minutes. Their blood-alcohol levels ranged from 0.02 to 0.12.

For example, the subject who had 2 ounces of alcohol had a blood-alcohol level of 0.02. Her score was 1:58 while sober and 2:10 after drinking.

Several of the subjects, including Follmer, expressed surprise that they had driven over cone markers but that they had no recollection of having done so.

In a separate interview . . . Hulbert said that type of reaction—the tendency not to see something while under the influence—ties in with his laboratory experiments at UCLA.

"The person most apt to be affected," he said, "is a beginning driver who is also an inexperienced drinker."

Controlling the Drinking Driver

Prevention, of course, could be the answer. Preventing the drinking person from driving is a task more of us should not be so hesitant to undertake.

"If we are correct in surmising that a great deal of intoxicated driving follows parties at which the host is socially obligated to maximize his guests' drinking," says Ph.D. Ira H. Cisin, "then these parties and the behavior required in the host role must be one of the primary targets for the control of drunken driving."

But just who, other than the drinker himself, is to set the measure of "control?"

One thing a host can do in the area of "control" is refrain from being an alcohol "pusher," and, out of consideration for his non-drinking guests, make soft drinks as available and socially acceptable as hard beverages. If alcohol is served, food of some kind should also be offered. Food in the stomach helps absorb the alcohol and slow its usually swift entrance into the bloodstream.

According to the report to the nation by the Cooperative Commission: ". . . tolerance for abstaining should be increased, with complete social acceptance of those who choose to abstain or who drink very little. An atmosphere should be created in which people feel genuinely free to 'take it or leave it.' The responsibility of the host to make available to his guests a choice of refreshments, nonalcoholic as well as alcoholic, needs to be stressed. Intoxication is not socially acceptable. It is no more amusing or stylish to be drunk in public than it is to throw up in public."

Insurance companies, too, are eager to decrease incidence of alcoholism, since accidents due to driving while intoxicated swell liability payments. Recent figures show that 50 percent of all drivers' premiums for automobile insurance is used to settle claims resulting from alcohol-related accidents.

Statistics show, also, that the cost to United States residents because of drunk driving exceeds the total amount paid annually to all doctors and dentists, and is more than twice that spent on private education. In terms of cold cash, alcohol-related accidents cost more than five billion dollars each year in losses.

"Actually, one person in every 50 operating motor vehicles of any kind at any given moment is drunk," says one expert—which should cause a chill to every nondrinking motorist as, on a highway or speedway, he watches cars flash by on either side.

There frequently arises among traffic safety experts the question as to whether new or improved automobile equipment devices can successfully deter the intoxicated driver from taking to the road. One such device is a psychological tester—that is, the drinking driver is tested before his car can move. Installed on the auto's dashboard, the device becomes operative when the driver switches on the ignition. A series of numbers (or symbols) flashes on for two seconds. The driver then has six seconds in which to push buttons that correspond to the dashboard series. With a correct response, the engine automatically starts. An incorrect response, and the engine will not turn over. Driving is impossible until the driver is sufficiently sober to pass the test.

One problem with devices of this type is that many nondrinking motorists who are excellent drivers might have difficulty with swift numerical (or symbol) recall. Their engines failing to start immediately, they would be angry not only with the device, but with the automobile manufacturer as well.

A Sense of Caring

A positive, nongadget way to decrease accidents is the so-called co-pilot arrangement. This arrangement might be considered a game. Here's how it works:

You and a friend are going out for the evening, perhaps to a house party. Though you both indulge in alcohol beverage, this

44

time your friend chooses to drive and not drink. Next time, you abstain and drive. With a foursome, only on one occasion out of four would any of the individuals not drink and do the driving.

In the final analysis, safety on the road, or the lack of it, involves a sense of caring—caring about the other fellow, and yourself, together with those who might be in the car with you. With a ton or more of steel under your command, the highway, freeway, or even the city street is a dangerous place to be even under optimum conditions.

4

YOUTH

". . . Alcohol education for youngsters
has been a dramatic failure."

—from the Hearings before the
Special Subcommittee on Alcohol
and Narcotics

4

How Many Young People Drink?

In a survey of 2,000 students in 3 high schools, Dr. George L. Maddox, chief of medical sociology at Duke University and editor of *The Domesticated Drug: Drinking Among Collegians*, states that 92 percent of high school students have at least sampled alcohol and that 23 percent use it occasionally.

The task force which collected and collated the data for the December 1971 First Special Report to Congress stated that in recent years about 57 percent of boys and 43 percent of girls aged 15 through 20 are drinkers of beverage alcohol, that 76 percent of those between 18 and 29 are drinkers, and that the highest proportion of heavy drinkers among women occurred at ages 21 to 24.

Increasingly, restrictions regarding the sale of liquor near schools are being overridden. In Westwood, California, for instance, the home of UCLA, previously no hard liquor was permitted to be sold within a mile-and-a-half radius. During 1965 this restriction was amended, passed by the State Senate, and signed by the Governor. Today "any intoxicating liquor", to quote Amendment 172h to bill No. 1398, is available a relatively few steps off campus.

A Johns Hopkins poll on the use of alcohol showed that among students in 48 four-year colleges, nearly 90 percent had tried an alcoholic beverage as compared with 74 percent for tobacco, 33 percent for barbiturates, 9 percent for LSD, and 6 percent for heroin. Only 9 percent of all students opposed drinking, while 33 percent were opposed to use of marijuana, 65 percent LSD, and 80 percent heroin. As to grade-school-age children, a 1971 Gallup report showed that 51 percent admitted to drinking in groups.

Following in-depth surveys, various investigators have concluded that the children of drinking parents are the more prone to drink. The Straus and Bacon survey of American college students, for instance, showed that:

> Where it was found parents abstained, 65% of sons and daughters abstained.
> If parents drank, 86% of sons and daughters drank.

In North Carolina, the results of a survey of college students showed that:

> If parents abstained, 88% of sons and daughters abstained.
> If parents drank, 88% of sons and daughters also drank.

Other surveys show that teenage drinkers are more likely to end their education at the high school level. Nondrinkers are more likely to plan for college. Drinkers do not participate in school and outside activities to the same extent as nondrinkers.

According to overall figures, it has been estimated that 20 to 30 percent of the nation's youth abstain.

Consumption of Alcohol by Youth

While it is true that the young rebel against adult hypocrisy, it also appears to be true that young people are consuming alcoholic beverages at virtually the same percentage rate as adults. Studies on drinking habits in Massachusetts and Mississippi indicate that teenagers with drinking problems comprise 2 to 5 percent of the adolescent population—the 5 percent being equal to their elders.

50

The rate for deaths from cirrhosis of the liver (a common ailment among heavy drinkers) is up 500 percent for males age 14 to 24. FBI crime statistics (1960-68) on drunk arrests are up 135 percent for males under 18, and up 206 percent for females of the same age.

A study at the Eagleville, Pennsylvania, center for treating addicts and alcoholics showed that the first "drug" used by thirteen-year-olds was almost invariably alcohol.

There is record of a West Coast boy attaining his tenth birthday and reporting that he had been sober for a single month. A girl alcoholic, now 14 and "dry" for 11 months, had her first drink when she was eight years of age, a drink handed her by an adult who "thought it was funny to see such a small girl get drunk."

". . . It is a far more serious problem than we ever imagined," stated a U.S. government medical authority. "It is not uncommon to see severe alcohol problems in kids nine, ten, twelve years old." The doctor added that statistics indicated that seven out of ten youngsters have had their first taste of alcohol by age 14, and 87 percent have tasted alcohol by age 16.

Prevention against alcohol addiction is the only way to turn this alarming tide. And prevention can be hoped for only if the young are educated to the dangers of drinking. They must be made aware that alcoholic beverages are not to be related to having a good time, but that such beverages can cause a very bad time. They must be given the opportunity to understand that alcohol has the power not only to incapacitate but to kill.

Prevention constitutes America's most challenging test, for how can any youngster be "prevented" from trying that first drink, or drinks? No agency, governmental or otherwise, can tell him not to take that drink. Depending upon his age, his parents have that right; yet it is in the home where most first drinks are taken, sometimes surreptitiously and sometimes with parental blessing.

There are those authorities who claim a child should be permitted, or even urged, to learn to drink at home. Based on what is known to date about alcoholism, this would seem a questionable contention, for these reasons: the taste for alcohol must be acquired and, at whatever age a human being takes the first drink, whether in the home or away from it, he or she has taken the initial step toward potential alcohol addiction. It is significant, in this regard, that in 1973 the National Council on Alcoholism found that the youngest alcoholics coming to their attention dropped from age 14 to 12!

The Young Driver

A serious problem that must be righted by youth is their tragic drinking-driver record. "The already disproportionate traffic death rate among young people is growing even further out of line from the rest of the population," states the National Transportation Safety Board, adding that highway accidents cause approximately half of all deaths among youth aged 15 to 24. "The highway death rate of that group has been pulling away from other age groups steadily since 1961, especially in the last four years," the Board further states. "Pulling away" might be considered mild terminology when one considers what has happened in Michigan. During the year since that state lowered the legal drinking age from 21 to 18, accidents involving drinking drivers 18 to 20 have skyrocked 119 percent. Accidents among 18-year-old drinking drivers increased 125 percent, whereas the rate among nondrinking youths the same age rose by only 17 percent.

Youth Drinking More

During 1972 and into 1973, reports from school authorities throughout the land indicated that young people were forsaking marijuana and the hard drugs for alcohol. "The latest fad in juvenile drug abuse is one that has a familiar ring to the older generation," stated *Newsweek*; "the choice of drug these days . . . is alcohol."

The magazine quotes a senior at a Brooklyn, New York, high school as declaring: "A lot of us used to smoke [grass] but we gave that up a year or two ago. Now my friends and I drink a lot . . . ."

The use of alcohol is now spreading down to children in lower grades. What these young people do not seem to understand is that alcohol is an addictive drug, and that it is in the early years that the boy or girl can get "hooked." It is in this period of his or her life that 1 out of 14 of those who try alcohol will have started on the road to alcoholism.

With respect to alcohol and other drugs, many communities have established programs aimed at helping the young addicts. In San Diego, California, for instance, there is DANE—Drug and Narcotic Education program. Roger Taylor, a counselor in that city's unified school-sponsored effort, claims that many students are giving up faddish drugs and returning to alcohol. "Lots of kids are going back to alcohol," Taylor said. "They want to get involved in other types of lifestyles. And at the junior high level, kids aren't afraid to say, 'Hey, I'm straight'."

[Author's note: It seems to be ironic that "going straight" is equated with drinking alcoholic beverages. Actually, the youngsters are merely switching from one drug to another.]

Now in its fifth year, DANE seeks to promote self-respect, pride in living, and more self-assurance in decision making. The program combats drug use of any kind within the school system through a number of methods—drug programs for credit, ex-addicts from the community as speakers, and a staff of 18 drug counselors who have teaching credentials and serve all schools in the district. Referrals are made by DANE counselors to drug rehabilitation centers for those students in need of rehabilitation.

Counselor Betty Blankenship said that marijuana and liquor are the two biggest problems with which DANE must deal. She added that a number of pupils wash reds down with wine to cover up their being [hard drug] stoned. They are thus mistaken as being drunk. In September, October, and November of 1971, 6 junior high and 72 senior high students were referred to rehabilitation agencies. During the same period of '72, 45 junior high and 85 senior high students were referred.

The program is sound and helpful and will show greater impact in the future, declares Russell Hencie, administrator of the Health Services Department for San Diego's city schools. "We've kind of pioneered the individual approach," Hencie says. "If we've learned anything it's that giving information in classroom instruction is not nearly as effective as getting into small, informal groups for discussions without trying to force information down kids' throats."

Whether the individual approach, the group approach, or education in school—or all three—are used, the facts regarding the deleterious effects of beverage alcohol must reach the youth of the nation. When it is considered that San Francisco alone has more alcohol-addicted persons than there are drug addicts in the entire United States, then it becomes quite clear that we must have even greater concern for alcohol-related problems than those problems which are caused by hard drugs.

Preventive Education

Since its December 1971 HEW Report, the U.S. government has promised national dissemination of information to youth and adults alike, backed by a $200,000 advertising campaign, to develop public awareness of the potential health hazards of beverage alcohol. "Programs of education about alcohol," states HEW, "its properties and effects, its potential for harm, and its responsible and irresponsible use, are now underway by the Federal Government and many local agencies. The aim is prevention of alcohol abuse, alcohol problems, and alcoholism, through developing public awareness of facts about alcohol."

[Author's note: Many involved with the alcohol problem take issue with the term "alcohol abuse." If alcohol has no redeeming qualities, then it is "alcohol use" which is the basic problem. The author is in agreement with the following quote from *Criteria for the Diagnosis of Alcoholism*, compiled by the Criteria Committee, National Council on Alcoholism, and printed in the August 1972 issue of *The American Journal of Psychiatry*:

> [Diagnostic terms that define conditions that fall short of alcoholism are necessary because of the effects of alcohol on behavior. Although the term alcohol abuse has wide currency, we prefer alcohol use, accompanying this term with a description of effect. This leaves the term "abuse" for such situations as child abuse, animal abuse, or self-abuse, where there is an animate object of the abuse, and does not anthropomorphize alcohol, which, after all, is a chemical (the "neutral spirit"). The term misuse, we believe, also carries an unnecessary moral implication.]

To develop public awareness HEW is disseminating a variety of educational materials, including films, television and radio spot announcements, newspaper and magazine advertisements, publications, and curriculum guides and materials. These have been, and are being created for use by the mass media, community groups, and schools.

54

The government's concern regarding schools and youth, among other places, was stated in the printed hearings before the Special Subcommittee on Alcoholism and Narcotics:*

"The goals of preventive alcohol education are to modify dangerous and potentially harmful drinking patterns . . . Alcohol education for youngsters has been a dramatic failure."

It is to be hoped that HEW and NIAAA, functioning under Public Law 91-616, will zealously and actively strive to overcome the "dramatic failure."

Two chief reasons for this failure have been the lack of trained teaching personnel and the antiquated, irrelevant teaching materials that have been available. While the DANE theory, to name but one, is admirable, teaching courses must be made mandatory for those chosen to educate the youth in our schools on the dangers of alcohol to health. Antiquated programs must be tossed aside and replaced with programs which have meaning and will give young people *the facts* in a form to which they can relate. Without knowledge, youth cannot hope to make a considered choice between drinking and abstinence. Prevention obviously makes rehabilitation unnecessary.

Al-Ateen

Because of the many variables present within family constellations, there is a growing tendency to help all family members rather than just the alcoholic. Al-Ateen, one of the offshoot organizations of Alcoholics Anonymous, has been effective in helping teenaged children of an alcoholic parent learn that they are not alone in their predicament. The organization is available to teenagers whether or not the alcoholic parent is a part of Alcoholics Anonymous or of some other rehabilitation program.

Through involvement, the Al-Ateen program allows teenaged children of alcoholic parents to learn from each others' attempts at adjustment. The great value derived from this organization, and from Al-Atots—a parallel organization for the still younger child— is the development of greater understanding within the family, which, in turn, may lead toward directing the alcoholic parent toward treatment and rehabilitation.

---

*A copy of these hearings—45-098-0—is available for 70 cents from the Superintendent of Documents, U.S. Government Printing Office, Washington, D.C., 20402.

Special Dangers for Youth

There seem to be even more serious dangers inherent for youth who drink alcoholic beverages than for adults, since young people—especially still-growing teenagers—have not achieved complete development. With the body attaining maturity between the ages of 15 and 25, the drug alcohol can kill new, tender cells or maturing cells.

Dr. Jorge Valles, director of Alcoholism Research and Treatment, Veteran's Administration Hospital, Houston, Texas, and professor of psychiatry at Baylor University Medical School, as well as author of the book *From Social Drinking to Alcoholism*, explains the result he has observed when but one part of the anatomy is affected:

"Primarily alcohol as a drug on the adolescent's imbalanced hypothalmus [the gland which helps form the floor of the median ventricle of the brain] obstructs his emotional maturation on both the psychological and physiological levels. As alcohol breaks the blood-brain barrier, it is responsible for permanent lesions in the hypothalmus. The younger the age at which youth starts to use alcohol, the greater the chances that he or she will develop into a chronic alcoholic."

Victories over typhoid fever, cholera, malaria, smallpox, whooping cough, diptheria, and polio were accomplished not through treatment but through preventive medicine. The Cancer Society has stated that the ultimate victory over cancer will come through preventive discoveries. Without prevention as a prime goal, the many exemplary purposes of NIAAA and law 91-616 will founder. Prevention must start where the drinking begins, with youth; and prevention has to mean not taking that first drink.

"We have to change our attitudes toward drinking and our drinking practices. It is part of our culture to think there is something wrong with a person if he doesn't drink," says Reverend Herman J. Kregal, the director of alcohol studies, Berkeley, California.

If youth becomes *fully informed* it is conceivable that they will question the use, by themselves and others, of the beverage which is the nation's No. 1 drug peril. If and when fully informed, they most probably will want to know why there are nine million alcoholics in America; why a commodity the government identifies as a drug is legal and easily procurable, with no warning whatever to the purchaser of its potentially addictive qualities; and why there has been no U.S. Surgeon General's health investigation and report on alcohol similar to the one on cigarettes.

Youth Questionnaire

How many drinking teenagers presently are hooked, or partly hooked, on alcohol cannot be known. For any young person who drinks—who, in fact, may be secretly troubled by his or her drinking—the Youth Information Branch of the Alcoholism Council of Greater Los Angeles has come up with a questionnaire that can prove helpful.*

The questions are patterned after the 20 questions used by Johns Hopkins University Hospital to decide whether or not a patient is a problem drinker or alcoholic.

As with the Johns Hopkins questions, it is suggested that if a young person answers Yes to even one question, it is a warning that he or she may be on the way to becoming an alcoholic. Yes to any two questions and the chances are that alcoholism is a distinct possibility. Three Yes answers mean definite alcoholism.

1. Do you lose time from school due to drinking?
2. Do you drink because you are shy with other people?
3. Do you drink to build up your self-confidence?
4. Do you drink alone?
5. Is drinking affecting your reputation—do you care?
6. Do you drink to escape from study or home worries?
7. Do you feel guilty or bummed after drinking?
8. Does it bother you if somebody says that maybe you drink too much?
9. Do you have to take a drink when you go out on a date?
10. Do you make out generally better when you have a drink?
11. Do you get into financial troubles over buying liquor?
12. Do you feel a sense of power when you drink?
13. Have you lost friends since you've started drinking?

---

*Listen Magazine, March, 1973.

14. Have you started hanging out with a crowd where stuff is easy to get?

15. Do your friends drink less than you do?

16. Do you drink until the bottle is done?

17. Have you ever had a complete loss of memory from drinking?

18. Have you ever been to a hospital or been busted due to drunk driving?

19. Do you turn off to any studies or lectures about drinking?

20. Do you think you have a problem with liquor?

LOOK INTO THE MIRROR:
The Generation Gap in Dialogue

Author's note: The following is printed as a possible theme for speakers on the subject of drug-and-alcohol use. It also should be of special interest to parents faced with the problem of communicating on the subject with their children. It is from an address by William H. Burgess to the Economic Round Table. The right to use the address in full or in part, verbally or in writing, is granted by Mr. Burgess and the publisher to anyone desirous of making such use. Credit is not necessary.

We all have had heart-to-heart talks with our children. Perhaps some of you have discussed the subject of drug abuse with your offspring. The following conversation might take place in any of our homes. I would like you to listen to it and then tell me if you agree with its premises.

> Son (or daughter), I have been aware that you and some of your friends have become drug users. As your father, sharing the responsibility for bringing you up, I want you to know that I think you are treading on dangerous ground. I would like to do everything in my power to convince you that being a drug user is not in your best interests.
>
> You have tremendous potential. If you can keep the use of your faculties unhampered by the effect of drugs, I know you will be a healthier, happier individual. Even seemingly innocuous drugs such as marijuana can lead to addiction. While pot may not be an addictive drug, research has shown that judgement can be clouded by its use. Under its effects you could do something you would be sorry for. For example, with your judgement impaired, you might even be tempted to get involved with addictive drugs.

58

You do not need to feel that drugs are necessary to build your self-confidence. In fact, the last reason in the world for using drugs is because you think you "need" them. I know that you have enough character and intestinal fortitude to rely on your own resources without depending on drugs. Your friends who use drugs are trying to buy enjoyment and escape the pain of facing themselves. You certainly have enough ingenuity to have a good time at a party or with your friends without resorting to drugs. Drugs at a party can actually be a handicap. Happiness is never a drug-induced state of mind.

As you grow into manhood, I would like you to know that there is a safer program of emotional control than by using drugs. No matter how unhappy or distressed you may be, reliance can better be placed on will power and self-discipline than on drugs. Renewal of the body, mind and spirit can be accomplished in a drug-free atmosphere with a positive program of relaxation.

If what I am saying makes sense to you, you also will have the satisfaction of knowing that your example can help prevent others from using drugs. What else is living if not living for someone else?

You are now old enough to realize that I cannot force you to do the things which I believe are for your own good. I can only give you the knowledge and hope that it will affect your attitudes and your behavior so that you will make a voluntary decision.

Our country needs more individualism, more stature, more moral fibre. As an individual you must not be timid about saying, "No, thank you."

If you would like my suggestions for a response when you are asked to use drugs, consider some of the following:

No, man, I'm off the bad scene.

Listen, child, I've outgrown grass.

Thanks, pal, I don't feel the need.

Nope, I don't use mind affecting drugs.

Or, if my conversation with you has had the desired effect and you want to blame your parents for being square, you can say:

Believe it or not, my parents convinced me . . . I'm off drugs.

If you decide not to use drugs, you will not lose your friends and no one will scorn you. You definitely will gain influence. I don't care what the drug user says to cover up. He has an inner respect for those who don't use drugs and won't compromise on the issue. Those who will not yield to pressure on that issue are not likely to yield to temptation or pressure on other issues, and everyone knows it. To not compromise with one's own self . . . that is the dignity of man. But to be one's own self in these days of tremendous social pressure, takes guts.

Drugs which knowingly degrade and demoralize are unworthy

59

of your heritage. Moderation is not the answer. I am not asking you to use drugs "responsibly." I am asking you to be a non-user. Furthermore, it would please me greatly if you are successful in helping to make non-use the thing to do and socially acceptable among your friends.

Do you agree that the foregoing conversation is one which might be used under the appropriate circumstances? Now let's test the attitudes on which your behavior is based by listening to the same conversation directed from son or daughter to father. Don't be surprised if your hair bristles and you take offense when your present attitudes are challenged.

Dad, I have been aware that you and some of your friends have been drug users. I want you to know that I think you are treading on dangerous ground. I would like to do everything in my power to convince you that being a drug user is not in your best interest. You have demonstrated tremendous potential. If you can keep the use of your faculties unhampered by the effect of an addictive drug, I think you will be a healthier, happier individual. Although pot is not addictive, alcohol, the seemingly innocuous drug, *is* addictive.

Research has shown, Dad, that judgement can be clouded by the use of alcohol. While under its effects you could do something you would be sorry for.

I realize, Dad, that alcohol is the most commonly used drug in the United States, and that among your generation who have acquired the taste for alcohol, virtually no one sees anything wrong in drinking. It is not against the law. It is not against social mores. "Everybody drinks," has become the cultivated attitude. But, Dad, you don't need to feel that alcohol is a necessity. In fact, the last reason in the world for using alcohol is because you think you need a drink. Your friends who use alcohol are trying to buy enjoyment and escape the pain of facing themselves. You certainly have enough character and intestinal fortitude to rely on your own resources without depending on alcohol. If anyone has enough ingenuity to have a good time at a party, or with his friends, without resorting to the use of alcohol, it's my Dad. Alcohol at a party can actually be a handicap. Happiness is never an alcohol-induced reaction.

You have demonstrated to me, Dad, the maturity of manhood. I am confident that you can depend on a safer program of emotional control than to use a drug such as alcohol. Renewal of the body, mind and spirit can be accomplished in an alcohol-free atmosphere by using a positive program of relaxation. No matter how vulnerable or distressed you may be, reliance can better be placed on will power and self discipline than on a drug.

You realize, Dad, that neither I nor the government can force you to do something for your own good. Laws attempting to control man's personal behavior, where the only victim is himself, are the most difficult to enforce.

Dad, I have learned that there is only one way for a person to know that he is completely free from the prospect or the fear of addiction . . . total abstinence. The act of refusing to use alcohol in a society where alcoholic beverages have become part of the culture requires a major decision, as well as will power, if you wish to abstain. However, is it easier for someone to kick the habit if he is addicted or not addicted? The answer is obvious. It should be easier to abstain if you are not addicted.

If you abstain, Dad, you will have an influence that extends beyond your own individual welfare. If what I am saying makes sense to you, Dad, you will have the satisfaction of knowing that your example has helped prevent others from using alcohol. What else is living if not living for someone else? Dad, you have such a strong social conscience that you govern your own activities not solely by your own likes and dislikes, but rather by the effect that you believe your actions will have on others.

While your friends may agree that an addictive drug can be used responsibly, Dad, drugs which knowingly degrade and demoralize are unworthy of your generation. There will always be those who conclude there is nothing wrong in using addictive drugs. If there is casual drinking on the part of the group who set the stage, the socially most acceptable, others will follow their example. Moderation is not the answer. I am hoping you will become a non-user. Furthermore, I hope you will help to make non-use the "thing to do." Why consume a beverage that contains a harmful drug when there are so many non-alcoholic drinks that are actually beneficial?

Our country needs more individualism, more stature, more moral fibre. As an individual and a father whom I respect, you, of all people, should not be timid about saying, "No thank you." When you are asked to have an alcoholic drink, why can't you say:

No, man, I'm off the sauce.

Listen, child, I've outgrown alcohol.

Thanks, pal, I don't feel the need.

Nope, I don't use mind affecting drugs.

Or, if my conversation with you has had an effect and you want to blame the younger generation, you can say:

Believe it or not, my son convinced me. I don't drink any more.

Perhaps Bill Cosby summarized both my position and yours, Dad, when he said, "I have no use for pot or booze . . . my wife and kids are my high."

ALCOHOLIC BEVERAGE CONTROL LAWS CONCERNING MINIMUM AGE REQUIREMENTS

State	Minimum Drinking Age Distilled Spirits	Wine	Beer	Legality of Providing & Allowing Minors To Drink Alcoholic Beverages
Alabama	21	21	21	Under No Circumstances
Alaska	19	19	19	Parent or Guardian, Licensed Physician or Nurse in giving Medical treatment.
Arizona	19	19	19	Under No Circumstances
Arkansas	21	21	21	Under No Circumstances
California	21	21	21	No Provision
Colorado	21	21	21	No Provision (18 for 3.2%)
Connecticut	18 (Eff. 10/1/72)	18	18	Parent or Guardian May Give permission to Minor.
Delaware	20	20	20	Permitted Within Private Home
D.C.	21	21 over 14% 18 under 14%	18	Physicians, Veterinarians or Dentists may administer Alcohol.
Florida	21	21	21	No Provision
Georgia	18	18	18	With Parent's Written Consent
Hawaii	18	18	18	No Provision
Idaho	19	19	19	Under No Circumstances
Illinois	21	21	21	Under No Circumstances
Indiana	21	21	21	Unlawful to have in possession unless accompanied by parent
Iowa	19	19	19	In private home with parent's or guardian's consent.

63

State	Minimum Drinking Age Distilled Spirits	Wine	Beer	Legality of Providing & Allowing Minors To Drink Alcoholic Beverages
Kansas	21	21	21	No Provision (18 for 3.2%)
Kentucky	21	21	21	No Provision
Louisiana	18*	18*	18*	Under No Circumstances
Maine	18	18	18	At Home in Presence of Parent
Maryland	21	21	21	No Provision
Massachusetts	18 (Eff. 3/1/73)	18	18	Parent, Guardian or Spouse May Procure.
Michigan	18	18	18	By Prescription of a Duly Licensed Physician
Minnesota	21	21	21	In Household of Parent or Guardian. (It is unlawful for anyone except a licensed Pharmacist to supply minor with liquor. 3.2% beer in presence of parents.)
Mississippi	21	18	18	No Provision
Missouri	21	21	21	With Parent's consent or for medicinal purposes
Montana	18	18 (Effective 7/1/73)	18	Parents may give for medicinal purposes. Physicians or Dentists may administer. Druggists may supply upon prescription of Physician. Wine may be consumed for sacramental purposes.
Nebraska	19	19	19	Parent may supply
Nevada	21	21	21	Parent, Guardian or Physician may supply.
New Hampshire	21	21	21	No Provision

* Louisiana: Under both ABC Board regulation and Criminal Code, permitted to sell all alcoholic beverages to 18 year olds.

| State | Minimum Drinking Age | | | Legality of Providing & Allowing Minors To Drink Alcoholic Beverages |
	Distilled Spirits	Wine	Beer	
New Jersey	18 (Eff. 1/1/73)	18	18	No Provision
New Mexico	21	21	21	Parent or Guardian may give.
New York	18	18	18	No Provision
North Carolina	21	18 (18 for wines not over 14% - 17 if minors are married)	18	Parents or physicians may give for medicinal purposes. Also may be taken in connection with the sacraments.
North Dakota	21	21	21	Parent may give
Ohio	21	21	21 (18 for 3.2%)	Parent, Guardian or Physician may give
Oklahoma	21	21	21 3.2 beer Male - 21 Female - 18 off-sale 21 on-sale	No Provision
Oregon	21	21	21	Parent, Guardian or other responsible relative may give in a private residence. May consume sacramental wine in a religious service.
Pennsylvania	21	21	21	Under No Circumstances
Rhode Island	18	18	18	Not Legal on Licensed Premises
South Carolina	21	18	18	May be consumed in home of parent or guardian, or in connection with religious service.
South Dakota	21	21 19 for non-in-toxicating	21 18 for 3.2%	By prescription; parent, spouse or guardian may give

| State | Minimum Drinking Age | | | Legality of Providing & Allowing Minors To Drink Alcoholic Beverages |
	Distilled Spirits	Wine	Beer	
Tennessee	18	18	18	Under No Circumstances
Texas	21	21	21	Minors are prohibited from consuming alcoholic beverages in any public place unless accompanied by a parent, guardian or adult husband, wife.
Utah	21	21	21	May be given for medicinal purposes by parent, guardian or doctor.
Vermont	18	18	18	Minors cannot be sold or furnished liquor by any person, licensee or other.
Virginia	21	21	21 (18 for 3.2%)	No Provision
Washington	21	21	21	Parent, Guardian or physician may give.
West Virginia	18	18	18	No Provision
Wisconsin	18	18	18	INTOXICATING LIQUORS -

Under no circumstances. No fermented malt beverage may be sold to any person under 18 unless accompanied by parent or guardian. No fermented malt beverage may be sold to persons under 21 who are not residents of Wisconsin and are residents of states bordering Wisconsin which prohibit such sales to persons under 21. Municipalities may by ordinance or regulation prohibit sales or gift of malt beverage to persons under 21.

Wyoming**	21	21	21	May be given by parent, guardian or Doctor when a medical patient.

This list, courtesy of Licensed Beverage Industries, Inc.

**Wyoming: Statutory provisions relating to minors & alcoholic beverages have been amended to make 18 years the age of majority effective 1/1/73 contingent on voter approval of constitutional amendment on November, 1972 permitting 18 year olds to vote in state elections.

5

INDUSTRIAL PROGRAMS

". . . this isn't merely a matter of a man's job. It is a matter of his life. We can save him if he'll let us."

—Dr. Howard Hess

5

The Need for Industry Programs

The annual loss to the economy of the United States resulting from alcohol use is estimated at $15 billion. As many as 5 percent of the nation's work force are addicted, and almost another 5 percent have serious problems related to alcohol.

The mass of alcohol-troubled drinkers among America's work force are estimated to be in their most productive years. According to the Cristopher D. Smithers Foundation of New York, "He is usually a skilled or semi-skilled person, varying in age between 35 and 50. He has been at least 7 years with the company, married, owns his own home, and usually has 2 or more children. In short, a responsible member of the community."

The alcoholic working employee averages a loss of 22 more on-the-job days a year and dies 12 years sooner than non-alcoholics working at his side. About 4.5 million workers suffer from alcohol-related problems.

In his series of *Valley News* articles, Cecil Carle, chairman of the public information committee as well as board member of the

Alcoholism Council of the San Fernando Valley, writes that surveys show that half of the nation's nine million alcohol addicted either attended or graduated from college, 87 percent completed high school, only 13 percent dropped out before high school. Forty-five percent, says Carle, are employed in professions or management, 30 percent do manual labor, and 25 percent are in white collar jobs. Only 3 percent of alcoholics are on any Skid Row. Actually only a fourth of all Skid Row derelicts are alcoholics, the rest being merely social misfits.

Since most cases of alcoholism usually require from 5 to 20 years to become chronic, help can come at any stage along the way if symptoms are heeded and assistance is asked for. It has been proved *that between 50 and 70 percent of on-the-job alcoholics who seek relief have successfully rehabilitated.*

It wasn't always so. Prior to World War II, no company is known to have had a rehabilitation program aimed at helping the employee problem drinker or alcoholic. Not until the organization of what is now known as Alcoholics Anonymous did business and industry finally recognize the need for such programs. One of the first was the Kemper Insurance Group of Chicago, whose help system was activated in 1946. E. I. du Pont de Nemours & Company instituted a program which by 1959 had screened and treated almost 1,000 of its workers.

Companies like the Consolidated Edison Company utilized a review board system which placed the initial responsibility with supervisors who were required to report declining job performance by an employee suspected of having an alcohol problem. In 1952, Consolidated established a consultation clinic in New York City which was used by more than 20 other companies. Allis-Chalmers in Milwaukee, Wisconsin, and the Eastman Kodak Company in Rochester, New York, also pioneered programs which were used as pilots by other companies. There are now more than 300 major companies that have established alcohol programs.

Organizing Company Programs

The average department head, lacking the support of a company program, does not have the experience to handle a subordinate who is a problem drinker. How shall he approach the worker? What does he say? Which course of action would be correct?

70

As Drs. Carl A. and Carmela M. Coppolino explain so well in their book *The Billion Dollar Hangover*, to his superior this employee "... presents a frustrating admixture of poor work and able performance, charming and disagreeable personality, hard work and rank negligence. The boss's-eye view is one of effective job performance mixed with an annoying, unpredictable loss of effectiveness and dependability. He never knows what to expect. But just when he believes his 'headache' is intolerable, his problem-drinking worker 'snaps out of it' and looks good again."

Upon the department head or supervisor falls the brunt of criticism from higher echelon concerning a subordinate's absenteeism, inferior job performance, increased accident rate, and poor morale. In most instances, the supervisor, who may have been covering up for his problem drinker, will want to help.

While the aid of Alcoholics Anonymous usually is arranged by most firms establishing a program, few employees are forced to become members of AA. This particular aid remains a matter of choice, since, as one company executive put it, "AA is . . . not for everyone." Obtaining community-sponsored therapeutic services as an adjunct to company programs is a necessary, and comparatively simple, procedure.

Advice in aiding to set up a company help program is available from the 80 National Council of Alcoholism, Inc. offices situated throughout the country. NCA's industrial counselors, specialists in their field, are available to cooperate in guiding interested top management to establish a program. "The single most important aspect of a successful recovery from alcoholism is the motivation to accept treatment," says Ross von Wergnand, director of labor management services for NCA. To be effective, a program must lack any overtones of being a crusade or a witch-hunt. Voluntary abstinence is a good method to obtain the heavy drinker's or the addicted drinker's cooperation to help himself.

There are also several private organizations which, for a fee, act as consultants to companies seeking to set up an employee-help program. These organizations institute up-to-date methods, including the training of personnel, to launch the program. One such consultant, Pharmacologic Approach Systems, Inc., of San Francisco, claims that "success rates as high as 85% are achievable."

That the worker considers his job and income the most important sustaining element in his life is strikingly borne out by an overall national study of adult employed men which showed that 80 percent, even if given the opportunity, would not quit work. Most evaluators claim that a man's work relationship is of prime importance. "A man will hang onto his job while he allows everything else around him to deteriorate," states the Reverend Vernon E. Johnson, director of the Johnson Institute, a counseling service in Minneapolis.

Some companies, such as Merrill Lynch, Pierce, Fenner, and Smith, which began its help program in 1971, advise their supervisors to confront employees with specific drinking problems when job performances are inadequate. Other companies, like Union Carbide Corporation, do not permit a specific confrontation. The supervisor may make no reference to the drinking. Instead, after pointing out the work difficulties, he tells the employee that continuation of the difficulties will lead to disciplinary action, up to and including termination. In most instances this is sufficient motivation to cause an individual to voluntarily take action.

"An employee may not be motivated by his wife and family or by fear of illness or disgrace, but he will be motivated by the threat to his livelihood," states Dr. John F. Welsh, Carbide's medical director.

Union Participation

Because of a sense of additional security, the employee whose union works in concert with a company program is more likely to conquer his drinking problem. According to Fran Winn of the United Automobile Workers, "Confronting the alcoholic with the reality that his affliction is endangering his economic livelihood and at the same time providing him with the opportunity for treatment and rehabilitation provides a method of motivation which has not been used in the past."

If the employee refuses to cooperate and his performance continues to decline, he knows he had better start seeking another job.

If he checks with his union, he invariably gets the same message as from his employer: help is available; it is freely offered in secret; his job is at stake, and if he can't reverse his present course dismissal is a distinct possibility.

"He has to get it through his head that he is in trouble," says Dr. Howard Hess, psychiatrist for two large organizations, who firmly believes in coordinating a program with an employee's union. "This isn't industrial relations. This is union and management getting together to try to help. It is an exciting cooperation.

"It is, of course, the union's job to protect men's jobs, but this isn't merely a matter of a man's job. It's a matter of his life."

Workers who fail to respond to management help offers eventually "lose their jobs . . . but, in effect, they have fired themselves," says Merle Gulick, co-chairman of a labor-management committee organized by the Community Council of Greater New York.

The majority of those who do respond, who realize that bottles and business don't mix, have an excellent chance to become respected employees.

The Ford Motor Company recently has instituted a program directed to alcohol-related "problems which adversely affect employee job performance and interfere with efficient Company operation." With the United Automobile Workers Union (UAW) participating in the program, the Ford Company has established a *Guide for Employee Emotional or Behavioral Problems*. The *Guide*, aimed at aiding supervisors detect those who are in need of help, offers three categories: Recognition, Referral, and Rehabilitation.

Under Recognition, the *Guide* suggests that "Characteristics usually associated with problem drinking or alcoholism include:

> Increased absence, particularly on Monday and Friday.
> Frequent unanticipated vacation days, especially following holidays or weekends.
> Loss of efficiency or unusual absence after lunch.
> Strong odor of alcohol or breath fresheners after return from lunch.
> Tremor of the hands.

The *Guide* further states in the section on Rehabilitation that "If the . . . program requires absence from work, the employee is entitled to an approved medical leave of absence and may receive appropriate insurance benefits. Any costs for medical treatment not covered by Company insurance benefits will be the responsibility of the employee."

The General Motors program—also in cooperation with the United Automobile Workers Union—keeps problem drinkers and alcoholics on the payroll as long as they continue to seek help. An estimated 1 in 20 G.M. employees drinks too much; the total of these and the dependent drinkers costs the company millions in lost production.

Success and Failure

Among business and industrial firms with established programs, there has been a "recovery" rate of over 50 percent. Allis-Chalmers, for example, reduced its absenteeism from 95 to 8 percent. The New York Transit Authority estimates that in sick pay alone it has saved almost $1 million annually because of its help program.

"The most expensive way to handle the problem drinker is to fire or ignore him. The most profitable and effective way is to help him recover," said James S. Kemper, Jr., president of Lumberman's Mutual Casualty Company, Kemper Insurance Group.

But there must be cooperation from the employee. The drinking employee who leaves that first or second interview feeling rebellious might remain determined to continue hiding his problem. "He is like an iceberg, with the biggest part hidden from management," said an executive of Anchor Hocking Corporation of Lancaster, Ohio.

"The job [of helping] is always difficult, often encouraging, and too frequently a failure," says Dr. Clyde Greene, Jr., medical director of the Pacific Telephone and Telegraph Company. "However, Pacific Telephone does believe that the program we have . . . is worthwhile . . . giving us a salvage rate of perhaps 40 to 45 percent."

The Standard Oil Company of New Jersey, with no formal policy for the handling of problem-drinking employees, makes use of available clinics and Alcoholics Anonymous. "Our success in rehabilitation is discouraging but not hopeless," states its assistant medical director, Dr. John M. Daily. "We hope that as community and company education grows, plus the continuing improvement in facilities for rehabilitation, our results will improve."

A program benefit often overlooked, points out Kenneth A. Rouse in *What to Do About the Employee With a Drinking Problem* "is the preventive influence on moderate drinkers against the development of dangerous drinking habits which may lead to alcoholism. In addition, an existing program will motivate some employees to undertake remedial action on their own, outside the scope of the company program."

The policy of most companies is to maintain privacy concerning the employee's problem. The large chain of banks which comprises the United California Bank, for instance, instructs its supervisors that every worker experiencing a drinking problem, male and female, be advised that an interview with the medical director is strictly confidential. No member of management ever sees the list of those who have conferred with the medical director or have been assisted by the program.

Based on available records, a mutual benefit accrues to both employee and employer once a program is conscientiously put into effect. "Our average alcoholic is 40 years old and has been with the Great Northern for 21 years," states C.L. Vaughan, Jr., in charge of Great Northern Railway's rehabilitation program. "If we were to let the man go, he'd have a difficult time getting a job in another business, and we'd be out 21 years experience."

Great Northern Railway's program is a highly personal facility, with assistance rendered by Mr. Vaughan's wife who works with the families of employees who are excessive drinkers. If a worker's behavior endangers safety, he is suspended or dismissed, but the company nevertheless continues to help him toward rehabilitation. If successfully rehabilitated, the worker is reinstated with full rights and seniority. "This system," says Vaughan, "has paid off with better than average performance and . . . grateful, loyal, and extremely dependable employees." That the system in no way adversely affects public safety is attested to by the fact that Great Northern has won a national safety award each year since instituting its program.

"Denial of the problem renders a disservice to all concerned," says Kodak's medical director, Dr. Gordon M. Hemmet, where 65 to 70 percent successful treatment is claimed. "We must remove the stigma and break through the denial . . . in order to open the doorway for recovery. The company medical department . . . as it exists at Eastman Kodak . . . does accept the fact that it must assume the primary responsibility for treatment and rehabilitation . . . We believe that industry has a unique opportunity to deal with the problem in its earlier stages while the employee still has a job."

An important trend on the part of many firms is the reduction in the number of company parties at which alcoholic beverages are served. One result of this change has been a consequent decrease in automobile accidents, sometimes fatal accidents, directly attributable to office parties. In increasing volume, appreciation for workers' on-the-job efforts is being rendered in the form of a holiday or vacation-time bonus instead of a company party.

Programs for Small Business

While the corporations and big companies have spearheaded the movement, smaller firms are also establishing help programs.* The smaller company has certain advantages. Fewer top-level individuals have to be convinced of the need. Once convinced, the procedure can be rapid. Often the smaller organization is owned and managed by one man or one family, perhaps two partners. The employees can be reached on a "family" basis. The "family" is more prone to listen and respond, more prone to accept what might be printed in the company house periodical.

Observe, for instance, how *Chinorama, The Magazine That Tells the Chino Story to Chino Employees*, relates an attitude to its personnel:

> Chino management wants to make clear that, in itself, an employee's drinking problem is not a reason for discipline, suspension or discharge. At the same time, it must be emphasized that every employee is accountable for his actions on the job . . . .
> Bluntly, to cease being a problem drinker one must stop drinking completely. An alcoholic can never become a social drinker. His disease will never allow him to control his drinking after he

---

*For information concerning possible U.S. Government aid in establishing a help program, contact the HEW Regional Office serving your area, or NIAAA, 5600 Fishers Lane, Rockville, Maryland 20852. Another important source for information and aid is your nearest National Council on Alcoholism (NCA) office.

has taken "the first drink." It doesn't matter if the first drink is beer, wine or whiskey; the results will be the same.

This is a big order. Is it too much to ask? The answer depends on how much the problem drinker's family, health, self-respect . . . and job . . . mean to him. At Chino there are several former problem drinkers. They are sober, reliable employees. They still have the urge to drink, but do not. They know the nature of their disease, and they avoid "the first drink" which would plunge them into active alcoholism again.

Executive Drinking

Supervisory and higher-echelon personnel are not magically free of alcohol-beverage difficulties. In a number of ways the problem-drinker executive represents a special case. He has better opportunity to hide his problem. His life style at home, at his club, at work, wherever he travels—the luncheon martini, the after-work cocktail, the drink in the office, on the commuter train or the plane—makes this man or woman susceptible to alcohol addiction.

The executive who drinks excessively can prove an extremely costly fixture. The sum spent to train him is considerable; his responsibilities are integrated into the firm's decision making; his time is valuable; and he is expensive to replace.

"A hidden problem drinker who signs contracts or makes investments can lose a million dollars in five minutes," is the evaluation of Dr. Seldon Bacon of the Rutgers Center of Alcohol Studies.

Image-conscious and invariably aware of his responsibility to his position, the executive usually will force himself to get to the office rather than "sleep it off at home," as his subordinate problem-drinker is likely to do. Somewhat less than clear-brained until midmorning, the executive can then use an outside appointment as an excuse, to himself as well as those who work close to him, to get away from his desk. Perhaps the appointment is actual, or perhaps he seeks the solace of a steam bath. Perhaps he has an early lunch with an executive buddy from another company, including a cocktail or two. By midafternoon there can be another bogus appointment at his club in town or in the suburbs.

The executive "works in a milieu where drinking is an acceptable part of his business day," states *Dun's Review*. "Little notice is taken of an executive who has three or four martinis during lunch, and the bar in the office is an accepted status symbol. These are not causes of alcoholism per se. But they can lead to heavy drinking, which, coupled with a tendency to alcoholism, can be lethal."

Aware that his spotty work performance can make him suspect, the executive who drinks too much often will give energetically of himself during his better hours in the office to offset the lost hours. There comes the time, however, when a few too many errors occur, and he is frequently unavailable when sought by peak-echelon management for an impromptu meeting.

Presuming that his company has a help program, the troubled executive, even more so than the average worker, might insist upon secrecy during treatment. An adjustment of hours is no insurmountable matter, however. If AA meetings are involved in the rehabilitation, they can be attended outside his business or home neighborhood.

Du Pont is one of the numerous corporate structures which adapts to the individual's needs, no matter the man's job plateau. "Whatever success we might have had in handling the drinking employee," says Frank Lawlor, Du Pont's Advisor on Alcoholism, "comes from not following too rigid a procedure, but rather the employment of flexibility and adapting the treatment according to the individual circumstances and needs."

Also included in the Du Pont program is a full-time employee, himself an ex-alcoholic and a member of AA, who operates under the guidance of a psychiatrist, gives talks to plant groups, and assists in handling cases.

Some Results of Industry Programs

Submitting testimony at Mt. Sinai Hospital in New York City, Du Pont's Dr. D'Alonzo pointed out, in October 1969 to the Senate Subcommittee on Alcoholism and Narcotics,* that problem-drinker and alcoholic employees lose more than 36 million working days a year; that annually one out of every 13 such men loses 22 working days more than the average employee.

Dr. D'Alonzo additionally stated that though the Du Pont rate of "salvage or rehabilitation has been about 65% in the past two

---

*One of the earlier hearings that ultimately led to enactment of Public Law 91-616.

78

years, as our experience matured, it has risen to 81%." The doctor then emphasized the program's humanitarian aspects. "How many children are properly raised, loved and educated as a result of a program to save the . . . employees? How many children suicides are prevented, marriages saved, and depressions forestalled? I do not have a figure to quote, but I have a high level of confidence that it would be substantial.

"I do have one figure of which we are proud because I think it tells a story from an objective viewpoint. Several years ago the mortality from cirrhosis of the liver in the United States was 12.2 per 100,000. The comparable figure for the Du Pont Company was 3."

The drinking employee who has learned how to control his problem "is a good employee," the medical director concluded, "and he is good for other employees. He is, in brief, worth saving. Our program is effective. There is nothing complicated about it. No large outlay of funds is necessary for it. We would certainly commend such a program to any other organization which employs people and which wishes to face a problem which is almost certainly there."

Concerned about the problem, Corning Glass Works and Ingersoll-Rand Company sponsor an Information Center at the Corning Hospital in Corning, New York.

The Kemper Group's help system, operating under behavioral-medical services, arranges for alcohol-troubled personnel to "receive the same consideration under the company's administrative benefits and medical procedures as employees who have other illnesses and who accept appropriate treatment."

All medical expenses incurred in treating its workers, whatever the illness, are covered by the Kemper Insurance Group and Health Plan, including income protection. Additionally, when a supervisor requests examination for diagnostic purposes by a physician, the company foots the bill.

Aware that excessive drinking by a member of a worker's family can affect job performance, Kemper management extends *through the employee* the same information and guidance as is available to the worker. Protecting the employee's privacy, supervisors are admonished not to place or allow to be placed into a worker's personnel record-jacket any document or memorandum bearing the diagnosis or supposition that the worker has alcoholism.

In Hartford, Connecticut, businessmen set up the Greater Hartford Council on Alcoholism which offers an educational course to supervisory personnel of regional companies. Surprised at the interest shown in such a community enterprise from the outset, Walter A. Stewart, executive director, explained that when the Council was still in the planning stages and "looking for people . . . we had 278 referrals from 77 companies."

The majority of programs within the business-industrial world seem to be successful. After establishing its program, Detroit Edison reduced absenteeism from twice company average to one-half company average. At Minnesota Mining, 80 percent of its former problem drinkers and alcoholics today show marked improvement in attendance, productivity, and family and community relationships.

People's Light and Coke Company reports that its program "has been effective in 50—60% of individuals involved."

The New England Electric System of Boston, Equitable Life Assurance Company, and the Hughes Aircraft programs also are considered successful company-savings, human-salvage programs, adding to the excellent overall prevention-treatment-rehabilitation record achieved by the majority of big-business companies.

That these companies, collectively, show an astonishing estimated 60 percent success must be attributed, in part, to the fact that the individual who chooses to drink alcoholic beverages is being educated to the fact that trouble lies ahead, serious trouble, if he or she cannot "take a drink or leave it."

Handling the Alcoholic

The American Management Association has stated that: "The business world now acknowledges four facts about alcoholism and the alcoholic:

1. Alcoholism is an illness, not a moral problem.
2. It can be treated.
3. The alcoholic is worth treating.
4. He himself is often the last to recognize or accept his problem.

Many of those who have experience in the handling of alcoholics and do recognize when a worker has a drinking problem are aware that alcoholics have certain personality traits, and that advice must be correctly rendered; i.e.:

A small reprimand for lateness or a hangover will not make the alcoholic mend his ways.

There should be no apology for bringing up the subject of his drinking. To get involved in discussing a man's "right to drink" is worthless. Urging him to be moderate is useless. Trying to scare him won't work. Predict that booze will kill him and he'll tell you about a friend who drinks more than a quart every day and functions just fine. If he too quickly agrees to see a psychiatrist, this could be but another evasion. He should not be given a chance to claim that if he finds out *why* he drinks too much he can adjust and return to drinking. He should be firmly advised that there can be relief in a sincere acknowledgement on his part that he cannot drink at all.

With this as a start, there is hope for rehabilitation and "cure."

The majority of drinking workers are not hopeless alcoholics. Few if any hopeless or almost-hopeless alcoholics can hold down jobs. Statistics show that 5 percent of all male employees' problems due to alcohol are readily detectable between five and seven years after their becoming addicted. Big-business programs are therefore effectively reaching problem and heavy drinkers who for the most part can, with help and guidance, quit before it is too late; business and industry are reaching those who realize it is better to quit, who still have the *will* to quit.

Thus a company can combine "a selfless social objective with a selfish profit motive," stated *Business Management* of the corporate help program, adding: "And to the combined applause of stockholder, government and community. What other corporate program can say as much?"

"This is one situation," echoes Lewis Presnell, NCA's Director in Industrial Services, "where hard-headed business sense and humanitarian interest can converge. It's not too often you get that kind of package."

It should be heartening to every firm in the nation that with the passing of Public Law 91—616, the Comprehensive Alcohol Abuse and Alcoholism Prevention, Treatment and Rehabilitation Act, the U.S. government finally has decided to bolster the "package" nationally. This law, through HEW and NIAAA, makes funds available to state and local agencies. This proferred aid should be of interest not only to the 39 states that presently operate departments or bureaus concerned with alcohol-related problems, but more particularly the 11 states which are without such bureaus.

In addition to private industry and government, so vital does the National Council on Alcoholism consider the detection and treatment of alcoholism within the business world that NCA annually holds 2-day seminars on alcohol-related problems in Detroit, St. Louis, Houston, Pittsburg, and Los Angeles.

SAMPLE POLICY PROGRAMS

The following programs are offered as guides to organizations interested in setting up their own alcoholism help programs.

UNION CARBIDE CORPORATION POLICY: ALCOHOLISM

Alcoholism is a disease in which alcohol consumption is interfering with an individual's normal process of behavior and living.

The supervisor must be alert to the earliest sign that alcoholism is interfering with work performance and insist that immediate corrective action be taken. He should avoid the sympathetic protection which carries many an alcoholic through the early phases of his illness to a rather obvious later phase which cannot be tolerated. At this point it is probably too late and the employee will have to be terminated.

Signs to watch out for are: absenteeism, lateness, overlong lunch hours, odor of alcohol, tremors, and poor work performance.

Supervisory Action

When a supervisor has reason to believe an individual has a problem, even though he may not be certain it is an alcohol problem, he should call the employee in and go over his reasons for concern item by item. The supervisor should tell the employee that:

Management feels he has a problem and he should do something about it. The supervisor need not leave his familiar role in dealing with the problem. However, if the employee admits to alcoholism or if the case is so flagrant that the supervisor has no doubt, it should be mentioned at this point.

Management wants to offer sympathetic participation in any program that appears appropriate to deal with the problem.

The employee is to report to the Medical Department for study and guidance. A medical examination and consultation are considered to be essential parts of any program of rehabilitation. The employee's willingness to cooperate in this respect will be taken as concrete evidence that he recognizes a problem and desires to correct it. Conversely, his failure to cooperate may make it necessary to take disciplinary action which might otherwise be avoided.

Repetition of behavior as discussed will lead to disciplinary action up to and including termination.

Local Management will be guided by the physician's opinion regarding the possibility of rehabilitation before actually terminating an employee. Before the decision is made by Management to terminate the employee for alcoholism, a committee may be appointed consisting of one or more supervisors, an industrial relations representative, the physician, and a member of Alcoholics Anonymous.

UNITED CALIFORNIA BANK POLICY ON ALCOHOLISM

We recognize that problem drinking is a progressive disease and not a moral problem and that it can be successfully treated.

We are concerned only with problem drinking. There is no interest in social drinking and no desire to intrude upon the employee's private life.

We recognize that a sympathetic and understanding attitude on the part of UCB is essential to recognition, diagnosis and rehabilitation.

We believe the disease must be handled, like any other non-occupational disease, by relying largely upon outside treatment facilities.

We believe that disciplinary action is taken only if the employee is not cooperative in making a conscientious effort to rehabilitate himself. Such policy is equally applicable to any other disease.

For the benefit of all levels of supervision—you should know: The criteria is job performance which includes behavior when in your home and business community and is not confined to just your behavior when on the actual physical premises of the bank.

The supervisor's role is to observe and discuss with the director poor job performance, particularly if he cannot definitely pin-point the reason for poor performance or job deterioration. Don't guess—"It may be the first signs of a drinking problem."

Discussion with the director is:

The mark of good responsible supervision

The mark of concern for the employee or his family

The mark of willingness to conform to bank policy

The mark of recognition that many of our dollar losses and losses of manpower are the direct result of drinking problems

We must at all levels of supervision know of our program and use it just as we use all other operating procedures and programs.

Last but of utmost importance—we must let every employee, both male and female, know that a talk with the director is strictly confidential. No member of management has ever seen or inquired as to the list of names of those who have talked to me [director of the employee alcoholism program] or been assisted by the program. My list . . . is known only to me and will remain completely confidential.

6

THE MILITARY

*"We as a nation . . . exercise pretty
heavy peer pressure on people at
times. And there, I feel, is where
we are contributing to the incidence
of alcoholism."*

*—Captain James A. Baxter
Director, Department of the Navy's
Alcohol Abuse Control Program*

6

The total number of alcoholics in the Armed Services is estimated by the United States General Accounting Office at over 150,000. Recognition by Congress of the growing import of the problem of alcoholism in the Armed Services culminated in the inclusion of alcohol as part of Public Law 91—129 which orders the Secretary of Defense to direct the various services to organize alcohol and drug prevention programs.

Title V

The master plans to combat alcohol addiction and to rehabilitate those in trouble with alcohol within the armed services operate under Title V of Public Law 92-129. The law was enacted by Congress on September 8, 1971, as an amendment to the Military Selective Services Act of 1967.

Public Law 92—129, Title V, was then followed, as of March 1, 1972, by Department of Defense (DOD) Directive 1010.2 which speeded the implementation of Title V by all of the military services. To help toward the administration of 1010.2 programs, the

DOD Directive set forth the following definitions* as related to those with alcohol-beverage problems:

Alcoholism—As used in this Directive alcoholism is psychological and/or physical dependency on alcohol.

Alcoholic—A general reference to individuals who suffer from alcoholism as defined above.

Alcohol Abuse—Any irresponsible use of an alcoholic beverage which leads to misconduct, unacceptable social behavior, or impairment of an individual's performance of duty, physical or mental health, financial responsibility or personal relationships. It may also lead to alcoholism.

Alcohol Addiction—A physiological condition in which there is a marked change in tolerance to alcohol and consumption of alcohol is necessary for the prevention of withdrawal symptoms.

Detoxification—The process of establishing physiological equilibrium to include the elimination of alcohol from the body. Elimination of alcohol occurs by means of natural metabolic processes to include excretion, and normally occurs within six to twenty-four hours from cessation of drinking in otherwise healthy individuals. Establishment of physiological equilibrium is a slower process and may require medical support to prevent the occurrence of severe withdrawal symptoms. Detoxification is the first step in the treatment process.

Intoxication—A state of impaired mental and/or physical functioning resulting from the presence of alcohol in a person's body. This condition does not necessarily indicate alcoholism as defined herein, nor does the absence of observable intoxication necessarily exclude the possibility of alcoholism.

Problem Drinker—A person who may or may not be an alcoholic but whose use of alcohol conforms to the definition of alcohol abuse herein.

---

*These definitions stated DOD, "are intended solely for the administration of the programs set forth in this Directive. They are not intended to modify or influence definitions applicable to statutory provisions and regulations which relate to determinations of misconduct and line of duty, disability benefits, and criminal or civil responsibility for a person's acts or omissions."

Recovered Alcoholic—A person whose alcoholism has been arrested. Normally this is accomplished through abstinence and is maintained through a continuing program of personal recovery.

Withdrawal Syndrome—A complication of detoxification in alcohol addition which is a potentially serious condition. It includes intense anxiety, degrees of mental and physical impairment, and may progress from tremors and convulsions through hallucinations and delirium to death. Recovery from the acute phase usually occurs two to five days after the onset.

Public Law 92—129's Title V, so important to any individual in the armed services with an alcohol-related problem, is composed of but two paragraphs and reads as follows:

TITLE V–IDENTIFICATION AND TREATMENT OF DRUG AND ALCOHOL DEPENDENT PERSONS IN THE ARMED FORCES

SEC. 501. (a) The Secretary of Defense shall prescribe and implement procedures, utilizing all practical available methods, and provide necessary facilities to (1) identify, treat, and rehabilitate members of the Armed Forces who are drug or alcohol dependent persons, and (2) identify those individuals examined at Armed Forces examining and entrance stations who are drug or alcohol dependent persons. Those individuals found to be drug or alcohol dependent persons under clause (2) of the preceding sentence shall be refused entrance into the Armed Forces and referred to civilian treatment facilities.

(b) The Secretary of Defense shall report to Congress within 60 days after the date of the enactment of this Act with respect to (1) the plans and programs which have been initiated to carry out the purposes of subsection (a) of this section, and (2) such recommendations for additional legislative action as he deems necessary to combat effectively drug and alcohol dependence in the Armed Forces and to treat and rehabilitate effectively any member found to be a drug or alcohol dependent person.

The Navy Program*

Under the direction of the Chief, Bureau of Naval Personnel, the Navy's Alcohol Abuse Control Program has been in existence since August 1971 as part of the Human Resource Development

---

*The Marine Corps is an integral part of the Department of the Navy.

Program. These interlocking programs offer assistance in such areas as race and intercultural relations as well as drug and alcohol use.

The Navy's Instruction 5300.20, issued May 19, 1972, states that when "not treated, alcoholism can lead to complications, e.g., alcohol addiction, withdrawal syndrome, psychiatric illnesses, and various organic illnesses. An alcoholic is not to be considered physically unfit for military service or employment on the basis of his alcoholism, because it can be arrested. However, an individual must actively seek and cooperate in treatment or rehabilitation efforts or he may be determined to be unsuitable for further military service or employment and may be separated."

The Navy has had an Alcohol Rehabilitation Center (ARC) in Long Beach, California, since June of 1967. The ARC program was expanded on January 1, 1972, with the establishment of a similar facility in Little Creek, Virginia. An additional ARC, to be completed during 1973, is planned at the Great Lakes Naval Station. Others possibly will be set up in the future.

The ARCs offer a comprehensive blend of medical and psychiatric treatment, education and counseling. At the Long Beach and Norfolk facilities the patient is informed concerning the nature of his problem and encouraged to develop a program of personal recovery. AA is very much a part of all of their programs, and all ARC counselors up to this time are recovering alcoholics. Since its inception, ARC Long Beach has treated over 1,000 patients and experienced a recovery rate of 72% (based on two years monitoring after discharge).

The Navy also is establishing Alcohol Rehabilitation Units in conjunction with the 14 Naval Hospitals throughout the world. The first ARU was opened on May 26, 1972 at the Naval Hospital in Philadelphia. Plans call for 13 additional openings in the near future, one of them at Guantanamo Bay, Cuba.

In addition to its Washington staff, the Navy has a core group of over 150 recovered Navy alcoholics (the list is ever growing) who have volunteered to work part time in local rehabilitation programs. These people will be most useful in the area of alcoholic prevention.

As of 1972 the Navy believes there are approximately 30,000

with alcohol-related problems among its personnel, less than 5% of whom have been given treatment.

It seems that the key factor in the Navy's alcohol-related treatment-rehabilitation program is prevention, since emphasis is placed on early identification. "We want to get people who are in the early stages of alcoholism before it begins to cause them problems and before their performance begins to suffer," says Captain James A. Baxter, an ex-alcoholic who heads the Navy's Alcohol Abuse Control Program. "We want to get them into our treatment programs, then back into resuming a productive Navy life."

While the Navy previously categorized alcoholism as misconduct, today every consideration is given to separating an individual's dependency on alcohol from his performance or misbehavior. The person afflicted is expected, however—and this factor must be viewed as of major importance in *any* effort to "cure" the alcohol addicted, no matter his profession or place in society—to accept the responsibility to help himself.

At its treatment centers at Little Creek and Long Beach, the patient is not looked upon as a moral degenerate or weak-willed neurotic or any of the various other labels society has hung on the alcoholic-addicted individual; rather that he is, in fact, suffering from something beyond his control. Those in charge of the Navy program are of the opinion that a recovered alcoholic is capable of returning to a job and doing it as well or better than his peers, and that he's just as reliable as anyone else, perhaps more so because he knows he has a problem.

The program at the Navy's first treatment-rehabilitation facility at Long Beach was designed by Captain J. J. Zuska of the Navy's Medical Corps. Both this facility and Little Creek have a relatively small 75-bed setup, with approximately 60 people on waiting lists. Philadelphia Naval Hospital, in the spring of 1972, instituted a program similar to those in California and Virginia.

Patients with alcohol-related problems who arrive for treatment at the centers have been dried out at naval hospitals. Confined to the center for a minimum of two weeks, they are required to attend daily rap sessions as well as six AA meetings each week. The patients take concentrated vitamins, but no tranquilizers because these, it is felt, can become as habit forming as alcohol.

Unless there is a physical impairment, patients must take Antabuse, which is dissolved in water prior to ingestion to thus make sure the tablet is not surreptitiously disposed of.

With Antabuse in their systems the patients, who range from seamen to captains, are cautioned against use of a variety of articles which contain alcohol; i.e., hair tonics, after-shave lotions, cough medicines, and others.

In Captain Baxter's estimation, "We as a nation, as a Navy, exercise pretty heavy peer pressure on people at times. And there, I feel, is where we are contributing to the incidence of alcoholism."

The Army Program

The Army's program, also open to civilian employees of the Department of the Army, has moved swiftly forward since enactment of Public Law 92—129 and the issuance of DOD's Directive 1010.2. According to Colonel L.R. Forney, Jr., Chief, Alcohol & Drug Policy Division, the Army has established decentralized alcohol and other drug facilities at major installations, with 29 halfway houses and 80 rap centers providing treatment and rehabilitation services.

The decentralized concept, the Army believes, provides services to the alcoholic as well as to his family and community, such a program allowing for the treatment of a greater number of individuals. The treatment program utilizes individual and group therapies, chemotherapy, and group living experiences. Various community groups, such as Alcoholics Anonymous, give adjunctive services.

The Department of the Army's DA Circular 600—85, dated June 1972, sets the basic policy, pattern, and regulations for its alcohol (and other drug) prevention and control program. This circular—a booklet, actually, which contains more than 100 pages—is directed chiefly to the attention of commanders and their immediate subordinates.

It is noteworthy that prevention is first on the list of Army objectives—the goal, to stop the "abuse" of alcohol and other drugs before it starts. Specific elements in this aspect of the program include education, law enforcement, and community action.

Prevention efforts are designed to reach all members of the Army community, including civilian employees, and also be coordinated with programs in the civilian community.

Volunteering for treatment is encouraged, and soldiers who do so are not subject to any disciplinary action. If a soldier cannot be effectively treated and rehabilitated in the service, any discharge resulting solely from his addiction to alcohol will not be under other than honorable conditions.

Direct help involves withdrawing the afflicted individual from acute intoxication and treating the symptoms that result. The Army's attitude is that how a soldier is detoxified strongly influences his participation in later treatment and rehabilitation. The time spent in detoxification varies with the individual; no individual is released from inpatient status until his withdrawal is complete and a medical assessment has been made.

The Army, like all other areas of society, has long sanctioned the use of alcoholic beverages. Only now is there an awareness of the high costs of alcohol use to the man and to the Army. It is inconsistent to recognize the need for a program to prevent alcoholism and at the same time to overlook the use of alcoholic beverages. Thus commanders are advised to structure military and social activities so that abstinence from alcohol is as acceptable as its use.

Since the use of alcohol is lawful and socially acceptable, the Army is not concerned with the private decisions of personnel to use or not use alcoholic beverages off the job. When such use, however, impairs work performance and physical or mental health or contributes to unacceptable social behavior or violations of the law, the commander or supervisor has a responsibility to take action.

Alcohol and Drug Prevention and Control Teams distribute information, give talks, lead group sessions, man "hot lines" and provide other services through rap centers. In addition, they coordinate with local civilian efforts and design and participate in programs for dependent wives and children, as resources permit. Team members insure that help is available 24 hours a day, seven days a week.

Since prevention is of major importance in any effort to successfully combat alcohol dependency, attention is called to *Appendix D,*

Prevention (from Department of the Army Circular 600—85) which is to be found at the end of the chapter. Much of this regarding prevention contains advice and suggestions which can prove of help to individuals and organizations outside, as well as those within, the armed services.

The Air Force Program

The U.S. Air Force (USAF) program for the rehabilitation of chronic alcoholics and those dependent upon alcohol has been accelerated in recent years, with help being rendered at both the base and away-from-base levels.

An alcohol treatment center was opened at Wright-Patterson Air Force Base (AFB), Ohio, in 1966, the operation of which will be discussed in subsequent pages. Additional treatment centers have since been established at USAF Regional Hospital, Eglin AFB, Florida; Wilford Hall USAF Medical Center, Lackland AFB, Texas; USAF Regional Hospital, Sheppard AFB, Texas; David Grant USAF Medical Center, Travis AFB, California; and USAF Medical Center, Scott AFB, Illinois. Overseas, treatment centers are located at the USAF Hospital, Lakenheath, England, and the USAF Hospital at Wiesbaden, Germany.

While these centers continue as important treatment and rehabilitation facilities, as of June 15, 1973 all commanders were instructed "to exert rehabilitative effort at the local level as the preferred alternative to immediate referral of a patient to a . . . treatment center." Transfer of a patient is not made to a treatment center until all local treatment-rehabilitation efforts have been exhausted.

When referral is made, a summary of the efforts undertaken at the base are rendered in detail to the center. Each summary includes the evaluation of the base medical officer and the base rehabilitation committee.

The program to rehabilitate the problem drinker or alcoholic at his home base rather than transfer him to a treatment center seeks "the dedicated support of all local agencies," ie: base medical services; chaplain programs, especially in the area of family counseling; off-base community mental health oriented programs; Al Anon, Al Ateen, and Alcoholics Anonymous groups either on

94

or off-base; local community inpatient treatment programs for individuals not eligible for the USAF alcohol treatment centers.

Detoxification and withdrawal, among other treatment factors, are, when necessary, accomplished at the base medical facility.

Primarily, the Air Force hopes the individual needing help will voluntarily enter the treatment program at his base. However, help is available to any USAF member referred by wife, friend, commander, or by a physician.

For those transferred to an area alcohol treatment center, the clinical program in its barest essentials consists of a 28-day in-house program. All programs are generally modeled on the Wright-Patterson program, although as programs develop and mature there may be variation between individual units. The Consultant in Psychiatry, Office of the Surgeon General, monitors all professional aspects of the program to insure that general objectives are met.

The 28-day program is designed to avoid the traditional hazards and pitfalls familiar to all physicians who have tried to deal with a person with a "drinking problem." Emphasis is on therapeutic relationship between the patient and the physician. The patients involved in the program live together in one room in the psychiatric ward of the hospital. The program is explained to them by fellow Air Force personnel who are in various stages of their hospital stay and who have had similar experiences. The physician acts as an objective, therapist-executive who modifies the treatment program according to each patient's individual needs. He does this within the broadly outlined requirements of the program. In order to reduce manipulations and power struggles to a minimum, the program has rules and regulations by which the patient must abide if he agrees to stay.

He is expected to attend Alcoholics Anonymous meetings, and he must participate in ward group meetings specifically oriented toward him and his problem. He participates in Recreational Therapy and Occupational Therapy or may choose to work in Hospital Industries as a substitute for the latter two therapies. The Occupational Therapy Department may provide a man with an opportunity to develop skills and interests he has abandoned since alcohol became an all-consuming part of his life.

He may discover talents or skills of which he was unaware. In addition, the patient may require psychological and metabolic testing to rule out organic changes secondary to alcohol.

The overall orientation of the program and message to the patient is that of a mutually exploratory educational experience. The treatment center attempts to expose the patient to all aspects of the medical profession's knowledge regarding alcohol, from the psychological to the sociological and interpersonal.

Wright-Patterson Program

The USAF Wright-Patterson Medical Center program, the basic model for other Air Force treatment centers, was created in 1966 with the encouragement and support of the Air Force Surgeon General.

In July 1969 Lt. Colonel Richard C. Scibetta and MSgt Lewis W. Dunlap assumed responsibility for the direction of the Wright-Patterson program. A comprehensive article written by Dr. Scibetta and Sgt. Dunlap, which appeared in the February 1971 *The Medical Service DIGEST*, published by the USAF's Surgeon General's office, stated that: "Although steadily expanding, the current program remains a modest, exploratory, operationally-oriented treatment program designed to assist selected alcoholics in a military setting. The intent of the program is to proceed slowly, in the hope that tomorrow's expansion will be guided by yesterday's successes. It is recognized that the survival and growth of such a program, if warranted, will depend on a record of effective rehabilitation and practical treatment techniques."

According to Dr. Scibetta and Sgt. Dunlap, while each patient is assigned to an individual physician, the patient's involvement with his physician is generally limited and varies from patient to patient and from doctor to doctor. Patients rarely require medication after withdrawal, although this too is individualized. Few patients have been treated with Antabuse, although there have been no policies governing this decision. The only standardized treatment approach is the attempt to provide an environment in which each patient must discover his own solution to his drinking problem. If a man finds that AA is his "answer" for mastering his difficulties, he receives support. If he feels his behavior is an "illness" requiring "treatment" according to the Jellinek model,* or if it is meaningful for him to see his behavior as sinful, necessitating a religious conversion or reaffirmation of his basic faith, that man's view of himself and his universe is respected and supported. The staff does not specifically encourage the man to call himself an alcoholic. However, after completing the program most men choose to use that term in describing themselves.

The discrepancy between the history available on admission and that revealed during hospitalization is dramatic, state the Scibetta-Dunlap team. Typical admission history from the patient, from the commander, and from medical records is that of moderate and periodic misuse of alcohol which has caused supervisory concern. With the support of group discussion and acceptance, the vast majority of patients later describe severe and progressive alcohol addiction of two or more years' duration. Symptoms typically include longstanding and routine blackouts, morning and daily shakes, vomiting and perhaps hematemesis while struggling to retain several "get well" drinks on arising, concealed drinking during the day, disguised but brief hospitalizations for alcoholism, degrees of withdrawal episodes including delirium tremens, several unsuccessful attempts to quit drinking independently or with outpatient treatment, recent or impending marital collapse, progressive social isolation and apathy, suicidal ruminations, driving accidents, and central nervous system impairment including forgetfulness and chronically "foggy" thinking.

Organic findings on admission include improving liver functions, sometimes severe but subsiding hypertention, and minor changes in red blood cell morphology. Of major significance is evidence of a residual organic brain syndrome which improves noticeably during the 28-day hospitalization and slowly for months thereafter. The impairment often is not detected by EEG, brain scan, x-rays, or routine neurological exam. It is readily demonstrable on selected psychometric testing. It is equally easily detected in the

---

*E.M. Jellinek, *The Disease Concept of Alcoholism*, College and University Press, New Haven, Conn., 1960.

mental status examination of the patient's ability to perform calculations, particularly serial subtractions, in which improvement directly parallels the rate of recovery.

Success Rates of the Three Services

The Navy claims a 75 percent success rate at their various treatment rehabilitation centers.

In the USAF Surgeon General's *DIGEST* article, Wright-Patterson states that as of July 31, 1970, they were surprised to discover that 87 percent of their patients have remained in the Air Force, even though fewer than half report total abstinence. However, two-thirds of the group report either total abstinence or controlled drinking. The overall impression is that the patients retained in the Air Force are doing well, which is supported by considerable collateral data as well as reports of promotions, awards, and other non-automatic recognition.

"The Army, at present, has no statistics concerning their success with Alcoholics," states Col. Forney. "Our program being highly decentralized . . . a 'success rate' . . . will vary widely between installations, depending on personnel resources, command, etc."

APPENDIX D
PREVENTION

Section I. GENERAL

D—1. Purpose. To prescribe policy, outline programs, and provide guidance for measures to prevent alcohol and drug abuse.

D—2. Objectives. The Army's objectives are to stop alcohol and drug abuse before they start and to minimize their effects when they exist.

D—3. Concept. a. In the broadest sense, any measures which enhance the quality of life in the military community assist in preventing abuse of alcohol and other drugs.

b. The three areas of the prevention portion of the Army's program are education, law enforcement, and community action.

Section II. EDUCATION

D—4. Purpose. To prescribe policies and provide guidance for the conduct of alcohol and drug abuse education.

D—5. Objectives. An effective educational program transmits credible information about alcohol and other drug abuse and associated problems and alters attitudes related to these problems. Education must be tailored to a variety of target audiences.

a. The Army has an obligation to insure that soldiers do not begin or continue the use of any drug out of ignorance of its effects. Those for whom alcohol and other drugs are not the problem, but the solution to other problems, must become aware of practical alternatives to escape through drug abuse.

b. Leaders and supervisors must know about the technical aspects of drugs, the drug culture, and the causes of alcohol and other drug abuse. In addition, they need to understand how to establish an environment that makes alcohol and other drug abuse less likely and provides the maximum opportunity for rehabilitation of soldiers with problems related to alcohol and other drug abuse. Leaders at all levels must learn how to use traditional principles of leadership in ways effective for reaching young soldiers.

c. Department of the Army civilian employees and military dependents must have ready access to factual and pertinent information.

d. Dependent school children deserve special attention, both because they are a high risk and because preventive efforts with them may be particularly productive.

D—6. Policy. Every installation will have an active educational program structured to meet local needs and designed to reach all target groups.

D—7. Concept. a. Getting facts across to troops is traditional in Army education. Facts include information about drugs, the reasons behind drug abuse, and ways of coping with the problems that result. Past programs have assumed that if men knew the possible physical and legal consequences of drug-taking, they would not abuse drugs. This assumption is wrong; knowing the facts is only a necessary first step.

b. Influencing attitudes and behavior is more difficult and more important. Whether or not a person abuses alcohol or other drugs depends to a significant extent on how he feels. Education must address the feelings that lead to drug-taking; drug abuse results from a series of decisions which to a considerable degree are emotional, not rational. In addition, education must modify the attitudes of those who regard alcoholics and other drug abusers as fundamentally different or evil men.

c. Education programs will need to make greater use of unconventional methods, in addition to the usual techniques. Examples are small group sessions, theatrical programs, and mixed media presentations. Recovered alcoholics and other ex-drug-abusers can be effective in education programs, but need to be chosen and supervised carefully.

d. Officers and noncommissioned officers should receive instruction in leading small group discussions on alcohol and other drug abuse.

e. Education efforts also should attempt to reach the natural leaders, those who strongly influence the behavior and attitudes of their associates. Men whose way of life is rewarding without drugs

100

should be encouraged to speak out about their beliefs as well as live them.

D—8. Implementation. a. Department of the Army, assisted by the Department of Defense, will provide general educational materials (pamphlets, posters, books, films, etc.) Section III contains a list of DA materials currently available.

b. Major commands and installations will supplement DA materials with locally developed items, including audio-visual materials and training aids. They may contract with local civilian agencies as funds are available.

c. Installation commanders will insure that an active education program reaches all personnel. The ADDIC can assist the commander with the supervision of education programs.

d. Each battalion and separate company should have at least one Drug Education Specialist, either an officer or enlisted man. It is desirable that he have some background in the social or behavioral sciences, experience in the drug culture, or both. It is essential that he be able to communicate easily with all members of the unit, especially the young soldier. He should help organize and develop unit drug abuse education activities. Drug Education Specialists should receive special training at the installation level.

e. Dependent schools under DA control will appoint a coordinator of Drug Abuse Education from the school staff who will assist in implementing a program involving educators, parents, students, and the military community. Where dependent schools are not under DA control, commanders will coordinate with school authorities and assist in the integration of drug abuse education in the curriculum.

f. Alcohol and other drug abuse education efforts should include civilian employees and dependents. Supervisors of civilian employees should be trained in this area. This training should be coordinated with the civilian personnel office to assure that it is made a requirement and part of the supervisory training program. See AR 600—300 for explicit instructions concerning alcoholism in civilian employees.

g. Commanders should encourage workshops, provide effective instructional materials, and periodically assess the effectiveness of the drug abuse education program.

Section IV. LAW ENFORCEMENT

D—21. Purpose. To prescribe law enforcement policies and provide guidance applicable to HQDA ADAPCP.

D—22. Concept. a. Direct enforcement primarily at eliminating the supply of illegal drugs and apprehending traffickers.

b. Establish programs to detect and apprehend those whose alcohol or other drug abuse interferes with their operating motor vehicles. Set up procedures to suspend or withdraw driving privileges of such persons.

D—23. Objectives. a. To stem the flow of illegal drugs to the military community.

b. To apprehend members of the Army community who illegally possess, use, or distribute drugs on Army installations.

c. Through joint military and civilian efforts, to prevent and control drug-related crimes and traffic accidents.

D—24. Implementation. Commanders will—

a. Maintain liaison and coordination with the Criminal Investigation Division (CID) and with appropriate international, federal, state, host-country, and local law enforcement and customs agencies on alcohol and other drug matters.

b. Establish oversea programs consistent with host-country agreements or treaties to prevent the importation of drugs. As a minimum, programs will include the inspection of individuals, mail, baggage, and household goods returning to the United States.

c. Refer to the Military Police or the Criminal Investigation Division offenses involving illegal possession, use, sale, or trafficking in drugs. In conjunction with CID, conduct periodic physical security inspections or crime surveys of facilities used for storage and handling of drugs subject to abuse. Review procedures for securing and accounting for drugs and other sensitive items during those inspections or surveys.

d. Develop programs to suppress trafficking.

e. Consult with local SJA, when possible, prior to employing search and seizure procedures.

Section V. COMMUNITY ACTION

D—25. Purpose. To indicate ways in which commanders can mobilize community resources to assist in their alcohol and drug abuse prevention and control programs.

D—26. Concept. a. Measures which improve the quality of life in the military community, especially those which provide meaningful alternatives to drug-taking, will help prevent the abuse of alcohol and other drugs.

b. Commanders have access to existing social agencies which can contribute to preventive actions. Experience has shown that representatives of these agencies make useful members of the ADDIC.

c. Many people in the Army community are willing to volunteer their ideas, time, and energies for the program.

d. Social pressure is a powerful force in determining behavior, especially with regard to using alcohol or other drugs.

e. Civilian communities near military installations often have resources which can supplement Army efforts.

D—27. Implementaion. a. Commanders should seek suggestions about prevention from various members of the military community, including the enlisted men, noncommissioned and junior officer councils, and wives and dependents.

b. The rap center can serve as a focus for community action. Its staff should distribute information, offer referral services, and maintain a "hot line". The center should provide a setting for group talks and rap sessions for soldiers and their dependents after normal duty hours. The officer in charge of the rap center is a suitable individual to develop and coordinate installation educational efforts. He is usually a member of the ADDIC. He and his staff should be encouraged to coordinate military efforts with those of the local civilian community.

c. Special Services should insure that adequate recreational facilities and equipment are available.

d. Army Community Services should provide information, assistance, and guidance to military families in obtaining help for alcohol and other drug related problems. ACS should convey to the ADDIC its experience on appropriate community problems.

e. The various Army clubs (wives, officers, NCO) should be encouraged to assist in the drug abuse prevention and control program, to include fund raising for local unfinanced requirements.

f. Military dependent children should be encouraged to attend education and training courses and mobilize peer pressure against alcohol and other drug abuse. '

g. A bulletin listing all recreation activities, including date, time, and place, should be published periodically and given the widest possible distribution to reach all members of the military community, especially lower grade enlisted men. The bulletin should show events scheduled on the installation and in the surrounding community.

h. Minority groups may well have special interest in prevention and can make significant contributions to community programs.

7

THE LICENSED
BEVERAGE
INDUSTRY

"The ideas are generated and the facts collected by LBI, through its staff of trained public relations experts, and 'sold' to the public by this staff . . . ."

—Licensed Beverage Industries, Inc.

7

Alcohol Beverage Industry Associations

According to the First Special Report to the U.S. Congress on Alcohol and Health, Public Law 91—616 aims "to dispel the many myths surrounding alcohol," to help problem drinkers and alcoholics stop drinking, and, in essence, to prevent Americans from drinking excessively.

The three propaganda arms of the alcohol-beverage industry— the Wine Institute, the United States Brewers Association, and the Licensed Beverage Industries, Inc. (LBI)—work to increase the consumption of alcoholic beverages.

Like public relations organizations of other major businesses, these of the wine, beer, and liquor industries were formed to promote sales. The primary function of LBI and companion organizations is to offset any private or governmental attempts at action that would prove in any way detrimental to the manufacture, distribution, and sales of alcohol beverages. They also aim to create an image that these beverages are good for the individual and to attribute an aura of glamour and good fellowship to all those who imbibe. These organizations are active lobbyists in all levels of

WHAT IS LBI?

HOW DOES THIS BENEFIT OUR INDUSTRY?

WHAT ARE ITS OBJECTIVES?

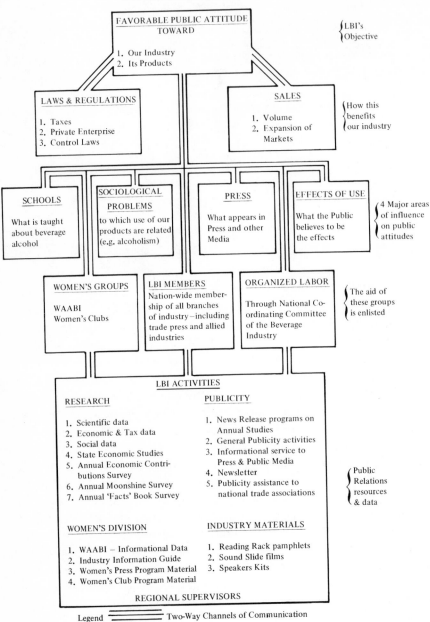

FAVORABLE PUBLIC ATTITUDE TOWARD

1. Our Industry
2. Its Products

{ LBI's Objective

LAWS & REGULATIONS

1. Taxes
2. Private Enterprise
3. Control Laws

SALES

1. Volume
2. Expansion of Markets

{ How this benefits our industry

SCHOOLS

What is taught about beverage alcohol

SOCIOLOGICAL PROBLEMS

to which use of our products are related (e.g. alcoholism)

PRESS

What appears in Press and other Media

EFFECTS OF USE

What the Public believes to be the effects

{ 4 Major areas of influence on public attitudes

WOMEN'S GROUPS

WAABI
Women's Clubs

LBI MEMBERS

Nation-wide membership of all branches of industry – including trade press and allied industries

ORGANIZED LABOR

Through National Coordinating Committee of the Beverage Industry

{ The aid of these groups is enlisted

LBI ACTIVITIES

RESEARCH

1. Scientific data
2. Economic & Tax data
3. Social data
4. State Economic Studies
5. Annual Economic Contributions Survey
6. Annual Moonshine Survey
7. Annual 'Facts' Book Survey

PUBLICITY

1. News Release programs on Annual Studies
2. General Publicity activities
3. Informational service to Press & Public Media
4. Newsletter
5. Publicity assistance to national trade associations

{ Public Relations resources & data

WOMEN'S DIVISION

1. WAABI – Informational Data
2. Industry Information Guide
3. Women's Press Program Material
4. Women's Club Program Material

INDUSTRY MATERIALS

1. Reading Rack pamphlets
2. Sound Slide films
3. Speakers Kits

REGIONAL SUPERVISORS

Legend ════════ Two-Way Channels of Communication

government. To cite but one example, in 1970 the United States Brewers Association moved its headquarters from New York City to Washington, D.C. to underline "the increasing importance of the industry's governmental relations."

The associations that champion the alcohol-beverage industry have done a remarkably successful job. Perhaps there is no better way to understand this than to examine the services of the Licensed Beverage Industries, Inc., as described by LBI itself. Following is a summary of an LBI pamphlet issued in 1970 to its membership, accompanied by the author's foot-noted analysis of various sections. The pamphlet opens with a chart (opposite page) of the LBI organization.

The pamphlet's Foreword states:
> Since 1946 the initials LBI have represented an important symbol, both to the American public and to the alcoholic beverage industry. To the mass communications media, LBI is the established source of accurate information on this major industry, and a respected voice on all subjects directly or indirectly involving its products.*
>
> To the industry, it is two things: the sole meeting ground for all segments of the industry, where mutual problems, policies and programs can be developed and implemented; and, the unified voice speaking for the 1.3 million Americans and the numerous firms and associations that make up this important member of the American industrial family.
>
> This booklet has been prepared to give you a specific and comprehensive account of LBI as a functioning organization, its broad range of activities and the manner in which it develops and achieves its objectives.

The booklet then continues (page 5):
> LBI is a familiar term to practically everyone in the liquor industry. Since 1946, LBI . . . that stands for Licensed Beverage Industries, Inc. . . . has been the nation-wide, all-industry public relations organization of the distilled spirits industry.
>
> Its job basically is to deal with all matters and problems affecting public attitudes toward the industry and its products.
>
> And that's an important job . . . because a favorable public attitude has more tangible value than simply creating a climate of

---

*While it is true that LBI provides an established source of information, its accuracy is open to question since information that is withheld may be more important than that which is made available.

opinion that affords a feeling of pride and satisfaction to those identified with our industry. In the long run, these public opinions and attitudes have a direct relationship to the laws and regulations relating to the way the industry's business is conducted . . . and to the volume of sales this industry enjoys.*

In many ways, LBI's job can be compared to the work of the companies and organizations it serves . . . the producing and selling of a product. The basic difference lies in the nature of the product.

LBI deals in facts and ideas . . . they are the product. The facts form the solid base for the opinions that every industry member knows the public should have about his industry, himself, and the product he sells. The ideas are generated and the facts collected by LBI, through its staff of trained public relations experts, and "sold" to the public by this staff . . . with a gigantic assist from LBI's nation-wide membership.†

Broadly speaking, there are three major "ideas" that LBI relates factually:

That the industry is of significance and importance to the economic and social life of our nation.

That the people of the industry play an important role in their communities, making important contributions to community life.

And that the industry's products have a definite, beneficial place in our society.**

The Licensed Beverage Industries, Inc. pamphlet's commentary continues:

Almost all of LBI's activity is built around the projection, to the widest possible audience, of facts which support these ideas. But the details of these activities, and how they are carried out, would fill several booklets. So for now, let's examine just a few of the highlights.

LBI membership includes practically all of the leading distillers, the major wholesale distributors throughout the country, rectifiers, importers, associations . . . national, state, and local . . . representing all branches of the industry, the trade press

---

*This frank admission of LBI's efforts to influence public opinion and thus directly affect laws and regulations should serve as a warning not only to consumers but also to legislators relying on the LBI for information.

†Perhaps the problems created by the use of alcohol in this country may indicate that the ideas generated by the LBI and "sold" to the public are not really in the public's interest.

**Note that the LBI does not specify any of the benefits which have won the industry's products "a definite, beneficial place in our society."

110

and a variety of important allied industries. Through its membership, LBI represents 60,000 licensees . . . and the hundreds of thousands of their employees . . . from coast to coast.

This membership is significant to both the structure and function of LBI. Because of this broad and comprehensive base, LBI is accepted by the public and the communications media as a qualified spokesman for the industry. Its views on matters of public interest concerning this industry, as well as supporting statistical and social research data, are sought daily by writers, commentators, editors, educators and others.*

On the other hand, LBI members who have had to face tax increase proposals, economic threats to their investments and continuance in business, and a variety of other compelling local problems that are part of the everyday hazard of licensees in this business, can attest to the invaluable helpfulness of LBI when the chips are down.

When these local problems develop, LBI members quickly turn to their public relations organization . . . equipped through long experience with the background knowledge and know-how to meet these challenges . . . for facts, ideas, programs and assistance in dealing with their special situation.

This LBI assistance takes several forms. Generally, such an activity starts with a thorough study of the problem, possibly in the form of an economic survey, to develop the true picture. During the past two years, for example, LBI has completed more than thirty such special state and local studies at the request of its members, covering a wide variety of subjects, and the results have been used in effective public relations campaigns.

On other occasions, the call may be for hurry-up action to fight a menacing "fire"† . . . and this brings LBI experts directly to the scene, to develop specialized public relations programs, help prepare the materials to be used, and provide guidance and assistance in carrying out a campaign to create a better understanding between the industry, the press and the public.

Long range or fire-fighting, its work with LBI members at the local level has been a dramatic hallmark of LBI activities. And throughout the year, LBI carries on a continuing industry information program, in many different forms, to keep its members up-to-date on public relations developments affecting the industry, its members and its products, and to provide them with

---

*The LBI's views on matters of "public interest" are understandably self-serving. It is imperative in this author's opinion, that an unbiased information service be at all times available to writers, commentators, editors, educators, and others.

†A "fire" is usually an attempt at local restrictions on the sale of alcoholic beverages, or a possible tax increase on a county or state level.

ideas and facts enabling them to act as local "salesmen" for LBI public relations policies and programs.

LBI also enjoys close working relationships with not only the press, through its membership in 38 state press associations, but with civic and public leaders as well.

A staff of eleven highly skilled regional supervisors maintain continuing contact with newspaper editors and publishers and with other community leaders who are influential in forming public attitudes. They also assist in developing and executing local programs of public relations in cooperation with industry groups, and maintain a continuous two-way liaison with the LBI membership on local and area industry problems.

LBI has been especially active with state control administrators, individually and through their associations ... the NCSLA and the NABCA ... and through the Joint Committee of the States to Study Alcoholic Beverage Laws, of which, incidentally, LBI's president is the only continuing member of the original Industry Advisory Committee.

From this brief outline, it is obvious that LBI is not a trade association in the customary sense, in that it has no function or responsibilities directly related to the trade, legal, merchandising, or competitive practices or problems of the industry or its members. It operates entirely in the field of public relations ... and on problems that are of mutual interest, concern and benefit to all segments and members of the industry.

As vitally important and necessary as the above-outlined "grass roots" activities and internal industry information work are, LBI's major efforts, of course, are on a broader, national scale ... the creation and maintaining of a good public image of the liquor industry. In this area, let's take a look at a few examples ...

Taxation ... For years, LBI has been the fountainhead of economic and statistical data and information used by the Industry Tax Council in opposing proposed increases in the already excessive and unfair tax levies, at the national, state and local levels, on our products. National and individual state studies are kept up-to-the-minute. Today, with the industry facing the biggest threat of "Prohibition-by-Taxation" since Repeal, the Tax Council is being reactivated and is already at work in various states. A National Council Against Illegal Liquor ... to combat the spread of the death-dealing, tax-evading, criminal-syndicate moonshine racket ... has also been set up by LBI, with State Councils already active in 16 states.*

---

*The high taxes paid by the liquor industry are, in fact, largely borne by the consumer and have become so important to governmental income, that they actually add to the bargaining power of the liquor industry in the matter of restricting laws and regulations.

Social Problems ... This is the area in which the industry is constantly under attack by anti-industry forces.

Page 17 of the LBI pamphlet continues with:

For example, in alcoholism the industry has long been recognized as a leader among the objective groups seeking better understanding of and greater scientific knowledge about this health problem. Through LBI, it has helped to develop the current public concept of alcoholism as a disease, of which the excessive use of alcohol is a symptom but not the cause, and for which prohibition is not the answer.* And it is recognized as a leader in the field of research through its $500,000 five-year grants-in-aid program, set up and administered by the Scientific Advisory Council to LBI, to assist nationally-known scientists and universities in seeking answers to the causes, treatment and possible cures for this illness. LBI's cooperation and participation is welcomed by other objective public and private organizations working to combat this disease.

LBI also sponsors research in highway safety, to put into proper perspective the relationship of drinking to safe driving, and to combat the unfounded concept that drunken drivers are responsible for a majority of fatal highway accidents. In this field, too, LBI works with objective public and private organizations in attempting to develop programs to reduce the incidence of drunken driving.†

Similar work is carried on, generally in cooperation with other objective groups, in the field of drinking by minors, where scientific studies have shown that while delinquents may drink, the drinking is a symptom of juvenile delinquency, not the cause.

The proper and beneficial uses of liquor ... through the use of authentic, objective information and statements from eminent scientists and doctors, researched from medical and other scientific journals and publications, LBI promotes such facts as [that] ...

To the individual the moderate use of liquor provides relaxaction and relief from the tensions of modern living, and promotes pleasant social intercourse, and ...

The moderate use of liquor by the normal adult is not harmful and actually can be beneficial. Through its Women's Division LBI also carries on activities to show that the proper and moderate

---

*Note the use of "prohibition" rather than "abstinence."

†Note the emphasis of this paragraph seems to indicate that the LBI is more interested in combating the statistics which show that drunk drivers are responsible for 50 percent of highway accidents than in working to reduce the number of accidents resulting from the use of alcohol.

use of alcholic beverages is a socially accepted part of today's gracious living.*

The pamphlet then moves into the area of education in the schools:

Alcoholic Education in the Schools . . . All 50 states require the teaching about alcohol in their schools. For almost a century, what has been taught has been largely Dry-inspired propaganda. LBI's Division of Educational Studies found out that most teachers want objective facts to teach. Shortly, two objective books . . . inaugurated by the Scientific Advisory Council to LBI and quickly taken over by a major textbook publishing firm . . . will be available for educators, replacing the obsolete concepts and Dry-inspired propaganda now in use and insuring a new perspective in alcohol education.†

The Economic Importance of the Industry . . . Continuing economic and statistical studies, showing our industry to be a major factor in the economic well-being of the country, are used in many forms . . . publicity, booklets, speeches and material for writers, its states and communities, educators, etc.**

These are just a few examples of the major activities being carried on by LBI, through its headquarters staff . . . including the Divisions of Economic Research, Social Research, Publicity, Publications and Trade Press, Educational Studies, Public Activities, Women's Activities and Regional Supervisors . . . with outstanding help from the National Women's Association of Allied Beverage Industries, Inc., and the National Coordinating Committee of the Alcoholic Beverage Industry, representing organized labor and industry groups, along with more than 200 volunteer industry members of the nationwide LBI Speakers Bureau.

Much has been accomplished . . . but there is still much to be done, and to this task, with the help of its members, LBI dedicates itself.††

---

*For a proper evaluation of the effects of alcohol, the reader might compare the "benefits" as listed by the LBI with the other "effects" shown on the chart on pages 134-135.

†It is LBI's job, of course, to use "wet-inspired" propaganda since the association feels that it will create more sales than "dry-inspired" propaganda.

**See chapter 8, "Alcohol's Cost to Society."

††Author's note: It will take equal dedication on the part of those interested in reducing the consumption of alcoholic beverages to match the efforts of the LBI in increasing consumption.

LBI chooses a highly paid and skillful agency to create the distilled spirits industry's advertising. In July 1970, *Time* and *Newsweek* magazines published an advertisement that many authorities considered to be a dangerous misrepresentation of fact.* The portion of the advertisement (following page) that particularly drew fire was the chart which shows the "Hours to wait [before driving] after start of drinking," with the inference that both the National Safety Council and the American Medical Association had sanctioned the chart's statistics.

The ensuing clash ultimately involved Chairman of the Board of the Preferred Risk Mutual Insurance Company, William N. Plymat, who was the first to take issue with the hours-to-wait chart, as well as the two magazines, the American Medical Association (AMA), the National Safety Council (NSC), and U.S. Transportation Secretary John A. Volpe.

On August 18th, Plymat wrote the NSC and the AMA concerning the advertisement and noted ". . . that this association appears to suggest that a man could have three shots of whiskey and still drive a car at once without waiting for any of the alcohol to oxidize . . . If you have any printed materials indicating the amount of alcohol that may safely be used by a driver within an hour of driving, we would appreciate having that information."

After receipt of a letter from the National Safety Council in which its president, Howard Pyle, concurred with Plymat's reaction, the latter wrote to *Time*'s Editor-in-Chief, Hedly Donovan. Donovan took the position that the magazine had not been "used" by LBI since the ad "was cleared in advance with the American Medical Association."

Plymat then, on October 6th, sent the editor a published item which stated that the AMA "attacked the Licensed Beverage

---

*U.S. Code, Title 15, Section 55, False advertising: Advertising, rather than labeling, which is misleading in a material respect, and in determining whether it is misleading there shall be taken into account among other things, not only representations made or suggested by statement, word, design, devise, sound, or any combination thereof but also the extent to which the advertising fails to reveal facts, materials in the light of such representation or material with respect to consequences which may result from the use of the commodity to which the advertisement relates under the conditions prescribed in said advertisement or under such conditions as are customary and usual.

The liquor industry vs. the drunk driver

We're the people who make distilled spirits. What is our stand on the issue of drinking and driving?

It's the same as the National Safety Council and the American Medical Association.

For years the Council said, "If you drink, don't drive." But unfortunately, it now says, too many don't heed this advice. "Drinking continues to be socially acceptable," it points out, "90 to 95 million Americans drink at least occasionally."

So the Council and the AMA are now taking a new tack—a nation-wide educational program aimed at helping social drinkers to know their limits. It also aims to build public support for dealing with "sick drivers" —alcoholics who misuse alcohol. Because experts agree that the biggest problem on highways is not the social drinker but the chronic alcoholic. Millions of Americans drink moderately and drive safely.

Getting personal for a minute—how much alcohol can *you* handle? To help you answer this question, we are offering a chart prepared by a nationally recognized authority. It tells in simple, factual form how many drinks over how long a time you can have before driving.

We'll be glad to send you as many copies as you would like. Just write Licensed Beverage Industries, Inc., 155 E. 44th Street, New York, N.Y. 10017.

We say that ideally, people should not drink before they drive. But this does not square with the facts of life. So if you do drink and drive, *know your limits*, use your head—use this chart.

Licensed Beverage Industries, Inc.

The operator of a motor vehicle is presumed by law to be impaired when the percent of alcohol in his blood is above a certain level. To drive legally the table below indicates how long a normal adult of given body weight must wait after drinking a given amount of whisky, to be safely within those limits. If the weight is between two of those shown use the lower one.

Drinks (1 ½ ounces) Consumed

Lbs. body weight	1	2	3	4	5	6	7	8
100	0	½	3½	6½	9½	12½	16	19
120	0	0	2	4½	7	9½	12½	15
140	0	0	1	3	5½	7½	10	12
160	0	0	0	2	4	6	8	9½
180	0	0	0	1	2½	4½	6½	8
200	0	0	0	½	2	3½	5	6½

Hours to wait after start of drinking

Prepared by Dr. Leon A. Greenberg
Rutgers University Center of Alcohol Studies

116

Industries" for the manner of its presentation of the advertisement.

"The chart shows what the legal limits are with respect to drinking and driving. The safe limits are something else," the Assistant Executive Vice President of AMA wrote in a letter to *Time* and *Newsweek* magazines.

Meanwhile, Plymat had contacted John A. Volpe, U.S. Secretary of Transportation. Volpe replied on December 3rd, stating that his department had obtained a commitment from Donovan not to repeat this ad. In his response on December 11th, Plymat urged the Secretary to "make it unmistakably clear by some public pronouncement that you endorse the statements of the National Safety Council that a driver should wait one hour for each drink he has consumed before driving a car."

Volpe then addressed the Licensed Beverage Industries in New York where he told representatives of the alcohol-beverage industry that "the legal limit is a far cry from the safe drinking [and driving] limit . . . The man who thinks he can safely drive with a blood alcohol content of up to 0.10 percent is the man who will jump a median strip to hit your car." (The legal blood-level percentages, depending on state laws, vary from 0.08 to 0.15 percent. See Chapter 3.)

The end result was that the American Medical Association and the National Safety Council demanded removal of its names from the LBI ad, and *Time* and *Newsweek* ceased publishing the advertisement. The Federal Trade Commission had been brought into the issue, but did not further pursue the matter when LBI promised not to repeat the ad. Nor did the FTC require LBI to advise the public of its misrepresentation, as is customary in such cases.

LBI's Recent Change

LBI and its companion propaganda arms are showing some change of attitude since enactment of Law 91—616. In the summer of 1972, for example, a billboard advertisement carried this message:

BEVERAGE BULLETIN
The Liquor Industry Says: If It's One For The Road—Make It Coffee.

That the Licensed Beverage Industry is susceptible to pressures is further attested to by the tone of its "If you choose to drink—drink responsibly" ad campaign.

Of course, that raises the point: how can one take an addictive drug and still be considered responsible? As the fact that alcohol is addictive reaches the public consciousness we can look for new slogans to rationalize the use of alcoholic beverages.

Not everyone should drink. But everyone who does should drink sensibly.

There are great numbers of people who have strong reasons for not drinking — religious, physical and personal reasons. And their desire to abstain should be respected by all.

It's a fact, however, that adult drinking is normal behavior in most circles today. The majority of people in this country choose to drink. And most who do so do not abuse the privilege.

They know that liquor is an adjunct of the good life. And that the enjoyment of liquor entails a responsibility to themselves and to society.

They know, too, that liquor is one of the most skillfully-made products in the world. And that to truly enjoy its quality and flavor, one should sip it slowly, consume it with food, take it in the company of others — all in relaxing, comfortable circumstances.

As the people who make and sell distilled spirits, we're pleased that most people drink our products just as carefully as we make them. Because the only way to fully appreciate what they're made of is to mix them with common sense.

We urge you to remember this the next time you're enjoying a friendly round with family or friends. And ask you to respect the wishes of anyone who'd rather have fruit juice or soft drinks instead.

If you choose to drink, drink responsibly.

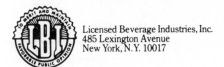

Licensed Beverage Industries, Inc.
485 Lexington Avenue
New York, N.Y. 10017

8

ALCOHOL'S COST TO SOCIETY

*". . . for every dollar of revenue received
by the State of Tennessee for consumption
of alcoholic beverages arising out of Memphis
and Shelby County, it cost the state $2.28 . . . ."*

—*Report on Alcohol*

8

Alcohol-Beverage Revenues

Evanston, Illinois, the home town of Frances Willard, founder of the World's Christian Temperance Union and "dry" for 116 years, lifted its ban on the sale of alcoholic beverages in January 1972. All but one of the city's Chamber of Commerce directors recommended to the council that liquor be sold in restaurants and hotels in this community. Said a director, "The city council needed revenue and a proposed hotel would not locate here if they could not get a liquor license."

In the minds of most people, revenue received from the sale of alcoholic beverages is among the chief cure-alls for financial distress. Even Abraham Lincoln, a total abstainer, said, "The people will drink and the government must have more money."

This thesis was not new in President Lincoln's day, and it certainly is not new today when the government needs more money than ever before in its history. When the consumer buys a bottle of distilled spirits for $4.75, $2.76 of the selling price is taxes. An estimated $8.2 billion was collected in alcohol-beverage taxes by local, state, and federal governments for the year 1971.

Of this sum $5.1 billion went to the federal government. Thus there is some validity to the statement that the federal government is in the liquor business, in partnership with the alcohol-beverage industry.

A number of studies indicate that the cost of drinking is rarely, if ever, recompensed by the tax dollars obtained from it. One recent study, made by Dr. Slater W. Hollis, professor at Memphis State University, Memphis, Tennessee, and Walter S. Krusich, vice president of the American Business Men's Research Foundation, to determine whether or not the economic cost to taxpayers and government from alcoholic beverages was greater than the revenue received, was published in the 1971 Fall and Winter issue of *Report on Alcohol.* Based on a dissertation by Dr. Hollis, the study covered the relationship between alcohol and crime; alcohol and transportation accidents; alcohol and accidents at home, at work, and at recreational areas; alcohol and disease; alcohol and divorce; alcohol and unemployment; and alcohol and pollution. The study's summary stated:

> . . . for every dollar of revenue received by the State of Tennessee for consumption of alcoholic beverages arising out of Memphis and Shelby County, it cost the state $2.28; for every dollar of revenue the county of Shelby received from consumption of alcoholic beverages it cost the county $11.08; for every dollar the city of Memphis received from the consumption of alcoholic beverages it cost the city $4.39.

Alcohol Consumption Increase

Every year of the past decade, the consumption of alcoholic beverages has increased. The per capita consumption (18 years of age and over) of alcohol beverages has now risen to 3.93 gallons of absolute alcohol, the all-time high. (In 1964, somewhat over $13 billion was spent for alcoholic beverages.) Of the 3.93 gallons per capita, HEW's December 1971 Report states: "This allows, for one drinker, about 44 fifths of whiskey; or 98 bottles of fortified wine; or 157 bottles of table wine; or 928 bottles of beer."

According to *Drug Use in America: Problem in Perspective*, the Second Report of the National Commission on Marihuana and

Drug Abuse (issued March 1973),* "The alcohol industry produced over one billion gallons of spirits, wine and beer for which 100 million consumers paid about $24 billion."

With the increase in consumption, the outlets for beverage alcohol also have increased. An August 1971 report by the U.S. Internal Revenue Service showed a rise in occupational licenses issued nation-wide to dealers during the preceding two years. The number of retailers increased by 7,539, to 418,231, which means that, based on the 1970 U.S. Census of persons over 21, there now exists one alcohol-beverage outlet for every 196 individuals who drink.

[Author's note: Pages 9 through 18 of the December 1971 HEW Report offer a particularly close examination of the nation's consumption of alcohol beverages.]

Though other cost-tax factors are involved, it is interesting to note that while Prohibition was the law of the land, with no alcohol-beverage taxes to help support the government, surpluses occurred in federal finances during 11 of those 13 years. In 22 of the 25 years after repeal of the Eighteenth Amendment, with liquor revenue available, there was a deficit in federal finances.

Alcohol—A Drain on the Economy

A series of news articles published after a two-week investigation, conducted with the help of a newly-opened branch of the National Council of Alcoholism for San Diego County, California, offered one local view of the cost-vs-gain of beverage alcohol.

". . . alcohol is the cause of heart-break for more than 180,000 San Diegans," a newspaper stated. "The real story lies in the cries for help over the phone; in the ultimate tragedy which forces six-year old children into self-help meetings. Tiny children of alcoholic parents are so affected by the problems at home that we had to form a group to help them. We call them the bubble-gum set. It's the first group like it in the United States."

The newspaper also declared that all levels of society appeared at the county's Alcoholism Rehabilitation Clinic ". . . housewives, top county officials, doctors, lawyers, skid row bums and society

---

*Excerpts from the Commission's Report are to be found beginning on page 217.

leaders, stewardesses, models, pilots and young businessmen not yet 26. Right now the case load includes the son of a San Diego millionaire, a formerly nationally-known rock musician, and a Navy captain."

The Navy, San Diego's biggest business, admitted that 10 percent of its personnel have alcohol-related problems, costing the Navy and taxpayers an estimated $45 million a year. Within San Diego's business world the cost was counted at $10 million, due, among other factors, to errors in job performance.

According to NIAAA, "alcohol and alcoholism drain the economy of an estimated $15 billion a year. Of this total, $10 billion is attributed to lost time in business, industry, civilian government, and the military . . . $2 billion is spent for health and welfare services provided to alcoholic persons and their families . . . and property damage, medical expenses, and other overhead costs account for another $3 billion or more."

The cost of alcohol is so extensive not only in dollars, but in health, lives, and basic food products—such as grain, fruit, and sugar—that the national government must vigorously pursue the intent of 91—616.

This editorial in *Business Week*, November 18, 1972, points up the need for continued public pressure on the government:

> . . . Although Congress earmarked $300 million for three years of alcoholism research and treatment when it passed the Hughes Act in 1970, President Nixon has allocated only $86 million of that amount to date, and most of the money has been used for treatment programs.
>
> There is no excuse for this sort of false economy. Congress clearly intended to involve the government in a large-scale, long-range commitment to solve the mysteries of alcoholism through basic research.

9

MEDICINE, SCIENCE, AND ALCOHOL

"All substances which exert an effect on the brain have the potential to be dangerous. This is true of alcohol."

—*NIAAA*

9

Is Alcohol "Healthful"?

To casual imbibers of wine, whiskey, and beer, it would be reassuring to know that, medically and scientifically, a few drinks will never hurt and might even do some good. The fact is that a few drinks might do your body some harm and will never do it any good. To the heavy drinker, alcohol does considerable harm. To the dependent drinker and alcoholic, this drug can prove disastrous.

In recent years, the myths about the "good" alcohol can do have been increasingly discredited. On a freezing day a jolt of hard liquor does *not* make the body warmer; it is *not* an antidote for frostbite. There is no evidence indicating alcohol to be helpful to the heart. The theory on which doctors have advised older people to "take a shot or two" as a cardiac stimulant has been disproven. Today liquor is rarely given to a person who has fainted or suffered shock.

Alcohol will not take the place of food. Alcohol does nothing to build tissue and cannot be stored for future use like sugar or fat. While beer and wine do contain small quantities of protein, starch, and sugar, their food value is negligible. The hazard of continually allowing alcohol to substitute for food can result in pellagra, cirrhosis of the liver, delirium tremens, polyneuropathy, alcoholic hallucinosis, Wernicke's disease, and Korsakoff's psychosis.

Unlike most other drugs, alcohol is a unique substance which can serve as a fuel (but not a food) for the body. It can be a source of energy, like sugar, but it also can act as a poison and derange the appetite mechanisms, thereby offsetting the desire for food.

Sludging

Recent evidence indicates that a wide variety of diseased conditions are brought about by a substance that coats the body's red cells, causing them to adhere to one another in clumps. These clumps, sometimes called "sludge," can be created by the ingestion of alcohol. Evidence has been advanced that every time a drink is taken even the moderate imbiber may incur some loss of irreplacable brain cells. There is also strong scientific medical information that alcohol-created sludge can deleteriously affect other parts of the human body, including the eyes. This data was the result of experiments at the Medical University of South Carolina by Professor Melvin H. Knisely and his associates, Drs. Herbert A. Moskow and Raymond C. Pennington.

The healthy heart, as we know, pumps the blood throughout the system via the arteries, veins, and capillaries. In the latter the red cells exude their oxygen which, with other factors, maintains healthy cells in the walls of the thread-like capillaries. If a diseased condition exists, for some as yet unknown reason a substance "coats" the red cells, uniting them into tiny clumps—sludge. Reaching the capillaries, the clumps often group together and may cause the blockage of a capillary. Should this condition proliferate, the cells of any of the body's organs can be starved for want of oxygen.

Failing to witness blockage in various body tissues which he examined, Dr. Knisely decided to search the network of capillaries underneath the eyeball. In more than 50 investigative sorties on humans suffering different diseases, he then witnessed variations of sludging and capillary blocking.

To further his investigations and findings, Dr. Knisely tried a number of substances to *create* sludging in healthy individuals, none of which worked. He then tried ethyl alcohol. Sludging and capillary blocking occurred just below the eyeball's transparent surface.

When alcohol in controlled quantities was given to rabbits every test showed blood-plugged capillaries due to sludging in each organ or tissue that could be viewed with illumination and microscope.

In some humans, experiments detected sludging after a single drink. Following a year and a half of experiments involving persons in various degrees of intoxication, the trio of doctors found that the higher the percentage of alcohol in the blood the higher the concentration of sludging. In a number of persons with extremely high alcohol percentages, it was discovered that eye-tissue hemorrhages doubtlessly occurred and adjacent cells died for lack of oxygen.

It is of particular interest to note that as a result of his findings Dr. Knisely, formerly a social drinker, has ceased drinking alcohol beverages of any kind.

Alcohol's Effect on the Brain

At death, the brain of the dependent drinker or alcoholic invariably will reveal enormous numbers of small areas of atrophy in which brain cells have been destroyed.*

Dr. Jorge Valles has attributed any acquired strong craving for ethyl alcohol to the hypothalamus. False impulses to this "control center" of the brain are caused by even the thought of alcohol, he said, creating "thirst" and "hunger" stimuli. This precept needs far more study than has been done to the present, Dr. Valles believes.

"Much of the assistance that my fellow psychiatrists try to give alcoholics is wasted," states the professor, "because they mistake results of the disease for its causes. They say a man drinks because he is discouraged over his divorce, over loss of his job, or other problems. But he got these problems because he drinks. And after that he used them as excuses for further drinking, whereas the real excuse is that he just can't stop and doesn't know why he can't.

---

*A member of NIAAA's medical staff has declared: "All substances which exert an effect on the brain have the potential to be dangerous. This is true of alcohol."

"We are creating alcoholics far more rapidly than we can ever treat them because people do not realize the danger in social drinking and fail to recognize the symptoms that indicate that compulsive alcoholism is beginning. They let it go on for years, and drink more and more, before finally they cannot escape the fact they have this disease—then it is very, very late to bring treatment and many times nothing can cure it."

The world of medical science, including privately-owned pharmaceutical companies as well as state and federal government research agencies, is involved in continuing research. Yet the reason or reasons *why* one individual who drinks beverage alcohol becomes addicted and the other 13 do not, remains a mystery.

The Brain Can Be Destroyed

Ernest Noble, M.D., professor of psychiatry, psychobiology and pharmacology at UC Irvine College of Medicine, has declared that brain damage caused by alcohol is not limited to hard drinkers or alcoholics.

The habitual consumption of alcohol, even in relatively small quantities, can affect the ability of brain cells to make proteins and RNA, or ribonucleic acids, one of two groups of complex acids found in every cell, according to Dr. Noble.

Proteins and RNA are essential for the function, metabolism and organization of all cells, as well as for their ability to duplicate themselves.

It has been realized, probably for centuries, that the chronic ingestion of large amounts of alcohol leads to brain dysfunction, manifested by the inability to adjust to situations and crises that occur in life, and also by what Dr. Noble calls "memory deficits."

Dr. Noble's studies have shown that the brain begins to shrink under the effects of alcohol.

"The physical size of the cortical mass decreases, showing that cells have been killed," he stated.

In extreme cases most of what is left may be nothing but connective and structural tissue. The neurons themselves, the cells that do the work of the brain, have been destroyed.

Because of findings of this kind, some scientists have prognosticated that 100 years from now, mind-altering drugs will be

132

virtually unknown. World leaders will have outlawed alcohol entirely in view of the increased need for brain power in society. By then, it is predicted, relaxation will be achieved by learned mind control rather than the use of chemicals.

The D.T.s

Probably the greatest single cause of convulsions in the United States today is not epilepsy, but alcohol.

Heavy and protracted drinking can raise the drinker's agitation so high that no amount of current sedation can possibly reduce it to a bearable level. Sudden cutting off of the intake (through a desperate desire to "get well" or running out of money) while agitation is high will leave an alcoholic without his favorite sedative. The withdrawal syndrome begun, alcoholic hallucinosis usually results. The brain is so irritable that it sees, hears and feels things that are not there.

From here, it is one small step to delirium tremens. A man with the D.T.'s is unable to stop moving. He lives in absolute terror. It is entirely possible this addicted drinker has cells in his central nervous system which will never regenerate. Brain cells, once destroyed, can never grow back.

Withdrawal Becomes Mandatory

The person whose protracted drinking has elevated his psychomotor-activity level extremely may suffer other unwanted effects such as shivering, shaking, pacing, sweating, palpitation, and he may show also great agitation and tremulousness. He has now reached the stage where "withdrawal" is virtually mandatory. Says one authoritative writer:

"The drinker who may feel some comfort in being addicted to alcohol rather than a hard drug should consider the scientific fact that narcotic withdrawal rarely, if ever, has caused death, whereas death from alcohol withdrawal is alarmingly common. It also is true that the narcotic addict can maintain a plateau with a stable amount of drugs for years but the progression of the disease of alcoholism forces the heavy drinker to keep reaching beyond his limits—and beyond."

He is "hooked" into a condition which can *never* get better, only worse—until he finds the way to abstain.

MAJOR DRUGS:

Drug Type	Name	Origin	Risk of Dependence Habituation (psychological)	Addiction (physical)	Tolerance (increasing amounts needed for same effect)	Average Amount Taken
Alcohol	Beer Distilled spirits Wine	Grain Grain Fruit	High	Moderate	Yes	12 ounces 1½ ounces 3 ounces
Barbiturates	Chloral hydrate Doriden Nembutal Phenobarbital Seconal	Synthetic	High	High	Yes	500 milligrams 400 milligrams 400 milligrams 50-100 milligrams 50-100 milligrams
Narcotics	Codeine Demerol Heroin Methadone Morphine Opium Percodan	Opium poppy Synthetic Opium poppy Synthetic Opium poppy Opium poppy Synthetic	High	High	Yes	15-50 milligrams 50-150 milligrams Varies 5-15 milligrams 10 milligrams Varies 15-50 milligrams
Cannabis	Hashish Marijuana THC	Cannabis plant Cannabis plant Synthetic	Moderate	None	No	Varies
Hallucinogens	DMT LSD Mescaline Nutmeg Psilocybin Scopolamine STP	Synthetic Synthetic Cactus Nutmeg tree Psilocybe mushroom Henbane plant/synthetic Synthetic	Low	None	Yes	Varies 150-200 micrograms 350 milligrams 1/3 ounce 25 milligrams .5 milligram 5 milligrams
Amphetamines	Benzedrine Dexedrine Methedrine Preludin	Synthetic	High	None	Yes	2.5-5 milligrams
Antidepressants	Elavil Ritalin Tofranil	Synthetic	Low	None	No Yes No	10-25 milligrams
Nicotine	Cigarettes Cigars Pipes Snuff	Tobacco leaves	High	None	Yes	Varies

DEPRESSANTS (Alcohol, Barbiturates, Narcotics)

PSYCHEDELICS (Cannabis, Hallucinogens)

STIMULANTS (Amphetamines, Antidepressants, Nicotine)

THEIR USES AND EFFECTS

How Taken	Short-Term Effects of Average Amount — Description	Duration	Short-Term Effects of Large Amount	Long-Term Effects (continued excessive use)	
Swallowed	Relaxation, breakdown of inhibitions, euphoria, depression, decreased alertness	2-4 hours	Stupor, nausea, unconsciousness hangover, death	Obesity, impotence, psychosis, ulcers, malnutrition, liver and brain damage, delirium tremens, death	**DEPRESSANTS**
Swallowed	Relaxation, euphoria, decreased alertness, drowsiness, impaired coordination, sleep	4-8 hours	Slurred speech, stupor, hangover, death	Excessive sleepiness, confusion, irritability, severe withdrawal sickness	**DEPRESSANTS**
Swallowed Injected Sniffed/injected Swallowed/injected Injected Inhaled/swallowed Swallowed	Relaxation, relief of pain and anxiety, decreased alertness, euphoria, hallucinations	4 hours	Stupor, death	Lethargy, constipation, weight loss, temporary sterility and impotence, withdrawal sickness	
Inhaled/swallowed Inhaled/swallowed Swallowed/injected	Relaxation, breakdown of inhibitions, alteration of perceptions, euphoria, increased appetite	2-4 hours	Panic, Stupor	Fatigue, psychosis	**PSYCHEDELICS**
Inhaled Swallowed/injected Swallowed Swallowed/sniffed Swallowed Swallowed Swallowed	Perceptual changes — especially visual, increased energy, hallucinations, panic	½ hour 10-12 hours 12-14 hours Varies 6-8 hours Varies 12-14 hours	Anxiety, hallucinations, psychosis, exhaustion, tremors, vomiting, panic	Increased delusions and panic, psychosis	**PSYCHEDELICS**
Swallowed/injected	Increased alertness, excitation, euphoria, decreased appetite	4-8 hours	Restlessness, rapid speech, irritability, insomnia, stomach disorders, convulsions	Insomnia, excitability, skin disorders, malnutrition, delusions, hallucinations, psychosis	**STIMULANTS**
Swallowed/injected	Relief of anxiety and depression, temporary impotence	12-24 hours	Nausea, hypertension, weight loss, insomnia	Stupor, coma, convulsions, congestive heart failure, damage to liver and white blood cells, death	**STIMULANTS**
Inhaled Inhaled Inhaled Sniffed	Relaxation, constriction of blood vessels	¼-2 hours	Headache, loss of appetite, nausea	Impaired breathing, heart and lung disease, cancer, death	**STIMULANTS**

Extracted from "Major Drugs: Their Uses and Effects"—a *Playboy* magazine chart; copyright © 1972 by *Playboy*.

Antabuse and other preventive medications are effective alcohol-ingestion arrestors, but only for as long or as short a period of time the drinker will continue to take them. With Antabuse in his system, the alcoholic or problem drinker knows he will become violently ill if he takes a drink. He also knows that by skipping Antabuse he can hit the bottle without the preventative hitting back.

Psychiatry has helped many dependent drinkers stay on the wagon. AA has played an important role in aiding the alcohol-addicted to desist. And we have seen how business and industry operates to attempt to aid dependent drinkers and alcoholics.

However, none of these methods can begin to work without the dependent drinker making the initial decision to abstain, to never again take another swallow of wine, beer, or whiskey. The addicted drinker must *want* to arrest his problem. Once this decision is made, it will be a fight to stay "clean." It will take an enormous amount of courage to make the decision and then stick to it. Unfortunately, despite determination, the depressing fact remains that not more than 50 percent of those who decide to quit manage to attain sobriety for the rest of their lives.

The percentage of those who achieve total arrest undoubtedly would be higher, claim most knowledgeable people in the field, if fewer of them would try to kick the habit on will power alone. As Marty Mann states in *Your Questions About Drinking and Alcohol*: "He can't stop drinking by simply willing to stop any more than a tubercular can stop coughing by willing to stop. In both cases he may be able to stop for short periods, but these don't last unless he has the help and treatment he needs. Some alcoholics have been able to stop for quite long periods simply through an effort of will, but all too often they return to uncontrolled drinking unless they get proper help. Recovery from alcoholism is a long and often complex process which very few individuals seem able to accomplish alone and unaided.

"First," says the noted authority, "he may need medical care to get the alcohol out of his system and to make him feel well again. Practicing alcoholics never feel well; most of the time, except when anesthetized by alcohol, they feel very sick indeed, and it's pretty hard to think straight or to do anything constructive when you feel that sick. Next, he needs to learn the nature of his illness, and to understand and accept it. Finally, he needs understanding support while he is learning to live without alcohol in a world where it is all around him. All this adds up to treatment, for alcoholism requires treatment just like any other illness."

Special Alcoholism Studies

The health professions need many more people who will direct their attentions to the problems caused by alcohol. In this area, NIAAA is appealing to the states and other recipients of financial aid under Public Law 91—616 to train persons not only to become doctors but to work in the field of alcohol addiction. With NIAAA aid, more in-depth studies presumably will be undertaken than in the past to probe the mystery: what makes an alcoholic (other than the fact of his drinking the substance)?

". . . carefully controlled experimental studies of alcoholic patients have been relatively rare," stated Michael Chandler at the 1971 National Council on Alcoholism's annual conference at the Disneyland Hotel, Anaheim, California. "Knowing where an individual is at any point in time does not, obviously, tell one how he got there . . . .

"I am aware of only three studies* in American literature which have attempted systematic, longitudinal followback studies of personality factors which predate the identifiable onset of problem drinking. In the case of alcoholism, one might anticipate following a population for a period of as much as 45 years to insure that drinking problems, if they are to emerge, will have had sufficient opportunity to express themselves. Premature termination in such a longitudinal study runs the risk of inaccurately treating as normal, persons whose pathology expresses itself only late in life.

". . . What would seem required, then, in order to unravel the apparently multiple-determined character of alcoholic etiology, is a detailed prospective follow-up study of children whose parentage places them at high risk in the development of problem drinking."

---

*The Oakland growth study of Mary Carver Jones (1968); the Cambridge-Sommerville study of McCord & McCord (1960); and the study of former child guidance clinic patients by Robins, Bates, and O'Neil (1962).

If France, the world's No. 1 alcohol-beverage drinking country, had conducted such a study it might have avoided its desperate plight of the 1950s and 1960s. The child crisis, as it was referred to, resulted from the tradition that "A little wine never hurt anyone." There were instances of babies suffering delirium tremens; at many schools pupils were drinking a pint or more a day; in school lunchrooms teachers were forbidden to dilute older. pupils' wine; 9 percent of the average family income went for drink while 2.8 percent was spent for housing and 4.2 percent for education. And in these circumstances the powerful French alcohol lobby disseminated free blotters advertising the nutritional claim: "A quart of wine is as nourishing as five eggs."*

Finally aware of the potential doom in store for France if this situation continued, laws were imposed to safeguard the young, including punishment for adults (mothers and fathers as well) who made minors drink. Replacing wine with milk was encouraged, and soft-drink companies were urged to more aggressively compete for the country's beverage business.

Though the overall situation in France remains difficult, by mid-1971 sale of bottled table waters and soda-type drinks increased by more than 8 percent a year since 1960, representing a growth 50 times faster than that of wine, and fruit drink sales increased 23 percent a year.

Physical Effects of Beverage Alcohol

Dependent drinkers and alcoholics run eight times the normal chance of being afflicted with cirrhosis of the liver. Many medical authorities, including Dr. Stanley E. Gitlow of the Mount Sinai School of Medicine, declare alcoholics are highly vulnerable to ulcers, chronic pancreatitis, gastritis, and complications affecting their blood and bone marrow. Heart disease, said Dr. Gitlow, may also be more common among alcoholics: "Alcohol diminishes cardiac function and increases blood fats, cholesterol, and blood pressure." It is well-known within the world of medicine that the

---

*The treatment of alcoholics, subsidies to the producers of alcohol beverages, and the indirect costs of alcohol addiction including working absenteeism, cost France around $500,000,000 a year while taxes on alcohol netted only one-third that amount.

alcohol-addicted individual also has lower resistance to numerous infections, and that his life span is shorter than nondrinkers.

Dr. Leon Greenberg of the Rutgers Center for Alcohol Studies insists that heavy drinking takes its toll on the human system. "Alcohol is an irritant," he said, "and every time someone takes a couple of martinis, he's whacking the inside of his stomach with a board."

"Alcohol has a definite effect upon . . . vital organs," stated alcohol authority Dr. Marvin A. Block. "As a matter of fact, every tissue and every organ is affected by it in one way or another since, when carried in the bloodstream, it reaches practically every tissue in the body . . . respiratory disease has been notoriously prevalent. About 25% of all alcoholics develop tuberculosis and, conversely, about 25% of all tuberculosis patients are alcoholic. [Also] they are more likely to develop bronchitis, pneumonia, pneumonitis, and other respiratory infections. [Another] most common problem is the inflammation of the stomach's lining, known as gastritis. Peptic ulcers, both gastric and duodenal, can be aggravated by the ingestion of alcohol."

Some of those who drink alcoholic beverages dismiss any possibility of ill effects or danger by reassuring themselves that it has been used as "a medicine" since time began. Although alcohol once was utilized medically, it no longer is. ". . . Prior to the discovery of the newer drugs and more efficient anesthetics, alcohol was wittingly employed as a hypnotic, sedative, and narcotic aid to surgery," said Dr. Block. However, "the newer drugs are more rapid in their action and produce anesthesia more quickly, passing through the various states in much less time than alcohol requires. The same states of induction, excitement, somnolence, deep anesthesia, and eventually paralysis are effectuated by alcohol quite as they are by every other such agent, except that the narcosis deepens far more slowly. For this reason, alcohol has been abandoned as a tool of anesthesiology. It is nevertheless still used by many laymen who, unaware of its basic potency, rely upon its drug effects for a variety of non-medical reasons."

Alcohol and Violence

To throw light on why alcohol drives some people to mayhem, a team of Stanford Medical Center researchers, headed by psychiatrist H. Keith H. Brodie, will combine a thorough evaluation of people who want to break the alcoholism violence cycle and a two-phased program of therapy.

The study is one portion of a $2 million, comprehensive research package awarded to the Stanford psychiatry department by the National Institute of Alcohol Abuse and Alcoholism for 16 alcoholism research projects.

In one study of 19 California youths 18 years old or younger, for example, eight of them had been under the influence of alcohol when they committed murder, assault or manslaughter.

More surprisingly, more than half of the murder victims examined in another study were found to have alcohol in their blood.

A survey of 588 murders showed that victims who had precipitated their own deaths by attacking first were under the influence to a significantly greater extent than victims of unprovoked attacks, said psychiatrist Brodie.

"A question is raised," psychiatrist Dr. Marvin Rosenzweig observed. "Does a person under the influence of alcohol tend to provoke an attack?"

The three-year study, which is intended to involve up to 100 alcoholic patients who have shown signs of violence is planned in such a way as to obtain a complete profile of the client—psychological, emotional and social.

The volunteers will keep track of their liquor intake and subsequent behavior to disclose, among other things, how drinking levels relate to violence levels and frequency.

Then four different kinds of drugs, all known to suppress aggressive impulses by different means, will be given to the patients at separate intervals.

If one of them is shown to reduce violent behavior in the subject, it reveals which physiological pathways alcohol may take to spur brutal behavior. The drug also becomes the treatment for that patient.

Once the drug therapy phase is completed, group therapy sessions also will be available to the participants as they grapple with the task of staying away from alcohol.

The study also will involve the patient's family, where possible, because the violence is most likely to be aimed at them. And surprisingly, a family is likely to tolerate violence and adjust to it. Because of family tolerance the level of liquor-linked violence can increase in a home until a neighbor, police, a trip to the hospital or the threat of losing one's job intervenes and exposes it.

Alcohol Addiction and Genetics

One of the more controversial issues related to alcohol is the part genetics play in addiction. For each evidence that the genes play a role—that the need, the craving, for alcohol is passed from parent to child, or from grandparent to grandchild—proof is also offered that genetics play virtually no part in the making of a dependent drinker.

No better example can be found of the yes-no attitudes on this particular issue than those expressed at the National Council on Alcoholism's medical and scientific conference where foremost investigators and practitioners gathered to read papers and exchange theories.

"My work suggests that addicts endow their children with a biological legacy which will make them good dope fiends or alcoholics under proper circumstances . . ." was the summary of the paper delivered by John R. Nichols, Ph.D., Professor of Social Science and Psychology, Pennsylvania State University.

Dr. Frank A. Seixas, Medical Director of NCA, stated: "In particular, the question has been raised, and is still unanswered, as to the contribution of the constitutional difference in the handling of alcohol by the individual (or its different effects on different individuals), and the effects of environment in predisposing choice of the use of alcohol as a method of problem solving."

Said Francis E. Camps of the London Hospital Medical College: ". . . contrary to our first throughts, it does not seem that people of a certain blood group and secretor status are predisposed to alcoholism. This may relieve the minds of some psychiatrists who treat alcoholics, since it divests patients of the chance to protest 'it is all in my genes.' On the other hand it does not give any aid to those who would like to have some means at their disposal of spotting the potential alcoholic."

"It is highly improbable that a preference for alcohol in man can be solved by any simple genetic or environmental explanation," declared H. Lennart Kain, M.D., Lund, Sweden.

141

Dr. Marc Alan Schuckit, a resident in psychiatry at Washington University School of Medicine in St. Louis said at the conference that while heredity "maybe is a chief cause leading to alcoholism," he would never again touch a drop of alcoholic beverage because of his findings.

Dr. Schuckit studied two groups of people, 98 in all. The first comprised men and women who had had a natural parent who was alcoholic but had been brought up by foster parents who were not. The second group was its opposite, people whose natural parents had not been alcoholics but were raised by a foster parent who was. To find persons with these exact family relationships, Dr. Schuckit interviewed patients in the alcoholic ward of a state hospital and learned which had half-brothers or half-sisters. It was the step-relations he studied, a high-risk group because all came from families that had drinking problems.

"We knew, though, that alcoholism runs in families. What we didn't know was whether it runs in families because of shared alcoholic environments at home, or because of shared genes," stated Dr. Schuckit.

"That's what the study was intended to clear up. The statistics show that in this small sample, having a real parent who was an alcoholic was a definite and more important influence on the development of alcoholism than was being brought up by an alcoholic parent-figure who is no blood kin," Dr. Schuckit said. "Having an alcoholic's genes is more important than being raised by one."

There may be as many as ten major factors in alcohol addiction, the doctor stated, and "heredity is one of them. That would be enough to keep me from drinking."

Some experts contend that when either parent drinks, the youngest boy is the one most likely to become alcohol addicted, and that the conflict between dependence and independence is more severe for this particular child. *Science News* in 1971, reporting on the work of Drs. Elliot S. Vesell and John G. Page at the National Institute of Health, stated that ". . . blatant individual variations in response to drugs vanish in identical twins but remain largely preserved in fraternal twins. The drugs they studied included ethanol . . . The results showed that large, individual differences in the rates at which the subjects metabolized drugs . . . were under complete genetic control."

Patrick J. Frawley, Jr., once a dependent drinker who today totally abstains, has remained intensely interested in the field of alcohol addiction. He claims that free will to drink or not drink must be based on adequate knowledge. In the booklet *Without Genetic Warning*, published by Frawley's Schick Laboratories in 1971, it is stated that: "Our young people must be given to understand that eating sugar, or drinking alcohol, even in moderation, are pleasures in which some, *but by no means all*, persons can safely indulge."

The pamphlet quotes Dr. Alton Ochsner concerning the matter of genetics: "There is no question that some ethnic groups have a higher incidence of physical susceptibility to alcohol. They have not been warned and therefore addiction does not appear to be a matter of character or intelligence, but instead occurs when such people try to drink moderately following the example of their neighbors. The American Indians, the fair-skinned Celts, and the Blacks from African rain forests should be counseled on the importance of genetic susceptibility and the danger of alcohol addiction."

An important part of the Frawley theory is that thirst plays a decisive role in addictive response. Without moving from his chair, the addict "develops a thirst like an athlete's"—a thirst for alcohol, in this instance. With this theory as the base for what is called "deep-sleep therapy," over 18,000 patients have been treated at the Schick-Shadel Hospitals in Seattle and Fort Worth. These hospitals claim a "cure" rate of over 60 percent, and claim furthermore that this more than 60 percent has remained totally abstinent after conclusion of treatment.

As researchers seek answers to the problems of 85,000 alcohol-related deaths each year, the enormous number of alcohol-related illnesses, as well as to alcoholism *per se*, the National Institute on Alcohol Abuse and Alcoholism has projected two principal goals.

1. The most immediate goal is to assist in making the best alcoholism treatment and rehabilitation services available at the community level. The long-range goal is to develop effective methods of preventing alcoholism and problem

143

drinking. To achieve these objectives, the NIAAA fosters, develops, conducts, and supports broad programs of research, training, development of community services, and public education.

2. Through a program of research grants, the NIAAA encourages and supports basic and applied investigations in universities, medical schools, and other institutions. Demonstration projects are also supported to develop and evaluate new techniques, approaches, and methods for the treatment and prevention of alcoholism and the rehabilitation of alcoholic persons and problem drinkers.

10

PROHIBITION

"... [we are] opposed to repeal of the
18th Amendment ... opposed to the restoration
in any manner of the legalized saloon ...
opposed to the federal or state governments
going into the liquor business."

—The Wickersham Commission

10

Early Use of Beverage Alcohol

Historical records offer proof that the consumption of beverage alcohol dates back to the earliest known civilizations. In 1100 B.C. laws related to the drinking of wine were enacted in China. King Solomon cautioned the ancient Hebrews about the effect of alcohol drinks, and Plato warned the Greeks. In 1535, alcohol beverage was imbibed, perhaps for the first time, in North America when the renowned French explorer Jacques Cartier introduced wine to the Indians at a feast held at the Island of Orleans on the St. Lawrence River.

In 1607—8 spirits and wine crossed the Atlantic Ocean with the settlers of the Virginia Colony. Distilleries were established. Beer was made in the colonists' homes. There was drinking at weddings, baptismals, funerals, and on other special occasions.

During the Virginia settlement, laws were passed in an effort to control and combat excessive drinking. When discovered drunk for the first time, a person was privately reprimanded by the minister. A second offense brought public censure. A third-time offender was placed "in halter" for twelve hours and, in addition, had to pay a fine. Each succeeding offense was to be dealt with by the Governor and the Council.

America's first brewery was built in 1637 in New England's Massachusetts Bay Colony. The Colony also meted out punishment, generally a whipping or a fine, to excessive drinkers. Drunkards were made conspicuous by being commanded to wear a red D, and were condemned by the clergy.

By the middle 1750s certain periodicals began advocating the elimination of wine and beer. The Society of Friends advised its members not to deal in spirituous liquors, claiming that, in contrast to prevailing common opinion, these beverages were deleterious to the health.*

Abstinence and Temperance

Dr. Benjamin Rush, a Friend and one of the signators of the Declaration of Independence, was the advocate of this "new thinking." A pamphlet he wrote in 1784, *An Inquiry into the Effect of Ardent Spirits on the Human Body and Mind*, was widely circulated and attracted the support of a large number of colonists. When Dr. Rush died in 1813, his work was assumed by Dr. Billy Clark and Reverend Lyman Beecher.

A group of prominent New Yorkers voluntarily decided to try abstinence for one year. So worthwhile did this New York group find the results that they remained abstainers and carried their, and Dr. Clark's, message to others. This was the first active movement for prohibition, and it ultimately led to the Eighteenth Amendment.

The abstinence-from-hard-liquor movement fanned westward through Illinois, Indiana, and Ohio. By 1826, the American Society for the Promotion of Temperance was founded, and within a few years the organization had a half-million members. By 1837, its name changed to the American Temperance Union (ATU), the conviction that only abstinence from spirituous beverages could ensure temperance was becoming increasingly accepted.

---

*Some denominations still require abstinence for membership. Among them are Christian Scientists, Seventh Day Adventists, and the Church of Jesus Christ of the Latter Day Saints (Mormons).

With the increase in consumption of intoxicating beverages in the United States, saloons were decried by many as a menace to family life. In 1895, the Anti-Saloon League of America was formed (today called the American Council of Alcohol Problems), eventually establishing branches in all the states and the District of Columbia. This League worked heavily in legislative and political areas to oppose Wet and to support Dry candidates.

As the movement grew, the ATU expanded the scope of its philosophy. Teetotalism—the elimination of wine and beer in addition to distilled spirits—was sought in the early 1900s. Despite the fact that the per-capita consumption of alcoholic beverages in 1910 had increased 26 percent over 1870, a number of states went dry. The temperance forces came to believe that the only real protection for the country would be a national law.

Federal Legislation

That some kind of national law would be put into effect became evident in 1917 when Congress enacted two wartime (World War I) restrictions: the sale of liquor was banned to soldiers; and the production and sale of wines, beer, and liquor was ordered decreased. Congress in that same year cleared the Eighteenth Amendment for submission to the states.

Within two years the Amendment had been ratified by the required 36 states, including 22 states which by now had enacted their own prohibition laws. Eventually every state, excepting Connecticut and Rhode Island, ratified.* The Volstead Act, providing the enforcement machinery for the Eighteenth Amendment, was passed over President Woodrow Wilson's veto in October of 1919. Prohibition went into effect January 20th, 1920, saloon keepers at midnight disposing of their unused wares, some emptying beer kegs into the gutters.

Defiance of the Volstead Act

". . . where [the Prohibition law] is not obeyed it will be enforced," stated Prohibition Commissioner John F. Kramer.

---

* The total vote in the Senates of the various States was 1,310 for, 237 against—84.6 percent dry. In the lower houses of the States, the vote was 3,782 for, 1,035 against—78.5 percent dry.

Twelve days later the first raid against lawbreakers occurred in New York City. This was the forerunner of 13 years of defiance, not only by those who lived outside the law but also by the majority of U.S. drinking citizens, thus creating a controversy that lasts to this day:

Was prohibition "good" for this nation or "bad?"

Was more beverage alcohol consumed, or less?

Did crime increase or decrease?

Did the "noble experiment," in fact, succeed or fail in its purpose?

There is ample proof that while Prohibition was in effect the bulk of Americans sought out bootleg whiskey, beer, and wine and, therefore, could be considered "criminals." They were breaking the law. Within the first year of Prohibition, Mr. Kramer's declaration notwithstanding, over 100 Prohibition agents in New York City alone were terminated from their jobs for accepting bribes. Corruption became rampant, a fact the Wets seized upon as they strove to have the Eighteenth Amendment repealed.

In any case, the enforcement processes, which became primarily the responsibility of federal authorities, were not only woefully inept but wide open to overtures from the gangster world. That 900 of the 943 federal agents assigned to Prohibition duties received salaries of from $1,200 to $2,000 a year certainly made them vulnerable to connivance with the underworld.

When Prohibition agents displaced T-Men to enforce the law, Ernest Gordon, writing in a Women's Christian Temperance Union (WCTU) periodical, declared:

"The Treasury Department had at its command the highly trained, highly efficient and thoroughly reliable corps of special agents which had made for itself so enviable a record in enforcing excise law. Authorities who intended to enforce the law would have retained it and would have been thankful for the chance. Instead of that, these men with their record, their reputation, and their experience, were dismissed. That in itself was notice to every lawbreaker that he was expected to break the laws."

There was immediate compliance with the law at the outset, the Governor stated, on the part of the alcohol beverage interests, because years of honest enforcement of the excise law by the

150

Federal Government had taught them to expect honest enforcement of the Eighteenth Amendment. "But almost at once they learned that the authorities in Washington did not respect it themselves and had no intention of enforcing respect from others."

Effects of Prohibition

Whether the Volstead Act was violated partly or chiefly by the public because they became quickly aware that many a politician "voted dry and drank wet," a common phrase of that day, cannot be accurately evaluated. However, enough politicians were arrested for violating the Volstead Act as to certainly have had some impact on the masses. To cite but a few, in a Florida city the mayor, police chief, and the city council president went to jail for violation. A midwest labor commissioner was convicted; a city magistrate was found guilty of accepting over $85,000 in bribes; the mayor of a New Jersey city, together with the police chief, two detectives, and a U.S. Customs inspector, were arraigned and convicted.

"That bootleggers operated under the Capitol dome," stated one reporter describing the activity in Washington, D.C., "to supply a clientele of Senators and House members was an open secret." Foreign embassies helped supply the National Press Club. Speakeasies, of course, did a landslide business. With an estimated 32,000 such hideaways in New York City, Mayor LaGuardia wryly declared that it would take a quarter of a million policemen to control the situation, and another 200,000 to keep the quarter of a million honest.

Much of the public drank perhaps as much out of rebellion to the law as to "have a good time." Bathtub gin was whipped up at home. At country club dances and football games the hip flask became a familiar object.

Statistics are available which show that there were fewer homicides and minor crimes, fewer Skid Row bums being taken to the tank, and fewer drinking-driver highway accidents.

One group of abstainer forces claimed that the thirteen dry years saw a general crime rate decline of between 35 and 40 percent.

151

A survey of institutions in his state by Henry W. Frannam, Professor of Economics at Yale, found that the number of prisoners in Connecticut jails charged with drunkenness fell from 7,314 in 1917 to 943 in 1920.

The nation's auto death rate decreased 40 percent.

Dr. H.M. Pollock, statistician for the New York State Hospital Commission, wrote: "In its mental disease record, in its crime record, in its drunkenness record, the year 1920 stands without an equal in the recent history of the country."*

One writer-researcher, who pointed out that no actual records were kept of alcohol-beverage consumption during Prohibition, used cirrhosis of the liver as his guide to determine whether the nation's drinking had increased or decreased. Utilizing U.S. Public Health Bureau data, he arrived at the conclusion that:

> During the prohibiton era the death rate from cirrhosis per 100,000 declined from a year average in the pre-prohibition years—[1900 through 1917]—of 13.11 to a prohibition yearly average—[1920 through 1932]—of 7.27. By 1965 the cirrhosis death rate had risen to 12.5, indicating (according to this reporter's scale) a 57% increase in the use of alcoholic beverages [after prohibition].

President Charles W. Eliot of Harvard University, one of the great educators in American history, had been a life-long opponent of prohibition but was completely converted to its support by his observation of the law's benefits. In a letter sent February 7, 1922, to a committee of the Massachusetts legislature (which was considering enactment of a law for concurrent enforcement of prohibition), he wrote: "Evidence has accumulated on every hand that prohibition has promoted public health, public happiness, and industrial efficiency. This evidence comes from manufacturers, physicians, nurses of all sorts (school, factory, hospital), and from social workers of many races and religions, laboring daily in a great variety of fields. Testimony also demonstrates beyond a doubt that Prohibition is actually sapping the terrible forces of disease, poverty, crime and vice; in spite of imperfect enforcement, it has eliminated the chief causes of crime, poverty, and misery among our people."

---

*Author's note: The records referred to showed a reduction of incidence in the categories cited.

The Eighteenth Amendment put out of business 236 distilleries, 1,090 breweries, and 177,790 saloons. Beverage alcohol advertising was eliminated. Many of the prominent distilleries and breweries converted to other products. Krugs in Omaha handled millions of bushels of grain; Willow Springs made Teto, a non-alcoholic beverage; Capitol Brewery of Washington became an ice cream factory; Squibbs Distilleries in Indiana made stock foods. Other firms converted to motorcycles, packed meat, and maple syrup. Before Prohibition these companies, combined, produced two and a half billion gallons of alcoholic beverages.

The Underworld

Crime increased among the underworld—due to the gangster's own private war over huge booty made possible by the illegal trade. The general public may have lived the war vicariously, in the press and through radio, but remained almost entirely unharmed. Gang leaders, in fact, were wary of upsetting the status quo. Enforcement officers, federal and local, thus could more easily look the other way. Also, as one bootlegger said: "It just don't make no sense to rough up our customers."

Dutch Schultz became the beer lord of New York. A young thug, arriving in Chicago from New York's Five Points gang to join Johnny Torrio, flashed a business card which advised he was: *Alphonse Capone. Second-hand furniture dealer. 2220 South Wabash Avenue.*

Quality liquor, obtainable during the first years of Prohibition, found its way chiefly to those who could pay the exorbitant prices. The virtually lethal stuff, concocted from denatured alcohol, was sent into the lower-class neighborhoods, sometimes giving the drinker a case of what was known as "the blind staggers."

Rumrunners became part of the night as schooners and landing launches ran without lights. One runner, Bill McCoy, an ex-shipyard owner, started at $100 a day to make the Nassau to New York run. Soon he had established headquarters in New York's Pennsylvania Hotel and was paying crew members a large bonus with every safe delivery of a cargo to the Long Island or New Jersey shore. Called "Captain Bill" before Prohibition, he became better known as "The Real McCoy," a testimonial to the quality of the illicit liquor being brought from the Bahamas. "Right off the boat" became a demand of those customers who could afford the best.

However, as Prohibition moved into its final years, there were subtle factors, rarely-discussed publicly, helping to doom it. Many people began to feel that the underworld was getting control of the country; the price of bootleg stuff had doubled; quality whiskey, wines, and beer were more difficult to obtain. An unspoken "we've had it!" began to pervade much of the populace.

By 1926, the Illinois and Massachusetts state legislatures had sought from Congress at least a modification of the Volstead Act. In Montana, the state enforcement statute was repealed. One nation-wide poll showed that over 31 percent favored repeal, with just under 50 percent indicating a wish for modification. Somewhat under 19 percent favored the law as it was.

The Wickersham Commission

Herbert Hoover had defeated the Wet, Al Smith, in the 1928 presidential race and had been in office one year when he felt there was sufficient evidence of a mounting public unrest against the Eighteenth Amendment to require his appointing a commission ". . . for a thorough investigation into the enforcement of the prohibition laws." Named for its chairman, George W. Wickersham, the Wickersham Commission—after 18 months of study and research concerning "the facts as to enforcement, the benefits and the abuses under the prohibition laws"—came up with nearly 4,000 pages of evidence and opinion. The Commission submitted, in addition to its several volumes of joint report, individual reports by each member.

The joint report stated that "it . . . is opposed to repeal of the 18th Amendment . . . is opposed to the restoration in any manner of the legalized saloon . . . is opposed to the federal or state governments going into the liquor business . . . is of the opinion that there is yet no adequate observation or enforcement . . . that for the present organization for enforcement is still inadequate; and . . . that the federal appropriations for enforcement . . . [are

154

not sufficient]." Suggestions were offered relative to better enforcement of the law.

Every member of the Commission believed that the Eighteenth Amendment was being poorly enforced. According to the Commission's evaluations, in 1930 there was but one federal enforcement officer for each 43,398 American citizens.

Of the 11 Commission members, all of whom submitted statements, 3 favored repeal; 6, including the Chairman, felt that national prohibition should be retained, with its enforcement improved. One member, Roscoe Pound, suggested a revision; and Henry W. Anderson decided that "We must not lose what has been gained by the abolition of the saloon."

In 1932, Franklin D. Roosevelt, a non-Dry, was elected to the highest office. He almost immediately prevailed upon Congress to legalize the sale of 3.2 percent beer. The Volstead Act was rescinded so the beer could be sold legally. Repeal followed on the 5th of December, 1933, when the Twenty-first Amendment to the Constitution was adopted. The following table shows a state-by-state vote concerning the adoption of the Twenty-first Amendment.

| State | Popular Vote | | Convention |
	For	Against	Date
1. Michigan	850,546	287,931	Apr. 10
2. Wisconsin	648,031	141,518	Apr. 25
3. Rhode Island	150,244	20,874	May 8
4. Wyoming	......	......	May 25
5. New Jersey	573,532	90,733	June 1
6. Delaware	45,615	13,505	June 25
7. Indiana	557,062	312,120	June 26
8. Massachusetts	436,356	97,702	June 26
9. New York	1,946,532	247,450	June 27
10. Illinois	1,227,668	341,773	July 10
11. Iowa	376,661	249,534	July 10
12. Connecticutt	236,742	34,816	July 11
13. New Hampshire	76,044	30,409	July 11
14. California	1,019,818	319,981	July 24
15. West Virginia	218,638	136,552	July 25
16. Arkansas	67,662	46,091	Aug. 1
17. Oregon	136,713	72,854	Aug. 7
18. Alabama	100,269	70,631	Aug. 8
19. Tennessee	126,983	119,870	Aug. 11
20. Maryland	503,642	156,961	Aug. 29
21. Arizona	37,643	11,323	Sept. 5
22. Nevada	......	......	Sept. 5
23. Vermont	41,182	20,714	Sept. 26
24. Colorado	133,066	62,969	Sept. 26
25. Washington	490,088	208,206	Oct. 3
26. Minnesota	390,179	209,049	Oct. 10
27. Idaho	56,652	40,977	Oct. 17
28. Maryland	205,130	45,776	Oct. 18
29. Virginia	99,459	58,517	Oct. 25
30. New Mexico	53,321	14,041	Nov. 2
31. Florida	98,247	24,439	Nov. 14
32. Texas	310,710	195,341	Nov. 27
33. Kentucky	386,653	234,417	Nov. 27
34. South Carolina	33,074	35,845	Dec. 4
35. Ohio	1,444,033	583,842	Dec. 5
36. Pennsylvania	1,864,411	583,513	Dec. 5
37. Utah	101,665	67,234	Dec. 5
38. Maine	114,975	53,000	Dec. 6
39. North Carolina	120,190	293,484	....
Total	15,279,216	5,333,992	

The *American Year Book*—1933

11

THE PUBLIC LAW

*". . . too often we think of this material
as a beverage and we know full well it is not."*

—Dr. Luther A. Cloud, President,
National Council on Alcoholism

*"It is a basic principle of medicine
that no condition is brought under
control by treating the casualties alone."*

—Dr. Morris E. Chafetz
Director, NIAAA

11

The "noble experiment" was repealed and, in 1933, 46 states set about establishing the administrative mechanics for alcohol beverages to again be manufactured and marketed; only Oklahoma and Mississippi maintained prohibition.

Twenty-nine of the 46 states decided to function under an open license system; 17 states settled on the monopoly system. In the former, private enterprise operates under state control and regulation through a licensing system. In the monopoly operation, the state assumes the place of private enterprise in the wholesale distribution and sale of distilled liquor, with licenses for the sale of beer and wine only available to private outlets.

Today none of the 50 states has prohibition. The 17 "monopoly" or "control" states sell distilled spirits exclusively through state-owned stores. The organization representing these 17 is known as the National Alcoholic Beverage Control Association. The Conference of State Liquor Administrators regulates the "free" states in an "open license system" in which licenses are rendered for a fee.

159

During World War II, many U.S. producers of distilled spirits converted their plants to the manufacture of industrial alcohol, a conversion which served over 40 percent of the nation's wartime military and industrial requirements. Directly after the war, grain was in such demand as a domestic and foreign food that not only hard liquor but all alcoholic beverages lagged in returning to full production. Beginning in the early 1950s, production and consumption of grain spirits, beer, and wine increased annually.

Social Pressures and Cultural Change

The ability to serve liquor or wine soon became a symbol of financial and social security. Drinking in the United States became culturally acceptable.

As the nation's consumption of distilled spirits alone spiraled from 2½ million gallons in 1919 to over 300 million gallons in 1970, having a drink before dinner, going to a cocktail party, ordering a luncheon martini, taking the champagne flight became a way of life for the majority of Americans.

In the home and outside it, the host went out of his way to make sure everyone was "happy;" and many a guest, not wishing to seem different, accepted an alcoholic beverage when he would have preferred not to. The person who chose to abstain was looked upon as asocial. That 32 percent of Americans today exercise their freedom not to drink is a very significant ratio considering the social pressures constantly being thrust upon them to imbibe.

Aware of these social pressures the NIAAA has created a series of very effective advertisements, one of which is reproduced here. It is hoped that these messages will trigger family and community action to help establish new social patterns.

Government Action

It took a long time for government to take a stand on the matter of alcohol *vs.* human ecology. The federal government and its Department of Health, Education, and Welfare (HEW) made a commitment, however, for human ecology with the passing of Public Law 91-616, the Comprehensive Alcohol Abuse and Prevention, Treatment and Rehabilitation Act, on December 31, 1970. A reproduction of Public Law 91—616 will be found at the end of this volume. Here is a summary:

If good old Harry is such a great host how come

...nobody remembers what happened at the party?
...Ron and Jean had such a terrible fight?
...Charlie drove into a tree on the way home?
...everybody felt so lousy the next day?

Maybe there's more to being a great host than pushing drinks. Maybe good old Harry is not a good host. Maybe good old Harry is

THE NEIGHBORHOOD PUSHER.

Alcohol is a drug. That's right, a drug. Ask your doctor. So if you serve alcohol, be a good host. Don't be a pusher. And when you're a guest, don't let good old Harry tell you how much to drink.

We have a free booklet about drinking. (Not for or against drinking, but *about* drinking.) It's filled with facts most people don't know. It's interesting. And it could help you help someone else.

Write: N.I.A.A.A., BOX 2045, ROCKVILLE, MARYLAND, 20852.

NATIONAL
INSTITUTE
ON ALCOHOL
ABUSE AND
ALCOHOLISM

U.S. DEPARTMENT OF HEALTH, EDUCATION, AND WELFARE · Health Services and Mental Health Administration

FEDERAL ALCOHOL ABUSE AND ALCOHOLISM PREVENTION TREATMENT, and REHABILITATION ACT OF 1970.

This legislation would establish the administrative structure and authorization for an unprecendented, massive, across-the-board federal attack upon the problem of alcoholism in this country. The legislation would:

(1) establish a National Institute for the Prevention and Control of Alcohol Abuse and Alcoholism within the National Institute of Mental Health of the Department of Health, Education, and Welfare. The Secretary of Health, Education, and Welfare, acting through the Institute, would be given a completely comprehensive range of responsibilities with respect to the prevention, treatment, and rehabilitation of alcoholics, including administrative, planning, coordination, statistical, research, training, education, classification, and reporting functions, all of which are set out in detail. These powers would be utilized and directed in accordance with a specific and comprehensive alcohol abuse and alcoholism control plan which would be drawn up and carried out by the Secretary, acting through the Institute, and which would be submitted annually to Congress for review;

(2) require the establishment of programs of prevention and the recognition and encouragement of treatment and rehabilitation programs for all federal employees and members of the armed forces. It would require the establishment of treatment programs for veterans and the inclusion of alcoholism in group health and disability insurance policies made available to federal employees. It also would require that, when necessary, emergency medical services be provided to alcoholic Federal offenders and that alcoholism treatment services be provided for such persons in Federal correctional institutions.

(3) require the recognition of alcohol abuse and alcoholism as a significant health problem in a broad range of programs affecting health matters, including vocational rehabilitation programs, the Economic Opportunity Act programs, welfare programs, highway safety planning programs, medicare, medicaid, and social security;

(4) authorize the Secretary of Health, Education, and Welfare, acting through the newly-created Institute, to make grants to and enter into contracts with State and local organizations, agencies, institutions, and individuals to carry out a comprehensive range of activities in the alcohol abuse and alcoholism prevention, treatment, and rehabilitation areas. These activities would include construction and staffing of facilities, development of model curricula, curricular materials, and curricular dissemination programs; training and education programs for medical schools,

162

outreach workers, and other professional and paraprofessional persons; support of community planning and educational programs; organization of community personnel; support of services to juveniles and young adults; and support of services in correctional institutions;*

(5) establish an independent Secretary's Advisory Committee on Alcohol Abuse and Alcoholism to advise and consult with the Secretary of Health, Education, and Welfare, to assist him in carrying out the purposes of this Act; and establish an Intergovernmental Coordinating Council on Alcohol Abuse and Alcoholism to coordinate all Federal prevention, treatment, and rehabilitation efforts dealing with problems of alcohol abuse and alcoholism.

Though the gears of government move slowly—due in part in this instance to the huge taxes that flow into federal, state, and local coffers from alcohol-beverage sales—progress has been made as this volume goes to press. One concrete instance is to be found in the December 1971 HEW First Special Report to the U.S. Congress on Alcohol & Health. The Report declared alcohol to be a drug, an addictive drug, and that alcohol beverages represented the nation's No. 1 drug peril. The federal government thus has assumed a long-needed leadership in combating ever increasing alcohol-related problems.

Government Action

The first indication that the federal government was aware of the seriousness of the alcohol problem came in a March 1966 Health and Education message delivered by the late Lyndon B. Johnson who, as the then President of the United States, went into some detail regarding the difficulties associated with alcohol. Senator Harold E. Hughes of Iowa, an ex-alcoholic, conducted hearings on Senate Bill S 3835 (to become Law 91—616 in its transition) as chairman of the Special Subcommittee on Alcoholism and Narcotics of the Committee of Labor and Public Welfare. All-important hearings were held on May 21 and 25, 1970.

---

*On June 21, 1973 the Senate passed by a voice vote S 11-25, and the expectation is that this bill will become a Public Law. The main purpose of S 11-25 is to extend the grant provisions of Public Law 91-616 for an additional three years. The bill also makes various other amendments to 91-616.

Testimony at Senate Hearings

The following exerpts from these Subcommittee hearings give a sampling of the testimony which resulted in the decision of Congress to pass Public Law 91—616 on the final day of 1970.

Luther A. Cloud, M.D., President of the National Council on Alcoholism (NCA):

> We have felt for a long time that the few federal programs in this field are buried so far down in the governmental structure that they are barely visible to the American people ... It is no exaggeration to state that S 3835 is truly an Emancipation Proclamation. Freed of servitude to alcohol, millions of our citizens can return to the mainstream of American life.

Asked what percentage of the elderly might be alcoholics, Dr. Cloud replied:

> I think it will run a bit less than the general population. We are dealing with a disease that in the last analysis is a killer . . . many do not survive till age 65. Speaking from my personal experience, many of my patients, despite all I can do, die in their 50s and 60s because of the various complications of alcoholism. The No. 1 drug being abused is alcohol . . . this needs to be reiterated wherever possible because too often we think of this material as a beverage and we know full well that it is not.

Marian Wettrick, member of the board of directors, North American Association of Alcoholism Programs:

> . . . recognition of a problem by the public and its elected leaders does not always lead to action to solve or remedy that problem . . . the character of S 3835 is not simply theoretical and long range, but pragmatic and immediate.

Dr. Marvin A. Block, M.D., member of the Committee on Alcoholism and Drug Dependence, American Medical Association (AMA):

> The attitude expressed in these provisions toward Federal employees is a forward-looking one, stressing as it does, continued employability predicated on acceptance of treatment. Major industrial firms already have similar practices but this policy by Congress could be a constructive influence on other companies and on state and local governments. Voluntary entry to diagnosis and treatment is an important point not only for the bill at hand but for subsequent legislation which may be devel-

164

oped later by States. No one should be forced into treatment against his will.

Asked by Senator Hughes how to distinguish between the so-called problem social drinker and the alcoholic, Dr. Block replied:

If excessive drinking were to bring about social ostracism, people would be very careful about it. Then the only ones who would drink excessively would be those who could not control it. How easily then we could pick out the alcoholic . . . this is a matter of education, understanding and propaganda. I think we could actually sell this to the American people if sufficient time, energy and money were spent on it.

Asked about the cost of the proposed law, Dr. Block declared:

I am not concerned about the cost at all. I am concerned with the treatment of those people and prevention. Prevention is the most important factor.

Dr. Morris E. Chafetz, who would become director of the National Institute on Alcohol Abuse and Alcoholism (NIAAA) on June 13, 1971, testified that:

This legislation cannot come too soon. Even those of us who have devoted most of our professional lives to dealing with alcoholic people are unaware of the severity of the problem and its ramifications. For decades most of us have used the oft-quoted figure of 4,500,000 to 5,000,000 alcoholic people in the country. A recently completed scientific study shows the figure to be beyond 9,000,000. The bill's emphasis on early identification and prevention is essential if we are to control the alcohol problem. It is a basic principle of medicine that no condition is brought under control by treating the casualties alone.

As to the complexity of the nation's drinking problem, Dr. Seldon D. Bacon, Ph.D., director of the Center of Alcohol Studies, Rutgers University, New Brunswick, New Jersey, stated:

Over the past 150 years it has been defined as a moral weakness and turned over to the churches; as an economic problem and turned over to market and price control authorities; defined as a youth learning problem and turned over to educators; defined as a crime problem and turned over to law enforcement and correction agencies . . . It is a condition which affects so many other people in so many aspects of life ordinarily considered to be beyond the direct responsibilities and know-how of medical and health professions, I can't allow it is only a disease. It is more than that.

At the second session of the hearings, Senator Jacob K. Javits of New York, who, with Utah's Senator Frank E. Moss, was co-sponsoring the bill with Senator Hughes, declared that they "had the backing of more than 40 senators from both parties," adding that he and the Senator from Utah had been campaigning for a bill since 1966.*

Next to be heard was Dr. Roger O. Egeberg, Assistant Secretary for Health and Scientific Affairs, HEW. Dr. Egeberg, who had often stated that alcohol beverages constitute the nation's No. 1 health problem, told the committee:

> There is tremendous need for more and better programs and materials including publications, films and TV and radio materials to educate the public about the problem.

One instance of the many in-depth studies on the subject of alcohol was given by Dr. Egeberg:

> They say that to book a man in Los Angeles County costs $100. If the man has been booked 100 times for acute alcoholism, he has cost the county a lot of money which could have been used to much better purpose if we had used a medical approach . . . I look to what they did in Norway and Finland . . . in the case of driving, they treat them very strongly. A person found guilty of driving with alcohol in his system in those countries is put to work making little rocks out of big rocks on the highway. We could, if we did something like that in this country, perhaps save half our traffic deaths.

Dr. Egeberg also pointed out:

> I think alcoholism . . . is far too important to hang onto the coattails of drug addiction . . . at the present time the public feel-ing is all on [other] drugs but we have many millions of alco-holics in this country and [hard drug] addicts are probably less than a half a million.

To this, Senator Hughes replied:

> I also believe that alcoholism should stand alone. I think it is of prime importance. There is a lot of stigma in both areas. Most

---

*Senators Javits and Moss introduced the Javits-Moss Alcoholism Care and Control Act of 1969, a substantial portion of which was enacted into Public Law 91-616.

people don't want to view alcohol as a drug for one thing and they don't want the stigma [of addiction] attached to that.

Congressional Action

In the weeks that followed the hearings' completion, Senators Hughes, Javits, and Moss amended the bill which was then read before the 91st Congress, 2nd session, August 3rd, 1970.

On December 31st, 1970, the Comprehensive Alcohol Abuse and Alcoholism Prevention, Treatment, and Rehabilitation Act became law (Public Law 91—616), the first major legislation of its kind ever enacted, with a total sum of $300 million allocated over a three-year period. Of this amount, $180 million was made available in grants to states, and $120 million was allocated to support organizations and activities at the community level.

The National Institute of Alcohol Abuse and Alcoholism was established within the framework of the Department of Health, Education, and Welfare to supervise the program. Assigned to direct NIAAA was Dr. Morris E. Chafetz, with the Secretary of HEW in supervisory command of the entire program.

12

VOLUNTARY ABSTINENCE

"It has been well said that drinking stops thinking. Now it is time to make thinking stop drinking."

—Congressman Harley O. Staggers

12

The Philosophy of Abstinence

Semantics play an important role in our lives. Words shape our attitudes and the way a word affects the collective subconscious of our society may dictate the success or failure of any advertising campaign, a political candidate or a public health program.

At first blush, the word "abstinence" may have negative connotations. Abstention seems analagous to deprivation, and none of us wishes to feel deprived.

But "abstain" is a transitive verb and abstention is meaningless unless we know from what we are abstaining. When we abstain from something negative and destructive, the act of abstention becomes not an act of deprivation, but an act of fulfillment.

None can better attest to the positive nature of voluntary abstinence than the recovered alcoholic and his family. They have learned the hard way that abstinence and deprivation are not one and the same; that indulgence can deprive and abstinence can be fulfilling.

For a variety of reasons (religion, health, recovery from alcoholism, personal tastes and a personal decision for the common good are those most cited), almost a third of our citizens have committed themselves to voluntary abstinence. By this one act of commitment, this segment of our society has freed itself from all the perils associated with the use of alcohol and improved its chances for a lifetime of mental and physical health and well-being.

To them, voluntary abstinence is a positive act. If all of us can be educated to think positively about voluntary abstinence we will open our minds to the possibility of creating meaningful and purposeful lives, not only for the nine million alcoholics in our present society, but for all those who will be afflicted with alcoholism in the future unless they abstain from taking that first drink.

Abstinence and the Alcoholic

Out of all the research and the conflicts of opinion relative to the effects of the use of alcohol on the human system, one hard fact has emerged: there is no known cure for the alcoholic other than total abstinence. In that respect, the recovered alcoholic can be likened to the heroin addict who has "kicked the habit" and who knows that just one "fix" may prove fatal to his hopes of remaining clean.

The act of refusing to drink alcoholic beverages in a society where they have become part of the culture requires both decision making and will power on the part of the person who wishes to abstain. Voluntary abstinence is the foundation of the Alcoholics Anonymous program and the success of AA has been in recognizing both the necessity and the difficulty of the decision to abstain.

The basic problem, however, is that there are more drinkers becoming alcoholics than there are alcoholics becoming recovered alcoholics (abstainers). It is estimated that not more than 50 percent of all the alcoholic addicted succeed in conquering their problem. Also, as previously set forth in these pages, it is somewhat discouraging to note that only 700,000 of the nation's nine million alcoholics have sought the help of Alcoholics Anonymous. With the increasing consumption of alcohol at earlier ages, it seems inevitable that there will be a rising tide of alcoholism and alcohol-related problems in this country. Abstaining "after the fact" does not prevent the creation of new alcoholics every day.

Abstinence and the Pre-alcoholic

Before a person is defined as an alcoholic, he is usually identified as a "problem drinker" or "heavy drinker." All alcoholics were heavy drinkers before they became totally addicted. It takes considerable evidence to convince someone that he is alcohol addicted, evidence that usually occurs as personal tragedy. It goes without saying that a recovered alcoholic would have preferred not to have undergone the damage to mind, body, and personal relationships that finally moved him to abstain because he realized he had no choice. What would it have taken to cause him to realize the misfortune he could have saved himself by making that same choice earlier? At the very least, an honest, educated evaluation of his drinking habits by those in a position to know (family, friends, business acquaintances) might have had an effect. To achieve that kind of social honesty, however, will require an educational program of such proportions as to make society understand that the plight of the alcohol-addicted individual is as serious as that of the user of any other addictive drug.

Some Questions about Voluntary Abstinence

In the end, there is only one way for a person to know that he is completely free from the fear of alcoholism: immediate abstinence. This may sound like an impossible decision for the average social drinker—and an unnecessary one. But let's ask some questions:

Is it easier for a person to "kick the habit" if he is addicted or if he is not addicted? The answer is obvious—it should be much easier to abstain if one is not addicted. However, there are hundreds of thousands of addicted drinkers, alcoholics, who are abstaining right now, and have abstained for a good part of their life, as the records of Alcoholics Anonymous and other agencies will attest. These recovered alcoholics were addicted *before* they chose voluntary abstinence; shouldn't it be easier, then, for others to choose voluntary abstinence *before* they are addicted?

What are your chances of becoming an alcoholic if you do not abstain? If you have never tasted a drop of alcohol in your life and took your first drink today, the chances are one in fourteen that you would eventually become an alcoholic. If you have already tasted alcohol and consider yourself a "light" or "social" drinker, the chances are one in ten that you will eventually become an alcoholic. If you consider yourself to be a "heavy drinker" and have had some problems related to your drinking, the chances are better than 50-50 that you will become an alcoholic.

Why voluntary abstinence instead of prohibition? Though the use of alcohol is basically self-destructive, it has been proven that laws attempting to control man's personal behavior where the only victim is himself are most difficult to enforce. (This is not to say that there should not be laws restricting acts while under the influence of alcohol which may be dangerous or harmful to others, such as drunk driving, violent behavior, etc.). Voluntary abstinence is a personal decision which, when made, will never have to be enforced. And it is one of those rare personal decisions which can result only in good. The acceptance of voluntary abstinence as a credo for our society would make all forms of prohibition meaningless and unnecessary.

The True Meaning of Prevention

The word "prevention" is used by all those interested in the many and complex problems stemming from the use of alcohol. "Prevention," however, has one meaning to the alcohol-beverage industry; another meaning to the government; and still a third meaning to those whose view of the problem is all-encompassing.

To the alcohol-beverage industry, prevention means preventing accidents stemming from the use of alcohol which have a negative effect on the industry's public image. To the government, prevention means preventing the high incidence of alcoholism which has become a public health problem. To those who believe that the basic problem is the use of alcohol as a beverage, prevention means total prevention of all the damage that results from the use of alcohol.

In terms of action to achieve "prevention," the three parties cited above have different goals. The liquor industry would encourage the use of alcohol by all, but would hope to have those who have consumed too much alcohol at one sitting police themselves so that they would commit no injurious acts; the government would not restrict the use of alcohol but would attempt to educate the consumer to be moderate in its use and to seek help if

174

he can not control his drinking; those interested in total prevention would educate the community to abstain from all consumption of alcohol in any quantity or in any form, with immediate emphasis on action to prevent young people from taking their first drink.

The Solution

At this point in history, the solution to this grave social problem is an individual one. Information, guidance and counseling is available from many sources.* No one will force any individual to make a decision. But each person who opts for abstinence will have an influence far beyond his individual welfare, or his family, his friends, and his erstwhile drinking partners.

For the future, the answer is early education which will convince the youth of today and tomorrow that the social structure of his world will be much stronger without the undermining influence of present society's most destructive drug. This educational effort cannot be confined to the school system. It must also be made at home where most social attitudes are developed. Unfortunately, this may pose a problem to the drinking parent who might be accused of hypocrisy. At that point, the parent may well have to decide for himself whether his own voluntary abstinence is too big a price to pay for the future of his children.

A Self-Help Program

To help the alcohol-addicted achieve abstinence it is imperative that the stigma be removed from the term alcoholic.

The estimated nine million alcoholics in this country have identified themselves as persons who are addicted, those to whom that first drink ultimately proved to be fatal.

Most recovered alcoholics have taken the painful step of self-identification and abstinence because of damage inflicted not only to themselves, but to their loved ones. It is, therefore, to the best interest not only of the recovered alcoholic but also to those around him that every effort be made to help him abstain.

---

*See list of organizations in Appendices.

Possibly the most important part of that effort is the elimination of the temptation of alcoholic beverages in the home.

The family and friends of the recovered alcoholic must understand that by helping him abstain, they help themselves; and by helping themselves, they help society.

APPENDICES

National Organizations Dealing with Treatment and/or Referral of Alcohol-Related Problems

North American Association of Alcoholism Programs

National Council on Alcoholism, Inc.

Public Law 91-616

Excerpts from *Drug Use in America: Problem in Perspective*—Second Report of the National Commission on Marihuana and Drug Abuse

HEW *First Special Report to the U.S. Congress on Alcohol & Health*

APPENDICE

NATIONAL ORGANIZATIONS DEALING WITH TREATMENT AND/OR REFERRAL OF ALCOHOL-RELATED PROBLEMS

Al-Anon—P.O. Box 182, Madison Square Station, New York, New York 10010.
Deals with family problems relating to alcoholism.

Alcoholics Anonymous—305 E. 45th Street, New York, New York 10017
Chapters in almost every city. Consult phone directory or nearest NCA office.

Al-Ateen (AA for teenagers)—Consult phone directory or nearest NCA office.

American Institute of Family Relations—44 E. 23rd Street, New York, New York 10010

American Medical Association—535 N. Dearborn Street, Chicago, Illinois 60610
Committee on Alcoholism and Addiction.

American Business Men's Research Foundation—599 North York Road, Elmhurst, Illinois 60126
Publishes quarterly "Reporting on Alcoholism."

National Council on Alcoholism—2 Park Avenue, New York, New York 10016
Operates under National Institute of Mental Health. More than 80 affiliated organizations providing information concerning local resources to combat alcoholism.

National Institute of Alcoholism and Alcohol Abuse—5600 Fisher Lane, Room 11A56, Rockville, Maryland 20852
Operates under HEW. Regional branches cover all areas of the nation.

North American Association of Alcoholism Programs—1130 17th Street, N.W., Washington, D.C. 20036

Project Health—Searle Education Systems, Inc., Chicago, Illinois
Health Education programs for industry.

Salvation Army—Local branches in almost all cities.

NORTH AMERICAN ASSOCIATION OF ALCOHOLISM PROGRAMS
1130 Seventeenth Street, N.W.
Washington, D.C. 20036

Augustus H. Hewlett, Executive Secretary
Phone: Office: 202—628—1585

Ruth Brock, Administrative Assistant

MEMBERSHIP LIST
As of September 1971

PROGRAM MEMBERS
(By states, in alphabetical order)

ALABAMA
Division of Community Services
502 Washington Avenue
Montgomery, Alabama 36104

ALASKA
Office of Alcoholism
Department of Health & Welfare
Pouch H
Juneau, Alaska 99801

ALBERTA
Alcoholism & Drug Abuse
Commission
Administrative Centre
9929 103rd Street
Edmonton, Alberta, Canada

ARIZONA
Alcohol & Drug Abuse Section
State Department of Health
1624 West Adams Street
Phoenix, Arizona 85007

ARKANSAS
Arkansas Commission on Alcoholism
109 West 12th Street
Little Rock, Arkansas 72202

BRITISH COLUMBIA
Alcoholism Foundation of B.C.
175 West Broadway
Vancouver, British Columbia,
Canada

CALIFORNIA
Alcoholism Programs
Office of Alcoholism Program
Management
Human Relations Agency
915 Capitol Mall, Room 278
Sacramento, California 95814

COLORADO
Alcoholism & Drug Dependence
Division
Department of Public Health
4210 East 11th Avenue, Room 319
Denver, Colorado 80220

CONNECTICUT
Alcohol & Drug Dependence
Division
Department of Mental Health
51 Coventry Street
Hartford, Connecticut 06112

DELAWARE
Alcoholism Services, Division of
Mental Health
3000 Newport Gap Pike
Wilmington, Delaware 19899

FLORIDA
Bureau of Alcoholic
Rehabilitation
Division of Mental Health
P.O. Box 1147
Avon Park, Florida 33825

GEORGIA
Community Alcoholism Programs
Community Services Branch
Division of Mental Health
State Department of Public
Health
47 Trinity Avenue, S.W., Room 534
Atlanta, Georgia 30334

ILLINOIS
Section on Alcoholism Programs
Department of Mental Health
401 South Spring Street
Springfield, Illinois 62706

INDIANA
Division on Alcoholism
State Department of Mental
Health
3000 West Washington Street
Indianapolis, Indiana 46222

IOWA
State Commission on Alcoholism
State Office Building
Des Moines, Iowa 50319

KANSAS
Governor's Advisory Committee
on Alcoholism
Room 400,KP & L Tower
Topeka, Kansas 66612

KENTUCKY
Office of Alcoholism
Department of Mental Health
P.O. Box 678
Frankfort, Kentucky 40601

LOUISIANA
Division of Alcoholism
State Department of Hospitals
P.O. Box 4215,Capitol Station
Baton Rouge, Louisiana 70804

MAINE
Division of Alcoholism Services
Bureau of Rehabilitation
Department of Health & Welfare
State House
Augusta, Maine 04330

MANITOBA
Alcoholism Foundation of Manitoba
124 Nassau Street
Winnipeg 13,Manitoba, Canada

MARYLAND
Division of Alcoholism Control
State Department of Mental
Hygiene
301 West Preston Street
Baltimore, Maryland 21201

MASSACHUSETTS
Division of Alcoholism
State Department of Public Health
755 Boylston Street, Room 616
Boston, Massachusetts 02116

MICHIGAN
Alcoholism Program
Division of Chronic Disease
Control
3500 North Logan
Lansing, Michigan 48914

181

MINNESOTA
Commission on Alcohol Problems
Room 19,State Office Building
St. Paul, Minnesota 55101

MISSISSIPPI
Alcohol Abuse & Alcoholism
Program Dev.
Division of Mental Health
Services
State Board of Health
P.O. Box 1700
Jackson, Mississippi 39205

MISSOURI
Alcoholism & Drug Abuse Program
722 Jefferson Street
Jefferson City, Missouri 65101

MONTANA
State Alcoholism Services Center
State Hospital
Warm Springs, Montana 59756

NEBRASKA
Division of Alcoholism
State Department of Public
Institutions
P.O. Box 94728
Lincoln, Nebraska 68509

NEVADA
Alcoholism Division, Department
of Health & Welfare
State Capitol
Carson City, Nevada 89701

NEW BRUNSWICK
Alcohol Education & Community
Services
Dept. of Health, Centennial
Building
Fredericton, New Brunswick,
Canada

NEW HAMPSHIRE
Program on Alcoholism & Drug
Abuse
Department of Health & Welfare
61 South Spring
Concord, New Hampshire 03301

NEW JERSEY
Alcoholism Control Programs
State Department of Health
John Fitch Plaza, South Warren
Street
Trenton, New Jersey 08625

NEW MEXICO
Commission on Alcoholism
P.O. Box 1731
Albuquerque, New Mexico 87103

NEW YORK
Bureau of Alcoholism
State Dept. of Mental Hygiene
44 Holland Avenue
Albany, New York 12208

NORTH CAROLINA
Division of Alcoholism
State Department of Mental Health
P.O. Box 9494
Raleigh, North Carolina 27603

NORTH DAKOTA
Div. On Alcoholism & Drug Abuse
State Health Dept., State Capitol
Bismarck, North Dakota 58501

OHIO
Alcoholism Program, Dept. of
Health
450 East Town Street, P.O. Box 118
Columbus, Ohio 43216

OKLAHOMA
Commission on Alcoholism
P.O. Box 201
Tulsa, Oklahoma 74102

ONTARIO
Addiction Research Foundation
33 Russell Street
Toronto 4,Ontario, Canada

OREGON
Alcohol & Drug Section
Mental Health Division
309 S.W. 4th Street
Portland, Oregon 97204

PENNSYLVANIA
Div. of Alcoholism Studies &
Rehabilitation
State Department of Health
P.O. Box 90
Harrisburg, Pennsylvania 17120

QUEBEC
L'Office de la Prevention et du
Traitement de l'alcoolisme et
des autres
Toxicomanies (OPTAT)
Edifice Ste-Foy 969 route
de l'Eglise
Quebec 10,P.Q., Canada

RHODE ISLAND
Division of Alcoholism, Dept.
of Social Welfare
Eaton Street
Providence, Rhode Island 02906

SASKATCHEWAN
Alcoholism Commission of
Saskatchewan
2134 Hamilton Street
Regina, Saskatchewan, Canada

SOUTH CAROLINA
Commission on Alcoholism
2414 Bull Street
Columbia, South Carolina 29201

SOUTH DAKOTA
Division of Alcoholism
State Building No. 2, Room 213
Pierre, South Dakota 57501

TENNESSEE
Alcoholism & Drug Dependence
Programs
Department of Mental Health
300 Cordell Hull Building
Nashville, Tennessee 37219

TEXAS
Commission on Alcoholism
808 Sam Houston State Office
Building
Austin, Texas 78701

UTAH
State Board on Alcoholism
770 East South Temple, Suite A
Salt Lake City, Utah 84111

VERMONT
Alcoholic Rehabilitation Board
59-63 Pearl Street
Burlington, Vermont 05401

VIRGINIA
Bureau of Alcohol & Drug Studies
State Health Department
109 Governor Street
Richmond, Virginia 23219

WASHINGTON
Department of Social & Health
Services
Division of Health
Alcoholism Section
P.O. Box 709,Olympia Airport
Olympia, Washington 98501

183

WEST VIRGINIA
Div. of Alcoholism, Dept. of
Mental Health
State Capitol
Charleston, West Virginia 25305

WISCONSIN
Bureau of Alcoholism & Drug Abuse
Dept. of Health & Social Services
1 West Wilson Street
Madison, Wisconsin 53702

WYOMING
Department of Alcoholic Treat-
ment Services
Wyoming State Hospital
Evanston, Wyoming 82930

NORTH AMERICAN ASSOCIATION OF ALCOHOLISM PROGRAMS

AGENCY MEMBERS WITHIN STATES
SEPTEMBER 1971

ARIZONA
St. Luke's Hospital Alcoholism
Treatment Center
525 North 18th Street
Phoenix, Arizona 85006

Alcoholism Prevention & Treatment
Program
P.O. Box 427
Sacaton, Arizona 85247

West Center of Tucson General
Hospital
3838 N. Campbell Avenue
Tucson, Arizona 85719

CALIFORNIA
Antelope Valley Rehabilitation
Centers
County of Los Angeles, P.O. Box 25
Acton, California 93510

Berkeley Center for Alcohol
Studies
Pacific School of Religion
1798 Scenic Avenue
Berkeley, California 94709

Alcohol Program, Co. of
Los Angeles
Health Department
5205 Melrose Avenue
Hollywood, California 90038

Los Angeles County Olive View
Hospital
14701 Foothill Boulevard, Box 403
Olive View, California 91330

Pasadena Community Program on
Alcoholism
25 South Euclid Avenue
Pasadena, California 91101

George LaFeve Associates
3701 Merrill
Riverside, California 92505

Alcoholism Clinic, Presbyterian
Hospital for Pacific Medical
Center
Clay & Webster Streets
San Francisco, California 94115

184

Center for Special Problems
199 10th Street
San Francisco, California 94103

COLORADO
Alcoholism Division, Mental
Health Center
Box 188
Fort Logan, Colorado 80115

DISTRICT OF COLUMBIA
Washington Area Council on
Alcoholism & Drug Addiction
1330 New Hampshire Avenue, N.W.
Suite 1
Washington, D.C. 20036

FLORIDA
Broward County Commission on
Alcoholism
Bennett Building, Room 219
4 North Federal Highway
Fort Lauderdale, Florida 33301

Brevard County Mental Health
Center
1770 Cedar Street
Rockledge, Florida 32955

Inter-Agency Law Enforcement
Planning Council
104 South Calhoun Street
Tallahassee, Florida 32304

GEORGIA
Southside Comprehensive Health
Center
1039 Ridge Avenue, S.W.
Atlanta, Georgia 30315

Central State Hospital
Milledgeville, Georgia 31061

HAWAII
Big Island Council on Alcoholism
P.O. Box 180
Hilo, Hawaii 96720

ILLINOIS
Alcoholism Inf. & Referral Center
Family Counseling Service
411 West Galena Boulevard
Aurora, Illinois 60506

Mercyville Institute of Mental
Health
1330 North Lake Street
Aurora, Illinois 60506

Central States Inst. of Addiction
Programs
126 North Desplaines Street
Chicago, Illinois 60606

Chicago's Alcoholic Treatment
Center
3026 South California Avenue
Chicago, Illinois 60608

Chicago Council on Alcoholism
6 North Michigan Avenue, Room 1422
Chicago, Illinois 60602

Martha Washington Hospital
2318 West Irving Park Road
Chicago, Illinois 60618

Community Concern for Alcohol
& Drug Abuse
20 North Grove Avenue
Elgin, Illinois 62002

Rock Island County Council on
Alcoholism
1630 5th Avenue, Suite 541
Moline, Illinois 61265

Alcoholism Rehabilitation Center
Lutheran General Hospital
1775 Dempster Street
Park Ridge, Illinois 60068

Illinois Alcoholism & Drug
Dependence Association
320 East Armstrong
Peoria, Illinois 61603

H. Douglas Singer Zone Center, ATU
Department of Mental Health
4402 North Main Street
Rockford, Illinois 61103

Northern Illinois Council on
Alcoholism
425 East State Street
Rockford, Illinois 61104

Division of Vocational
Rehabilitation
623 East Adams Street
Springfield, Illinois 61101

Sangamon County Council on
Alcoholism
Suite 1008, 500 East Monroe St.
Springfield, Illinois 62701

INDIANA
Fairbanks Memorial Home &
Hospital
1575 Northwestern
Indianapolis, Indiana 46202

IOWA
Harrison Treatment & Rehab.
Center
725 Sixth Avenue
Des Moines, Iowa 50309

University of Iowa Treatment Unit
Oakdale, Iowa 52319

Northwest Iowa Alc. Treatment Unit
Spencer Municipal Hospital
115 East 11th Street
Spencer, Iowa 51301

KENTUCKY
Alc. Information Center
9911 LaGrange Road
Louisville, Kentucky 40223

KANSAS
Shawnee Community Mental Health
Corp.
1615 West 8th Street
Topeka, Kansas 66606

Veterans Administration Hospital
2200 Gage Boulevard
Topeka, Kansas 66622

LOUISIANA
Comm. on Alc. & Drug Abuse for
Greater New Orleans
410 Chartres Street, Room 200
New Orleans, Louisiana 70130

MAINE
Bangor Counseling Center
43 Illinois Avenue
Bangor, Maine 04401

MARYLAND
Baltimore Area Council on
Alcoholism
22 East 25 Street
Baltimore, Maryland 21218

Baltimore County Health Dept.
105 West Chesapeake Avenue
Towson, Maryland 21204

Hidden Brook Treatment Center
for Alcoholism
Thomas Run Road
Bel Air, Maryland 21204

MASSACHUSETTS
Washingtonian Center for Addictions
41 Morton Street
Jamaica Plain (Boston), Mass. 02130

MICHIGAN

Greater Detroit Council on
Alcoholism
6131 West Outer Drive
Detroit, Michigan 48235

NCA-Greater Flint Area, Inc.
202 E. Boulevard Drive, Suite 300
Flint, Michigan 48503

Kent County Council on Alcoholism
1619 Walker Avenue, N.W.
Grand Rapids, Michigan 49504

Kalamazoo Committee on Alcoholism
350 South Burdick
Kalamazoo, Michigan 49006

Michigan Alcohol & Addiction Assn.
P.O. Box 61
Lansing, Michigan 48902

MINNESOTA

Hazelden, Box 11
Center City, Minnesota 55012

Hennepin Co. Alc. & Inebriety
Program
605 4th Avenue South
Minneapolis, Minnesota 55415

Lynville Metropolitan Office
230 Oak Grove
Minneapolis, Minn. 55403

Alc. & Chemical Addiction Service
St. Cloud Hospital
1406 6th Avenue North
St. Cloud, Minnesota 56301

Alcohol & Drug Addiction Unit
State Hospital
Willmar, Minnesota 56201

MISSOURI

Greater KC Council on Alcoholism
Room 210, 2 West 40th Street
Kansas City, Missouri 64111

Jackson Co. Public Hosp. Detox.
Rehab.
Little Blue & Lee's Summit Roads
Kansas City, Missouri 64139

Alcoholism Treatment & Research
Center
Malcolm Bliss Mental Health Center
420 Grattan Street
St. Louis, Missouri 63104

NEBRASKA

Alcoholic Rehab. Center, State
Hospital
Ingleside, Nebraska 68953

NEVADA

Washoe County Council on Alcoholism
Suite 412, 10 State Street
Reno, Nevada 89507

NEW HAMPSHIRE

N.H. State Liquor Commission
Storrs Street
Concord, New Hampshire 03301

N.H. Div. of Vocational Rehab.
64 North Main Street
Concord, New Hampshire 03301

NEW JERSEY

Center of Alcohol Studies
Rutgers-The State University
New Brunswick, New Jersey 08903

NEW MEXICO

Jicarilla Apache Alcoholism Project
P.O. Box 312
Dulce, New Mexico 87528

NEW YORK
Alcoholic Clinic, Downstate
Medical Center
State Univ. of New York
600 Albany Avenue
Brooklyn, New York 11203

Committee on Alcoholism, CCGNY
225 Park Avenue South
New York, New York 10003

Men's Social Service Dept.
Salvation Army
120 West 14 Street
New York, New York 10011

Bureau of Shelter Services, Dept.
of Soc. Serv.
325 Lafayette Street
New York, New York 10013

NORTH CAROLINA
Educ. Div., Bd. of Alcoholic
Control
Parkway Office
Asheville, North Carolina 28801

Lee-Harnett Mental Health Center
Box 457
Buies Creek, North Carolina 27506

Alamance County Council on
Alcoholism
802 N.C. National Bank Building
Burlington, North Carolina 27215

Charlotte Council on Alcoholism
1125 E. Morehead Street, Suite 101
Charlotte, North Carolina 28204

The Randolph Clinic, Inc.
1804 East 4th Street
Charlotte, North Carolina 28204

Center for Alc. Rehab. Educ.
Services
709 Battleground Avenue
Greensboro, North Carolina 27401

Walter B. Jones, ARC
Box 5066
Greenville, North Carolina 27834

Alcohol Education Center
P.O. Box 348
Jamestown, North Carolina 27282

Sandhills Mental Health Center
Pinehurst, North Carolina 28374

Wilson County Council on Alcoholism
Room 208 Woodard Building
116 S. Goldsboro
Wilson, North Carolina 27893

Alcoholism Program of Forsyth
County
804 O'Hanlon Bldg., 105 W. 4th St.
Winston-Salem, North Carolina 27201

NORTH DAKOTA
Alcoholism Program, State Hospital
Jamestown, North Dakota 58401

Heartview Foundation
Mandan, North Dakota 58554

OHIO
Alcoholism Program, Dept. of
Public Health
702 Municipal Building
Akron, Ohio 44308

Alcohol & Drug Abuse Section
Div. of Health
601 Lakeside Avenue
Cleveland, Ohio 44114

Cleveland Center on Alcoholism
2071 East 102 Street
Cleveland, Ohio 44106

Div. on Alcoholism, Dept. of
Health
181 South Washington Boulevard
Columbus, Ohio 43215

Dayton Area Council on Alc. &
Drug Abuse
184 Salem Avenue
Dayton, Ohio 45406

Greene County Council on Alcoholism
120 North Detroit Street
Xenia, Ohio 45385

OKLAHOMA
Tulsa Council on Alcoholism
2121 S. Columbia, Suite LL 1
Tulsa, Oklahoma 74114

ONTARIO
Employee Serv. Branch, Dept. of
Civil Serv.
1200 Bay Street, Suite 208
Toronto 181,Ontario, Canada

OREGON
Lane Co. Council on Alcoholism
P.O. Box 582 ·
Eugene, Oregon 97401

Eastern Oregon Alcoholism
Foundation
304 S.W. Hailey
Pendelton, Oregon 97801

Alcoholic Rehabilitation Assn.
915 S.E. Hawthorne
Portland, Oregon 97214

Oregon Council on Alc. Problems
1704 N.E. 32nd Avenue
Portland, Oregon 97212

PENNSYLVANIA
Eagleville Hospital & Rehab. Center
P.O. Box 45, Montgomery County
Eagleville, Pennsylvania 19408

Off. of MH, Dept. of Public Wel.
Health & Welfare Bldg., Room 303
Harrisburg, Pennsylvania 17120

United Steelworkers of America
1500 Commonwealth Building
Pittsburgh, Pennsylvania 15222

SOUTH CAROLINA
Dept. of MH, Div. of Alc. &
Drug Addiction
P.O. Box 485
Columbia, South Carolina 29202

Mid-Carolina Council on Alc.
1900 Hampton Street
Columbia, South Carolina 29201

Palmetto Center, P.O. Box 1567
Florence, South Carolina 29501

TENNESSEE
Jackson Area Counc. on Alc.
P.O. Box 1031
Jackson, Tennessee 38301

TEXAS
Alcoholism Program, Amarillo
Hospital Distr.
Northwest Texas Hospital
P.O. Box 1110
Amarillo, Texas 79105

Dept. of MH & MR, Box 12668
Capitol Station
Austin, Texas 78711

Coastal Bend Council on Alc.
310 Jones Building
Corpus Christi, Texas 78401

McLennan Co. Counc. on Alc.
110 S. 12th Street
Waco, Texas 76701

UTAH
Ute Tirbe Alc. Inf. & Counseling
Program
P.O. Box 69
Fort Duchesne, Utah 84026

Utah Alcoholism Foundation
2875 South Main
Salt Lake City, Utah 84115

Kennecott Copper Corporation
Ind. Rel. Dept., P.O. Box 11299
Salt Lake City, Utah 84111

WASHINGTON
King Co. Commission on Alc.
Courthouse No. 2
100 Crockett Street, Room 334
Seattle, Washington 98101

WEST VIRGINIA
AIC, Appalachian MH Center
201 Henry Street
Elkins, West Virginia 26241

WISCONSIN
Alc. Inf. & Referral Center
210 Monona Avenue, Room 313D
Madison, Wisconsin 53709

Dept. of Soc. Work, U. of Wisc.
Exten.
606 State Street
Madison, Wisconsin 53706

DePaul Rehabilitation Hospital
4143 South 13th Street
Milwaukee, Wisconsin 53221

Racine Counc. on Alc. at the
A Center
2000 Domanik Drive
Racine, Wisconsin 53404

WYNOT ATC Rehab. Fdtn., Route 1
Weyerhauser, Wisconsin 54895

ADDENDUM
Agency

Chit Chat Foundation, Box 418 *
Robesonia, Pennsylvania 19551

Program

Change UTAH to:
Division of Alcoholism & Drugs
2875 South Main
Salt Lake City, Utah 84115

NATIONAL COUNCIL ON ALCOHOLISM, INC.
2 Park Avenue
New York, N.Y. 10016
(212) 899-3160

AFFILIATE DIRECTORY
March 1972

ALASKA
Anchorage — Anchorage Council on
Alcoholism
P.O. Box 506
Anchorage, Alaska 99501
Tel: (907) 272-6211

ARIZONA
Phoenix — NCA-Greater Phoenix Area
Community Service Building
1515 East Osborn Road - Room No. 43
Phoenix, Arizona 85014
Tel: (602) 264-6214

CALIFORNIA
Carmel — Monterey Peninsula Council
on Alcoholism
P.O. Box 1058
Carmel, California 93921
Tel: (408) 624-2256

Los Angeles — Alcoholism Council of
Greater Los Angeles
2001 Beverly Boulevard
Los Angeles, California 90057
Tel: (213) 380-0332

Oakland — NCA-Alameda County
431 30th Street
Oakland, California 94609
Tel: (415) 834-5598

Pasadena — Pasadena Council on
Alcoholism
201 North El Molino, Suite 107
Pasadena, California 91001
Tel: (213) 795-9127

San Diego — NCA-Greater San Diego
Area
P.O. Box 20852
San Diego, California 92190
Tel: (714) 234-7381

San Francisco — NCA-San Francisco
Area
2340 Clay Street - Suite 407
San Francisco, California 94115
Tel: (415) 346-1480

Santa Barbara — NCA-Santa Barbara
Area, Inc.
804 Santa Barbara Street
P.O. Box 28
Santa Barbara, California 93102
Tel: (805) 966-6474

COLORADO
Colorado Springs — NCA-Pikes Peak
Region, Inc.
P.O. Box 395
Colorado Springs, Colorado 80909
Tel: (303) 634-3487

Denver — NCA-Mile High Area
United Way Service Center - Room 506
1375 Delaware Street
Denver, Colorado 80204
Tel: (303) 623-6146

Grand Junction — NCA-Mesa County,
Inc.
610 Rood
Grand Junction, Colorado 81501
Tel: (303) 243-3140

CONNECTICUT

Cos Cob — Alcoholism Council of
  Southern Connecticut, Inc.
521 Post Road
Cos Cob, Connecticut 06807
Tel: (203) 661-9011

DISTRICT OF COLUMBIA

Washinton, D.C. — Washington Area
  Council on Alcoholism and Drug
  Abuse
1330 New Hampshire Avenue, N.W.
Washington, D.C. 20036
Tel: (202) 466-2323

ILLINOIS

Chicago — Chicago Council on
  Alcoholism
6 North Michigan Avenue   Suite 1422
Chicago, Illinois 60602
Tel: (312) 726-1368

IOWA

Des Moines — NCA-Des Moines Area, Inc.
1223 Bankers Trust Building
Des Moines, Iowa 50309
Tel: (515) 244-2297

KANSAS

Topeka — NCA-Kansas Division, Inc.
2044 Fillmore
Topeka, Kansas 66604
Tel: (913) 235-2339

LOUISIANA

Shreveport — Caddo-Bossier Council
  on Alcoholism and Drug Abuse
Commercial Building - Room 9
509 Market Street
Shreveport, Louisiana 71101
Tel: (318) 425-1403

MARYLAND

Baltimore — Baltimore Area Council on
  Alcoholism
22 East 25th Street
Baltimore, Maryland 21218
Tel: (301) 366-5555

MICHIGAN

Detroit — Greater Detroit Council on
  Alcoholism
6131 West Outer Drive
Detroit, Michigan 48235
Tel: (313) 864-4065

Flint — NCA-Greater Flint Area, Inc.
202 E. Boulevard Drive - Suite 300
Flint, Michigan 48503
Tel: (313) 235-0639

Lansing — Tri-County Council on
  Alcoholism and Addictions
300 No. Washington Avenue - Suite 304
Lansing, Michigan 48914
Tel: (517) 482-3392

Muskegon — Muskegon County Council
  on Alcoholism
308 Michigan Theatre Building
Muskegon, Michigan 49440
Tel: (616) 722-1931

MINNESOTA

St. Paul — Family Service of St. Paul
300 Wilder Building
5th and Washington Street
St. Paul, Minnesota 55106
Tel: (612) 222-0311

MISSOURI

Kansas City — NCA-Kansas City Area
6155 Oak Street
Kansas City, Missouri 64113
Tel: (816) 361-5900

192

St. Louis – Greater St. Louis Council
on Alcoholism
1210 Locust Street - Room 101
St. Louis, Missouri 63103
Tel: (314) 231-9600

NEBRASKA
Lincoln – Lincoln Council on
Alcoholism
217 Lincoln Center
215 South 15th Street
Lincoln, Nebraska 68508
Tel: (402) 475-2695

NEW JERSEY
Montclair – NCA-North Jersey Area,
Inc.
Council of Social Agencies Bldg.
Room 211
60 South Fullerton Avenue
Montclair, New Jersey 07042
Tel: (201) 783-9313

Red Bank – Alcoholism Council of
Monmouth County, New Jersey,
Inc.
54 Broad Street - Room 225
Red Bank, New Jersey 07701
Tel: (201) 741-5203

NEW MEXICO
Albuquerque – Albuquerque Area
Council on Alcoholism, Inc.
229-B Truman Street, N.E.
Albuquerque, New Mexico 87110
Tel: (505) 268-6216

NEW YORK
Buffalo – Buffalo Area Council on
Alcoholism
1 West Genesee Street
723 Genesee Building
Buffalo, New York 14202
Tel: (716) 853-0375

Corning – Corning Area Council on
Alcoholism, Inc.
Corning Hospital
176 Denison Parkway East
Corning, New York 14830
Tel: (607) 962-5051 (ext. 311)

Elmira – Chemung County Council on
Alcoholism
114 East Gray Street
240 Elmira Theater Building
Elmira, New York 14901
Tel: (607) 734-1567

Garden City – Long Island Council on
Alcoholism
350 Old Country Road
Garden City, Long Island, New York
11530
Tel: (516) PI7-2606

New York City – National Council on
Alcoholism - New York City
Affiliate
225 Park Avenue, South
New York, New York 10003
Tel: (212) 777-5752

Rochester – NCA-Rochester Area-
Health Association of Rochester
and Monroe County, Inc.
973 East Avenue
Rochester, New York 14607
Tel: (716) 271-3540

Utica – NCA-Oneida County, Inc.
167 Genesee Street
Utica, New York 13501
Tel: (315) 732-1072

White Plains – Westchester Council on
Alcoholism
129 Court Street
White Plains, New York 10601
Tel: (914) 946-1358

OHIO

Cincinnati — Council on Alcoholism of
the Cincinnati Area
2400 Reading Road - Room 202
Cincinnati, Ohio 45202
Tel: (513) 721-2905

OKLAHOMA

Tulsa — Tulsa Council on Alcoholism
2121 South Columbia Avenue
Suite LL 1, Parkland Plaza Building
Tulsa, Oklahoma 74114
Tel: (918) 747-8891

PENNSYLVANIA

Bethlehem — Bethlehem Council on
Alcoholism
Community Chest Building
520 East Broad Street
Bethlehem, Pennsylvania 18018
Tel: (215) 867-3986

Lancaster — NCA-Lancaster County,
Inc.
630 Janet Avenue
Lancaster, Pennsylvania 17601
Tel: (717) 299-2831

Philadelphia — NCA-Delaware Valley
Area, Inc.
3401 Market Street
Philadelphia, Pennsylvania 19104
Tel: (215) 387-0590

Pittsburgh — Alcoholism Program -
United Mental Health Services of
Allegheny County, Inc.
4026 Jenkins Arcade
Pittsburgh, Pennsylvania 15222
Tel: (412) 391-3820

Reading — NCA-Berks County, Inc.
300 North Fifth Street
Reading, Pennsylvania 19601
Tel: (215) 372-8917-18

RHODE ISLAND

Providence — "Hope" Council on
Alcoholism, Inc.
P.O. Box 2451
Providence, Rhode Island 02906
Tel: (401) 421-2027

TENNESSEE

Chattanooga — Chattanooga Area
Council on Alcoholism and Drug
Abuse
1212 Dodds Avenue
Chattanooga, Tennessee 37403
Tel: (615) 267-3354

Memphis — Memphis Alcohol and Drug
Council
1349 Monroe Avenue - Room 302
Memphis, Tennessee 38104
Tel: (901) 272-1757

Nashville — Mid-Cumberland
Council on Alcohol and
Drugs
814 Church Street
Nashville, Tennessee 37203
Tel: (615) 254-6547

TEXAS

Houston — Houston Council on
Alcoholism
601 Medical Towers
Houston, Texas 77025
Tel: (713) 526-1791

San Antonio — NCA-San Antonio Area
5307 Broadway - Suite 209
San Antonio, Texas 78209
Tel: (512) 828-3742

VIRGINIA

Norfolk — Virginia Council on
Alcoholism & Drug Dependence -
Tidewater Area
Suite 520 - Professional Arts Building
142 West York Street
Norfolk, Virginia 23510
Tel: (703) 625-5838

WASHINGTON
Seattle — Seattle-King County Council
on Alcoholism
3109 Arcade Building
1319 Second Avenue
Seattle, Washington 98101
Tel: (206) 623-8380

Vancouver — Clark County Council on
Alcoholism
207 Central Building
1206½ Main Street
Vancouver, Washington 98660
Tel: (206) 696-1631

Yakima — Yakima Valley Council on
Alcoholism
202 Miller Building
Yakima, Washington 98901
Tel: (509) 248-1800

WISCONSIN
Milwaukee — Milwaukee Council on
Alcoholism, Inc.
135 West Wells Street - Suite 416
Milwaukee, Wisconsin 53203
Tel: (414) 276-8487

NATIONAL COUNCIL ON ALCOHOLISM, INC.
2 Park Avenue
New York, N.Y. 10016
(212) 889-3160

ASSOCIATE DIRECTORY
March 1972

ALABAMA
Mobile — Southwest Alabama Council
on Alcoholism, Inc.
1950 Government Street - Room 202
Mobile, Alabama 36606
Tel: (205) 471-3977

ALASKA
Kodiak — Kodiak Council on
Alcoholism
P.O. Box 627
Kodiak, Alaska 99615

ARIZONA
Tucson — Alcoholism Council of
Southern Arizona
Box 4845, University Station
Tucson, Arizona 85717
Tel: (602) 325-6074

Yuma — Yuma County on Alcoholism
& Drug Abuse
2222 Avenue A, Wing D, Room 8
Yuma, Arizona 85364

CALIFORNIA
Placerville — El Dorado Council on
Alcoholism
P.O. Box 246
Placerville, California 95667

Riverside — Committee on Alcoholism
& Drug Abuse for Inland Empire
3701 Merrill Avenue
Riverside, California 92506
Tel: (714) 682-4644

San Luis Obispo — National Council on
Alcoholism San Luis Obispo Area,
Inc.
1987 Wilding Lane
San Luis Obispo, California 94301
Tel: (805) 543-2723

Santa Ana — Orange County Council
on Alcoholism
1913 East 17th Street - Suite 103
Santa Ana, California 92703
Tel: (714) 835-3830

195

Santa Rosa – Sonoma County Council
on Alcoholism
P.O. Box 2661
Santa Rosa, California 95404
Tel: (707) 544-7544

CONNECTICUT
Groton – Southeastern Council on
Alcoholism & Drug Dependence,
Inc.
242 North Road
P.O. Box 962
Groton, Connecticut 06340
Tel: (403) 455-8511

New Haven – The Alcohol Council of
Greater New Haven
412 Orange Street
New Haven, Connecticut 06511

FLORIDA
Fort Lauderdale – Broward County
Commission on Alcoholism
Bennett Building - Room 219
4 N. Federal Highway
Fort Lauderdale, Florida 33301
Tel: (305) 525-0206

Miami Beach – City of Miami Beach
Court Alcoholic Rehabilitation Program
1001 Ocean Drive
Miami Beach, Florida 33139

Sarasota – Sarasota Rehabilitation Program, Inc.
727 So. Orange Avenue
Sarasota, Florida 33577

GEORGIA
Waycross – Area Drug Alcoholism
Council
102 Gilmore Street
Waycross, Georgia 31501

ILLINOIS
Aurora – Mercyville Institute of
Mental Health
1330 No. Lake Street
Aurora, Illinois 60506

Peoria – Peoria Area Council on
Alcoholism
Allied Agencies Center
320 East Armstrong Avenue
Peoria, Illinois 61603
Tel: (309) 676-4681

INDIANA
South Bend – Alcoholism Council,
Inc. of St. Joseph County
521 W. Colfax Avenue
South Bend, Indiana 46601
Tel: (219) 234-3136

IOWA
Sioux City – Siouxland and Council
on Alcoholism
St. Vincent Hospital - Rooms 210 - 215
624 Jones Street
Sioux City, Iowa 51104
Tel: (712) 279-2123

KENTUCKY
Anchorage – Alcoholic Information
Center
9911 La Grange Road
Anchorage, Kentucky 40223

Harlan – Upper Cumberland and
Alcoholism & Drug Abuse Council,
Inc.
c/o Bank of Harlan
Box 919
Harlan, Kentucky 40831

LOUISIANA
Baton Rouge — Baton Rouge Area
Council on Alcoholism & Drug
Abuse
2035 Wooddale Blvd.
Suite E
Baton Rouge, Louisiana 70806
Tel: (504) 924-6630

Monroe — Twin Cities Council on
Alcoholism
P.O. Box 332
2400 Louisville Avenue
Monroe, Louisiana 71201
Tel: (318) 323-0231

MARYLAND
Easton — Eastern Shore Council on
Alcoholism, Inc.
P.O. Box 351
Easton, Maryland 21601
Tel: (301) 822-4133

Hagerstown — Washington County
Council on Alcoholism
310 Professional Arts Bldg.
Hagerstown, Maryland 21740

MASSACHUSETTS
Salem — North Shore Committee on
Alcoholism, Inc.
5 Broad Street, Health Center
Salem, Massachusetts 01970

Worcester — Worcester County Council
on Alcoholism, Inc.
9 Walnut Street
Worcester, Massachusetts
Tel: (617) 757-1423

MICHIGAN
Ann Arbor — The Washtenaw County
Council on Alcoholism
218 North Division Street
Ann Arbor, Michigan 48106
Tel: (313) 971-7900

Kalamazoo Alcoholism and
Addiction Council
350 South Burdick Street
Kalamazoo, Michigan 49001
Tel: (616) 381-6642

Munising — Alger County Alcoholism
Council
Box 87
Munising, Michigan 49862
Tel: (906) 387-3210

MINNESOTA
Minneapolis — Minnesota Council on
Alcohol Problems
122 West Franklin Avenue
Minneapolis, Minnesota 55404

Minneapolis — Lynnville, Inc.
230 Oak Grove
Minneapolis, Minnesota 55403

MISSISSIPPI
Parchman — Department of Alcoholic
Rehabilitation
Mississippi State Penitentiary
Parchman, Mississippi 38738
Tel: (601) 745-2411

NEBRASKA
Grand Island — Central Nebraska
Council on Alcoholism
208 Masonic Building
Grand Island, Nebraska 68801
Tel: (308) 384-7365

NEVADA
Las Vegas — Southern Nevada
Council on Alcoholism
13 Harvard Street
Las Vegas, Nevada 89107
Tel: (702) 384-9009

NEW JERSEY

Burlington — Burlington County
Community Action Program
9 West Union Street
Burlington, New Jersey 08016

Flemington — Hunterdon Council on
Alcoholism
c/o Hunterdon Medical Center
Flemington, New Jersey 08822

NEW YORK

Ithaca — Alcoholism Council of
Tompkins County
223 Fayette Street
Ithaca, New York 14850

Johnson City — Broome County
Committee on Alcoholism, Inc.
44 Harrison Street
Johnson City, New York 13790
Tel: (607) 798-9971

Niagara Falls — Niagara County
Council on Alcoholism, Inc.
727 Main Street
Niagara Falls, New York
Tel: (716) 282-1002

Saranac Lake — St. Joseph's Rehabili-
tation Center
P.O. Box 470
Saranac Lake, New York 12983
Tel: (518) 891-3950

Schenectady — Alcoholism Council of
Schenectady County, Inc.
277 State Street
Schenectady, New York 12305
Tel: (518) 372-3371

Syracuse — Onodaga Council on
Alcoholism
Community Chest Building - Room 405
107 James Street
Syracuse, New York 13202
Tel: (315) 471-1359

Watertown — Jefferson County
Committee on Alcoholism, Inc.
Hotel Woodruff - Suite 118
Watertown, New York 13601

NORTH CAROLINA

Charlotte — Charlotte Council on
Alcoholism, Inc.
100 Billingsley Road
Charlotte, North Carolina 28211
Tel: (704) 375-5521

Durham — Durham Council on
Alcoholism
606 Snow Building
Durham, North Carolina 27701
Tel: (919) 682-5227

Morganton — Burke County Council on
Alcoholism, Inc.
211 North Sterling Street
Morganton, North Carolina 28655
Tel: (704) 433-1221

OHIO

Hamilton — NCA-Butler County, Inc.
Gonzaga Memorial Hall
Mercy Hospital
111 Buckeye Street
Hamilton, Ohio 45011
Tel: (513) 869-6471

OREGON

Portland — Council on Alcoholism
Portland Tri-County Area
538 S. E. Ash
Portland, Oregon 97214
Tel: (503) 255-6649

198

PENNSYLVANIA
Allentown — Lehigh County Council on
Alcohol and Drug Abuse
34 North Fifth Street
Allentown, Pennsylvania 18101
Tel: (215) 437-0801

Erie — Erie Council on Alcoholism
110 West 10th Street
Erie, Pennsylvania 16501

Johnstown — Conemaugh Valley
Council on Alcoholism
418 Lincoln Street
Johnstown, Pennsylvania 15906
Tel: (814) 535-6211

Pittsburgh — Community Action
Pittsburgh, Inc.
107 Sixth Street
Pittsburgh, Pennsylvania 15222
Tel: (412) 355-6333

Scranton — Alcoholism & Drug Abuse
Council of Northeastern
Pennsylvania
Suite 404 - Chamber of Commerce
Building
Scranton, Pennsylvania 18503
Tel: (717) 346-7309

Washington — Washington County
Council on Alcoholism, Inc.
18 West Wheeling Street
Washington, Pennsylvania 15301
Tel: (412) 222-7150

SOUTH CAROLINA
Charleston — Trident Council on
Alcohol & Drug Abuse
P.O. Box 2682
Charleston, South Carolina 29403

TEXAS
Austin — Austin Council on
Alcoholism
411 Littlefield Building
Austin, Texas 78701
Tel: (512) 472-2461

Orange — Orange Council on
Alcoholism
P.O. Box 635
408 North 5th Street
Orange, Texas 77630
Tel: (713) 883-4532

VIRGINIA
Abingdon — The Progressive
Community Club
118 Wall Street
Abingdon, Virginia 24210

Richmond — The Middle Atlantic
Institute for Alcohol and other
Drug Studies
3202 W. Cary Street
Richmond, Virginia 23221

WASHINGTON
Longview — Lower Columbia Council
on Alcoholism
835 15th Avenue
Longview, Washington 98632

Olympia — Thurston-Mason Counties,
Inc. Alcoholism Information &
Referral Center
110 West State Street
Olympia, Washington 98501
Tel: (206) 943-8510

Seattle — The Studio Club
9010 13th Avenue N.W.
Seattle, Washington 98107

Tacoma — Pierce County Council on
Alcoholism
109 North Tacoma Avenue
Tacoma, Washington 98403
Tel: (206) 383-3311 ext. 761

WISCONSIN
Baldwin — Tri-County Council on
Alcohol-Drug Abuse
Box 64
Baldwin, Wisconsin 54002

Kenosha — Kenosha County Council on
Alcoholism
16-17 Isermann Building
616 56th Street
Kenosha, Wisconsin 53140

Green Bay — Brown County
Educational & Information
Center on Alcoholism
Room 300 - Courthouse Annex
Green Bay, Wisconsin 54301
Tel: (414) 432-1959

La Crosse — West Central Council on
Alcoholism
1312 Winnebago Street
La Crosse, Wisconsin 54601

HEW — NIAAA REGIONAL OFFICES

The regional referral offices, which cover all areas of the U.S., can be contacted at the following phone numbers:

REGION I   (Conn., Me., Mass.,
N.H., R.I., Vt.))
Boston, Mass.
Phone: Code 617, 223-6824

REGION II   (N.J., N.Y., P.R.,
V.I.)
New York, New York
Phone: Code 212, 264-2567

REGION III   (Del., Md., Pa., Va.,
Wash., D.C., W. Va.)
Philadelphia, Pa.
Phone: Code 215, 597-9135

REGION IV   (Ala., Fla., Ga., Ky.,
Miss., N.C., S.C., Tenn.)
Atlanta, Georgia
Phone: Code 404, 526-5231

REGION V   (Ind., Ill., Minn.,
Ohio, Wis., Mich.)
Chicago, Illinois
Phone: Code 312, 353-5226

REGION VI   (Ark., La., N.M.,
Okla., Texas)
Dallas, Texas
Phone: Code 214, 749-3426

REGION VII   (Iowa, Kans., Mo.,
Nebr.)
Kansas City, Missouri
Phone: Code 816, 374-5291

REGION VIII (Colo., Mont., N.D.,
S.D., Utah, Wyo.)
Denver, Colo.
Phone: Code 303, 837-3177

REGION IX   (Ariz., Calif., Hawaii,
Nev., Guam, A.S., W.I.)
San Francisco, Calif.
Phone: Code 415, 556-2215

REGION X   (Alaska, Idaho, Ore.,
Wash.)
Seattle, Wash.
Phone: Code 206, 442-0524

200

PUBLIC
LAW 91-616

Public Law 91-616
91st Congress, S. 3835
December 31, 1970

An Act

84 STAT. 1848

To provide a comprehensive Federal program for the prevention and treatment of alcohol abuse and alcoholism.

Be it enacted by the Senate and House of Representatives of the United States of America in Congress assembled,

Comprehensive Alcohol Abuse and Alcoholism Prevention, Treatment, and Rehabilitation Act of 1970.

SHORT TITLE

Section 1. This Act may be cited as the "Comprehensive Alcohol Abuse and Alcoholism Prevention, Treatment, and Rehabilitation Act of 1970".

TITLE I—NATIONAL INSTITUTE ON ALCOHOL ABUSE AND ALCOHOLISM

ESTABLISHMENT OF THE INSTITUTE

Sec. 101. (a) There is established in the National Institute of Mental Health, the National Institute on Alcohol Abuse and Alcoholism (hereafter in this Act referred to as the "Institute") to administer the programs and authorities assigned to the Secretary of Health, Education, and Welfare (hereafter in this Act referred to as the "Secretary") by this Act and part C of the Community Mental Health Centers Act. The Secretary, acting through the Institute, shall, in carrying out the purposes of section 301 of the Public Health Service Act with respect to alcohol abuse and alcoholism, develop and conduct comprehensive health, education, training, research, and planning programs for the prevention and treatment of alcohol abuse and alcoholism and for the rehabilitation of alcohol abusers and alcoholics.

82 Stat. 1006;
Ante, p. 59.
42 USC 2688e.
58 Stat. 691;
79 Stat. 448.
42 USC 241.

(b) The Institute shall be under the direction of a Director who shall be appointed by the Secretary.

REPORTS BY THE SECRETARY

Sec. 102. The Secretary shall—

(1) submit an annual report to Congress which shall include a description of the actions taken, services provided, and funds expended under this Act and part C of the Community Mental Health Centers Act, an evaluation of the effectiveness of such actions, services, and expenditures of funds, and such other information as the Secretary considers appropriate;

Reports to President and Congress.

203

(2) submit to Congress on or before the expiration of the one-year period beginning on the date of enactment of this Act a report (A) containing current information on the health consequences of using alcoholic beverages, and (B) containing such recommendations for legislation and administrative action as he may deem appropriate;

(3) submit such additional reports as may be requested by the President of the United States or by Congress; and

(4) submit to the President of the United States and to Congress such recommendations as will further the prevention, treatment, and control of alcohol abuse and alcoholism.

TITLE II—ALCOHOL ABUSE AND ALCOHOLISM PREVENTION, TREATMENT, AND REHABILITATION PROGRAMS FOR FEDERAL CIVILIAN EMPLOYEES

ALCOHOL ABUSE AND ALCOHOLISM AMONG FEDERAL CIVILIAN EMPLOYEES

Sec. 201. (a) The Civil Service Commission shall be responsible for developing and maintaining, in cooperation with the Secretary and with other Federal agencies and departments, appropriate prevention, treatment, and rehabilitation programs and services for alcohol abuse and alcoholism among Federal civilian employees, consistent with the purposes of this Act. Such policies and services shall make optimal use of existing governmental facilities, services, and skills.

(b) The Secretary, acting through the Institute, shall be responsible for fostering similar alcohol abuse and alcoholism prevention, treatment, and rehabilitation programs and services in State and local governments and in private industry.

(c) (1) No person may be denied or deprived of Federal civilian employment or a Federal professional or other license or right solely on the ground of prior alcohol abuse or prior alcoholism.

(2) This subsection shall not apply to employment (A) in the Central Intelligence Agency, the Federal Bureau of Investigation, the National Security Agency, or any other department or agency of the Federal Government designated for purposes of national

security by the President, or (B) in any position in any department or agency of the Federal Government, not referred to in clause (A), which position is determined pursuant to regulations prescribed by the head of such agency or department to be a sensitive position.

(d) This title shall not be construed to prohibit the dismissal from employment of a Federal civilian employee who cannot properly function in his employment.

TITLE III—FEDERAL ASSISTANCE FOR STATE AND LOCAL PROGRAMS

PART A—FORMULA GRANTS

AUTHORIZATION

Sec. 301. There are authorized to be appropriated $40,000,000 for the fiscal year ending June 30, 1971, $60,000,000 for the fiscal year ending June 30, 1972, $80,000,000 for the fiscal year ending June 30, 1973, for grants to States to assist them in planning, establishing, maintaining, coordinating, and evaluating projects for the development of more effective prevention, treatment, and rehabilitation programs to deal with alcohol abuse and alcoholism. For purposes of this part, the term "State" includes the District of Columbia, the Virgin Islands, the Commonwealth of Puerto Rico, Guam, American Samoa, and the Trust Territory of the Pacific Islands, in addition to the fifty States.

Appropriation.

"State."

STATE ALLOTMENT

Sec. 302. (a) For each fiscal year the Secretary shall, in accordance with regulations, allot the sums appropriated for such year pursuant to section 301 among the States on the basis of the relative population, financial need, and need for more effective prevention, treatment, and rehabilitation of alcohol abuse and alcoholism; except that no such allotment to any State (other than the Virgin Islands, American Samoa, Guam, and the Trust Territory of the Pacific Islands) for any fiscal year shall be less than $200,000.

(b) Any amount so allotted to a State (other than the Virgin Islands, American Samoa, Guam, and the Trust Territory of the

Pacific Islands) and remaining unobligated at the end of such year shall remain available to such State, for the purposes for which made, for the next fiscal year (and for such year only), and any such amount shall be in addition to the amounts allotted to such State for such purpose for such next fiscal year; except that any such amount, remaining unobligated at the end of the sixth month following the end of such year for which it was allotted, which the Secretary determines will remain unobligated by the close of such next fiscal year, may be reallotted by the Secretary, to be available for the purposes for which made until the close of such next fiscal year, to other States which have need therefor, on such basis as the Secretary deems equitable and consistent with the purposes of this part, and any amount so reallotted to a State shall be in addition to the amounts allotted and available to the States for the same period. Any amount allotted under subsection (a) to the Virgin Islands, American Samoa, Guam, or the Trust Territory of the Pacific Islands for a fiscal year and remaining unobligated at the end of such year shall remain available to it, for the purposes for which made, for the next two fiscal years (and for such years only), and any such amount shall be in addition to the amounts allotted to it for such purpose for each of such next two fiscal years; except that any such amount, remaining unobligated at the end of the first of such next two years, which the Secretary determines will remain unobligated at the close of the second of such next two years, to any other of such four States which have need therefor, on such basis as the Secretary deems equitable and consistent with the purposes of this part, and any amount so reallotted to a State shall be in addition to the amounts allotted and available to the State for the same period.

(c) At the request of any State, a portion of any allotment or allotments of such State under this part shall be available to pay that portion of the expenditures found necessary by the Secretary for the proper and efficient administration during such year of the State plan approved under this part, except that not more than 10 per centum of the total of the allotments of such State ιor a year, or $50,000, whichever is the least, shall be available for such purpose for such year.

206

STATE PLANS

Sec. 303. (a) Any State desiring to participate in this part shall submit a State plan for carrying out its purposes. Such plan must—

(1) designate a single State agency as the sole agency for the administration of the plan, or designate such agency as the sole agency for supervising the administration of the plan;

(2) contain satisfactory evidence that the State agency designated in accordance with paragraph (1) (hereafter in this section referred to as the "State agency") will have authority to carry out such plan in conformity with this part;

(3) provide for the designation of a State advisory council which shall include representatives of nongovernmental organizations or groups, and of public agencies concerned with the prevention and treatment of alcohol abuse and alcoholism, to consult with the State agency in carrying out the plan;

(4) set forth, in accordance with criteria established by the Secretary, a survey of need for the prevention and treatment of alcohol abuse and alcoholism including a survey of the health facilities needed to provide services for alcohol abuse and alcoholism and a plan for the development and distribution of such facilities and programs throughout the State;

(5) provide such methods of administration of the State plan, including methods relating to the establishment and maintenance of personnel standards on a merit basis (except that the Secretary shall exercise no authority with respect to the selection, tenure of office, or compensation of any individual employed in accordance with such methods), as are found by the Secretary to be necessary for the proper and efficient operation of the plan;

(6) provide that the State agency will make such reports, in such form and containing such information, as the Secretary may from time to time reasonably require, and will keep such records and afford such access thereto as the Secretary may find necessary to assure the correctness and verification of such reports;

(7) provide that the Comptroller General of the United

States or his duly authorized representatives shall have access for the purpose of audit and examination to the records specified in paragraph (6);

(8) provide that the State agency will from time to time, but not less often than annually, review its State plan and submit to the Secretary any modifications thereof which it considers necessary;

(9) provide reasonable assurance that Federal funds made available under this part for any period will be so used as to supplement and increase, to the extent feasible and practical, the level of State, local, and other non-Federal funds that would in the absence of such Federal funds be made available for the programs described in this part, and will in no event supplant such State, local, and other non-Federal funds; and

(10) contain such additional information and assurance as the Secretary may find necessary to carry out the provisions and purposes of this part.

State plans, approval.

(b) The Secretary shall approve any State plan and any modification thereof which complies with the provisions of subsection

PART B—PROJECT GRANTS AND CONTRACTS

GRANTS AND CONTRACTS FOR THE PREVENTION AND TREATMENT OF ALCOHOL ABUSE AND ALCOHOLISM

80 Stat. 1009;
Ante, p. 59.
42 USC 2688e
note.

Sec. 311. Section 247 of part C of the Community Mental Health Centers Act is amended to read as follows:

"GRANTS AND CONTRACTS FOR THE PREVENTION AND TREATMENT OF ALCOHOL ABUSE AND ALCOHOLISM

"Sec. 247. (a) The Secretary, acting through the National Institute on Alcohol Abuse and Alcoholism, may make grants to public and private nonprofit agencies, organizations, and institutions and may enter into contracts with public and private agencies, organizations, and institutions, and individuals—

"(1) to conduct demonstration, service, and evaluation projects,

"(2) to provide education and training,

"(3) to provide programs and services in cooperation with schools, courts, penal institutions, and other public agencies, and

"(4) to provide counseling and education activities on an

individual or community basis, for the prevention and treatment of alcohol abuse and alcoholism and for the rehabilitation of alcohol abusers and alcoholics.

"(b) Projects for which grants or contracts are made under this section shall, whenever possible, be community based, provide a comprehensive range of services, and be integrated with, and involve the active participation of, a wide range of public and nongovernmental agencies, organizations, institutions, and individuals.

"(c) (1) In administering the provisions of this section, the Secretary shall require coordination of all applications for programs in a State. `Applications.`

"(2) Each applicant from within a State, upon filing its application with the Secretary for a grant or contract under this section, shall submit a copy of its application for review by the State agency designated under section 303 of the Comprehensive Alcohol Abuse and Alcoholism Prevention, Treatment, and Rehabilitation Act of 1970, if such agency exists. Such State agency shall be g iven not more than thirty days from the date of receipt of the application to submit to the Secretary, in writing, an evaluation of the project set forth in the application. Such evaluation shall include comments on the relationship of the project to other projects pending and approved and to the State comprehensive plan for treatment and prevention of alcohol abuse and alcoholism under such section 303. The State shall furnish the applicant a copy of any such evaluation. `Filing.` `Ante, p. 1850.`

"(3) Approval of any application for a grant or contract by the Secretary, including the earmarking of financial assistance for a program or project, may be granted only if the application substantially meets a set of criteria established by the Secretary that— `Approval, criteria.`

"(A) provide that the activities and services for which assistance under this section is sought will be substantially administered by or under the supervision of the applicant;

"(B) provide for such methods of administration as are necessary for the proper and efficient operation of such programs or projects;

"(C) provide for such fiscal control and fund accounting procedures as may be necessary to assure proper disbursement of and accounting for Federal funds paid to the applicant; and

"(D) provide reasonable assurance that Federal funds made available under this section for any period will be so used as to supplement and increase, to the extent feasible and practical, the level of State, local, and other non-Federal funds that would in the absence of such Federal funds be made available for the programs described in this section, and will in no event supplant such State, local, and other non-Federal funds.

Appropriation.

"(d) To carry out the purposes of this section, there are authorized to be appropriated $30,000,000 for the fiscal year ending June 30, 1971, $40,000,000 for the fiscal year ending June 30, 1972, and $50,000,000 for the fiscal year ending June 30, 1973."

PART C—ADMISSION TO HOSPITALS

ADMISSION OF ALCOHOL ABUSERS AND ALCOHOLICS TO PRIVATE AND PUBLIC HOSPITALS

Failure to comply, termination of Federal assistance.

Sec. 321. (a) Alcohol abusers and alcoholics shall be admitted to and treated in private and public general hospitals, which receive Federal funds for alcoholic treatment programs, on the basis of medical need and shall not be discriminated against solely because of their alcoholism. No hospital that violates this section shall receive Federal financial assistance under the provisions of this Act; except that the Secretary shall not terminate any such Federal assistance until the Secretary has advised the appropriate person or persons of the failure to comply with this section, and has provided an opportunity for correction or a hearing.

Hearing opportunity.
Judicial review.

77 Stat. 298.
42 USC 2694,

(b) Any action taken by the Secretary pursuant to this section shall be subject to such judicial review as is provided by section 404 of the Community Mental Health Centers Act.

PART D—GENERAL

COMPREHENSIVE STATE HEALTH PLANS

80 Stat. 1184;
Ante, p. 1241.
42 USC 246.

Sec. 331. Section 314(d) (2) of the Public Health Service Act is amended—

(1) by striking out "and" at the end of subparagraph (J);

(2) by striking out the period at the end of subparagraph (K) and inserting in lieu thereof "; and"; and

(3) by adding after subparagraph (K) the following new subparagraph:

"(L) provide for services for the prevention and treatment of alcohol abuse and alcoholism, commensurate with the extent of the problem."

SPECIALIZED FACILITIES

Sec. 332. Section 243(a) of the Community Mental Health Centers Act is amended (1) by inserting "or leasing" after "construction", and (2) by inserting "facilities for emergency medical services, intermediate care services, or outpatient services, and" immediately before "post-hospitalization treatment facilities".

82 Stat. 1008
42 USC 2688h.

CONFIDENTIALITY OF RECORDS

Sec. 333. The Secretary may authorize persons engaged in research on, or treatment with respect to, alcohol abuse and alcoholism to protect the privacy of individuals who are the subject of such research or treatment by withholding from all persons not connected with the conduct of such research or treatment the names or other identifying characteristics of such individuals. Persons so authorized to protect the privacy of such individuals may not be compelled in any Federal, State, or local civil, criminal, administrative, legislative, or other proceeding to indentify such individuals.

Research and treatment populations.

TITLE IV—THE NATIONAL ADVISORY COUNCIL ON ALCOHOL ABUSE AND ALCOHOLISM

ESTABLISHMENT OF COUNCIL

Sec. 401. (a) Section 217(a) of the Public Health Service Act is amended—

64 Stat. 446.
42 USC 218.

(1) in the first sentence thereof, by inserting "the National Advisory Council on Alcohol Abuse and Alcoholism," immediately after "the National Advisory Mental Health Council,";

(2) in the second sentence thereof, by (A) inserting "the National Advisory Council on Alcoholic Abuse and Alcoholism," immediately after "the National Advisory Mental Health Council,", and (B) inserting "alcohol abuse and alcoholism," immediately after "psychiatric disorders,"; and

(3) in the fourth sentence, (A) by inserting "(other than the members of the National Advisory Council on Alcohol Abuse and Alcoholism)" after "the terms of the members"; (B) by striking out "and" before "(2)"; and (C) by striking out the period at the end and inserting a semicolon and "and (3) the

terms of the members of the National Council on Alcohol Abuse and Alcoholism first taking office after the date of enactment of this clause, shall expire as follows: Three shall expire four years after such date, three shall expire three years after such date, three shall expire two years after such date, and three shall expire one year after such date, as designated by the Secretary at the time of appointment."

64 Stat. 446.
42 USC 218.

(b) Section 217(b) of such Act is amended, in the second sentence thereof, by inserting "alcohol abuse and alcoholism," immediately after "mental health,".

(c) Section 217 of such Act is further amended by adding at the end thereof the following new subsection:

"(d) The National Advisory Council on Alcohol Abuse and Alcoholism shall advise, consult with, and make recommendations to, the Secretary on matters relating to the activities and functions of the Secretary in the field of alcohol abuse and alcoholism. The Council is authorized (1) to review research projects or programs submitted to or initiated by it in the field of alcohol abuse and alcoholism and recommend to the Secretary any such projects which it believes show promise of making valuable contributions to human knowledge with respect to the cause, prevention, or methods of diagnosis and treatment of alcohol abuse and alcoholism, and (2) to collect information as to studies being carried on in the field of alcohol abuse and alcoholism and, with the approval of the Secretary, make available such information through appropriate publications for the benefit of health and welfare agencies or organizations (public or private) or physicians or any other scientists, and for the information of

58 Stat. 709.
42 USC 219.

the general public. The Council is also authorized to recommend to the Secretary, for acceptance pursuant to section 501 of this Act, conditional gifts for work in the field of alcohol abuse and alcoholism; and the Secretary shall recommend acceptance of any such gifts only after consultation with the Council."

APPROVAL BY COUNCIL OF CERTAIN GRANTS UNDER PART C OF COMMUNITY MENTAL HEALTH CENTERS ACT

Ante, p. 62.

Sec. 402. Section 266 of the Community Mental Health Centers Act is amended (1) by inserting "(other than part C thereof)" immediately after "this title", and (2) by adding immediately after the period the following: "Grants under part C

of this title for such costs may be made only upon recommendation of the National Advisory Council on Alcohol Abuse and
Alcoholism established by such section."

TITLE V—GENERAL

Sec. 501. If any section, provision, or term of this Act is
adjudged invalid for any reason, such judgment shall not affect,
impair, or invalidate any other section, provision, or term of this
Act, and the remaining sections, provisions, and terms shall be
and remain in full force and effect. Separability.

Sec. 502. (a) Each recipient of assistance under this Act pursuant to grants or contracts entered into under other than
competitive bidding procedures shall keep such records as the
Secretary shall prescribe, including records which fully disclose
the amount and disposition by such recipient of the proceeds of
such grant or contract, the total cost of the project or undertaking in connection with which such grant or contract is given or
used, and the amount of that portion of the cost of the project or
undertaking supplied by other sources, and such other records as
will facilitate an effective audit. Recordkeeping.

(b) The Secretary and Comptroller General of the United
States, or any of their duly authorized representatives, shall have
access for the purpose of audit and examination to any books,
documents, papers, and records of such recipients that are pertinent to the grants or contracts entered into under the provisions
of this Act under other than competitive bidding procedures. Records,
accessibility.

Sec. 503. Payments under this Act may be made in advance or
by way of reimbursement and in such installments as the Secretary may determine. Payments

Approved December 31, 1970.

LEGISLATIVE HISTORY:

HOUSE REPORT No. 91-1663 accompanying H. R. 18874 (Comm. on Interstate
          and Foreign Commerce).
SENATE REPORT No. 91-1069 (Comm. on Labor and Public Welfare).
CONGRESSIONAL RECORD, Vol. 116 (1970):
     Aug. 10, considered and passed Senate.
     Dec. 18, considered and passed House, amended, in lieu of H.R. 18874.
     Dec. 19, Senate agreed to House amendment.

Excerpts from

Drug Use
in America:
Problem in
Perspective

Second Report
of the National
Commission on
Marihuana and
Drug Abuse

Drug Abuse: Synonym for Social Disapproval

Drug abuse is another way of saying drug problem. Now immortalized in the titles of federal and state governmental agencies (and we might add, in our own), this term has the virtue of rallying all parties to a common cause: no one could possibly be *for* abuse of drugs any more than they could be *for* abuse of minorities, power or children. By the same token, the term also obscures the fact that "abuse" is undefined where drugs are concerned. Neither the public, its policy makers nor the expert community share a common understanding of its meaning or of the nature of the phenomenon to which it refers.

The Commission has noted over the last two years that the public and press often employ drug *abuse* interchangeably with drug *use*. Indeed, many "drug abuse experts," including government officials, do so as well.

Tobacco and Alcohol

. . . cigarette smoking increases with age until it reaches a peak of nearly half the population in the 26—34 age bracket and decreases after that time. Although there are no differences by sex among young smokers, higher proportions of men than women are current cigarette smokers'. . . .

As shown in Table II—3, 53% or 74,080,000 adults 18 years and over, and 24% or 5,977,000 youth 12 to 17 years of age had consumed some type of alcoholic beverage within the week prior to the survey.†

Numerous social and demographic differences exist with respect to alcohol consumption. On the variable of sex, males, both adult and youth, are considerably more likely than females to be alcohol consumers. With regard to age, use begins its steep climb during the middle teens, reaches its highest point (66%) in the 22—25 year age group and gradually levels off thereafter to about 39% of the 50 years and over age group.

†The "past seven days" was arbitrarily established to define "use" because it provides more reliable data on consumption of beer, wine and liquor than does a longer reporting period.

Alcohol consumption also increases with years of formal education; only 38% of adults with some high school education as compared with more than 71% of those with some college education had consumed alcohol within the past week.

The highest proportion of adult consumers resides in the Northeast (65%) and the lowest proportion (37%) live in the South. Among youth, consumers are more equally distributed throughout the country, but again the smallest proportion is found in the South (15%). In both age groups, consumption is more prevalent in metropolitan than rural areas but the differences according to community type are not as pronounced among youth as they are for the adult population. (See Table II-3.)

Incidence of Student Drug Use

Among junior high school, senior high school and college students, alcohol is, by far, the drug of choice. Figures extrapolated from student surveys show that by 1972, approximately 56% of the junior high school students, almost three-fourth (74%) of the senior high school students and 83% of the college students have used alcohol at least once. (See Figures II-2, 3 and 4)

Examination of the figures on the growth rate of alcohol use relative to the incidence of other drug use for the period 1969 to 1972, reveals three separate and distinct patterns. Among junior high school students, although alcohol maintained its substantial lead over all other drug types in the incidence of use, the gap was beginning to close. Over the four year period, the percentage increase in the incidence of use of all drugs, except tobacco and inhalants, was equal to or greater, in several cases, much greater, than the percent increase in the incidence of alcohol use.

Among senior high students, a very different picture emerged. The large increase in the incidence of alcohol use (+90%) over the four year period was surpassed only by the larger percent increase in hallucinogen use (+133%), but was trailed fairly close by the increase in marihuana use (+74%). All other drug types show percentage increases far below that of alcohol, and the incidence of tobacco use actually decreased.

Table II-3.—Alcoholic Beverage Consumption by Consumer Characteristics
[In percent]

Consumers of alcoholic beverages	Adults (N=2411)	Youth (N=880)
Consumers of alcoholic beverages	53	24
Sex:		
Male	>65	27
Female	>42	21
Age:		
12—13		16
14—15		21
16—17		35
18—21	65	
22—25	66	
26—34	62	
35—49	57	
50 and over	>39	
Education:		
Less than high school graduate	38	
High school graduate	52	
At least some college	>71	
Region:		
Northeast	65	28
North central	55	28
South	>37	>15
West	52	28
Community type:		
Large metro area	65	24
Other metro area	54	28
Nonmetro area	>39	20

Figures are not additive; thus they do not total 100 percent

For the college students, yet a third pattern emerged. Relative to the incidence of alcohol, which showed a percentage decrease, use of all drug types except tobacco and inhalants increased. The incidence of hallucinogen use showed the highest rate of growth (+133%), followed by marihuana (+56%) and still further behind were the opiates, depressants and stimulants, in that order.

Present Social Impact

Turning now to the social impact of dependence on various substances in the United States today, we find first that public perception of the problem is not related either to the prevalence of dependence or to the environmental and pharmacologic aspects of the issue.

Alcohol dependence is without question the most serious drug problem in this country today. Alcohol users far outnumber those of all other drugs and are found along the entire continuum of dependence. The reinforcement potential of alcohol and its potential for behavioral disruption are high. Use of the drug is pervasive within the general population, and its ready availability facilitates the development of high degrees of dependence among vulnerable populations. The prevalence of intensified and compulsive use among the entire alcohol-using population is roughly 10%, and a serious decrement in social functioning is noticeable in half of this group.

While there are many abstainers and the number of non-dependent users is large, alcohol use nonetheless carries a substantial social cost. The risk of individual involvement is accentuated also by the pervasive sentiment which tends to exclude alcohol from classification as a drug, thereby eliminating it from the concept of "drug abuse" and the social problems which go by that name. As noted in Chapter One, according to the National Survey, alcohol is regarded as a drug by only 39% of the adult population and 34% of the youth population. Twice-daily use of the drug is viewed as drug abuse by only 36% of the adults and 37% of the youth in contrast to the use of heroin "once in a while," which is regarded as drug abuse by 82% and 80% of these populations. Finally, only 7% of the public mentioned alcoholism as a serious social problem, as compared with the 53% who mentioned drugs.

Behavorial Effects

The major behavioral effects of alcohol derive from its depressant action on the central nervous system, also affecting the function of peripheral nerves, skeletal, smooth and cardiac muscle and other body tissues. Any behavioral stimulation which is observed is probably attributable to the suppression of inhibitory control mechanisms in various parts of the brain. Among the commonly observed acute effects of alcohol use are a reduction of anxiety, mild euphoria, some lack of muscular coordination, slurred speech, enhanced conviviality and assertiveness.

Low doses of alcohol, although said to improve functioning with regard to some simple motor or cognitive tasks, reduce the level of performance of such complex tasks as driving. When taken in moderate doses, alcohol has been found to reduce substantially motor skills as well as orderly thought processes and speech patterns. Higher doses of this substance may cause the user to become highly irritable and emotional and displays of anger and crying are not uncommon. Exceptionally high doses are known to cause stupor, unconsciousness and sometimes death.

The standard setting, dose-response function and personal expectations of the individual with regard to alcohol are, in part, responsible for his behavior while under its influence. When loss of control, whether physical or emotional, is an expected and recurrent reaction to alcohol use, the individual often feels justified in his belief that it was the drug which was responsible for his behavior.

Some researchers have advanced the theory that alcohol reduces anxiety related to sexual behavior and enhances sexual aggression; in fact, however, scientific opinion is split on the validity of this proposition.

Various empirical studies on the relationship between the use of alcohol and the commission of violent crime have shown that, in the case of homicide and other assaultive offenses, alcohol was used by at least half of the offenders directly prior to the crime (Shupe, 1964; Wolfgang, 1958; MacDonald, 1961; Voss and Hepburn, 1968). These studies also show that in alcohol-related violent crime, the violence is most often directed at relatives or friends who were drinking together.

Sex crimes have also been attributed to the use of alcohol. In a survey of sex offenders conducted by the Kinsey Institute for Sex Research, alcohol was reported as a factor in 67% of the sexual crimes against children and 39% of sexually aggressive acts against women (Gebhard, et al., 1967).

Molof (1967) found that youth who used alcohol were responsible for significantly more crimes of assault than their nondrinking counterparts, and Goodwin and his colleagues (1971) reported that the use of alcohol was significantly associated with other forms of antisocial behavior including poor school attendance, an unfavorable work record and excessive fighting.

Finally, some researchers have stated that a criminal may be prone to excessive drinking in order to increase courage in preparation for the commission of a crime.

The Population of Heavy Alcohol Users

The problems associated with drinking and alcoholism have been demonstrated by many researchers. In a national survey conducted by Cahalan, et al., (1969), for example, 31% of the sample indicated some problem with drinking within the last three years. Forty percent of the men and 15% of the women claimed some psychological dependence on alcohol while 12% of the men and 8% of the women reportedly experienced some health problem associated with drinking during the three years preceding the survey.

The Cahalan, et al., 1969 survey of drinking practices found that 28% of the male drinkers and 8% of the female drinkers were heavy drinkers and that half of the heavy drinkers (6% of the general population) were heavy-escape drinkers who drank excessively in an effort to avoid social pressures and personal problems. Although such heavy-escape drinkers included most of those termed "alcoholics," they may also include excessive drinkers who have avoided much of the long-term psychological and physical effects of alcoholism.

In any case, Cahalan, et al., (1969) found that most important predictors of heavy drinking to be sex, age, city size and social position. The proportion of male heavy drinkers, for example, was found to be about three and one-half times higher than the proportion of female heavy drinkers (28% vs. 8%).* Among drinkers, the highest proportion of heavy drinkers (30%) are men in the

---

*The U.S. Department of Health, Education and Welfare found in 1965 that at least five times as many men as women were "alcoholics."

30—34 and 45—49 year age groups; in women the highest proportions (10%) are found in the 45—49 and 21—24 year age groups. For sexes, the prevalence of heavy drinking declined rapidly after age 50. Residents of large urban areas consistently evidenced higher rates of heavy drinking than did residents of smaller towns.

Economic Loss

The available data indicate that most heroin-dependent persons are males, under 26 years of age with a tenth-grade education or less, whose age at first arrest for heroin use was generally between 16 and 19 years. To a great extent, the heroin-dependent individual suffers the loss of his youth, his most formative and important years for healthy growth and development, which can never be regained or recouped. And the community simultaneously suffers the loss of its most valuable natural resource.

Because alcohol dependence develops gradually, economic losses do not generally occur among younger populations, in marked contrast to those associated with heroin use. However, once alcohol dependence develops, its impact on economic functioning is devastating.

Gillespie (1967) found that between 27 and 81% (median 52%) of alcoholics are unemployed. Fifty-two percent of the hospitalized alcoholics in Glatt's sample (1967) lost their jobs because of drinking, while Robbins, et al. (1969) discovered that 56% of alcoholics had job difficulties directly attributable to drinking. Among alcohol-dependent persons who remain employed, the decrement in job performance is substantial. For example, the American Society for Personnel Administration (1972) has estimated that "there are 4.4 million employed people in the country who are alcoholics; 90% of them have been on the job 10—20 years; they're costing employers $8—10 billion per year."

Although the precise amount of absenteeism, accidents and economic losses attendant to alcohol use is difficult to assess, its impact is clearly considerable. Zentner (1969) found that the cost to industry primarily in absenteeism and inefficient job performance among employed alcoholics is nearly $2 billion per year. Trice (1965) found that alcoholics use two to five times more sick

223

time than non-alcoholics and receive three times the amount of disability payments. Trice and Roman (1972) note that sickness payments for problem drinkers was three times greater than those for the normal worker.

A review of the existing literature indicates that most observers generally agree that drug and alcohol dependence contribute to increased insurance rates, industrial accidents, increased absenteeism, theft, problems of morale and discipline, impaired job performance, security risks, retraining costs and other associated problems.

Death

Death is a particularly finite measure of the social cost of drug dependence. The correlation between unnatural or premature death and drug dependence is an astounding one. Because the data regarding alcohol-related death is national in scope and reliable, while that regarding other drugs is regional and sketchy, we will have to present this information separately. It does appear in general, however, that drug-dependent persons and heavy non-dependent users are more likely than the rest of the population to die by their own hand, either intentionally or accidentally, or by the hand of others.

Robbins, et al. (1959) reported that 26% of suicide victims were reported to be chronic alcoholics. On the basis of a study made one year later, 31% of the suicides were found to be alcoholics (Palola, et al., 1962). The suicide rate for hospitalized male alcoholics was reported by Kessel and Walton (1965) to be 86 times the rate expected for the general population; and 75% of the suicide victims studied by Murphy and Robins (1967) were found to suffer from either alcoholism or depression.

In addition to suicide, the excessive drinker of alcohol risks death and injury in various other ways. Alcoholics are 2.5 to 3 times as likely to die during any given time period as the general population (Tashiro and Lipscomb, 1963; Brenner, 1967). The most frequent causes of death are violence 24% (9% in general population), heart disease 23% (40% in general population), and cirrhosis of the liver 14% (3% in general population). Alcoholics are seven times as likely to die in fatal accidents as non-alcoholics (Tashiro and Lipscomb, 1963).

Waller (1968) found that 71% of persons who died of accidental poisoning had a blood alcohol content of .10% or higher. The same was true of 58% of those killed by fire and 45% of those who drowned. In contrast, only 7% of the victims of death by natural causes had significant levels of blood alcohol.

Accidents in the home, on the job or on the road show very few factors in common other than human carelessness. It is striking, therefore, to note how closely alcohol use is correlated with accidental injury. By subjecting non-fatal accident victims to the breathalyzer test, Wechsler et al., (1969) found that 22% of home accident victims, 30% of transportation accident victims, and 15.5% of those with occupational injuries had positive blood alcohol readings. Victims of fights or assaults showed significantly higher alcohol involvement, with 56% showing positive blood alcohol readings.

As we noted earlier in this chapter, a drinker is less likely to survive than a non-drinker even when both are involved in the same two-vehicle automobile accident. In a study of such crashes in which one driver survived, it was the non-drinking driver who survived in 59 of 67 cases (U.S. Department of Transportation, 1970b).

The Commission's review of presently available data indicates that property damage, insurance costs and medical services consequent to alcohol-related motor vehicle accidents ran to $1 billion in 1971 (National Clearinghouse for Alcohol Information, 1972). A review of highway fatalities since 1966 shows that each year approximately one-half are related to accidents involving alcohol. From a public welfare standpoint, the impact is considerable when one considers the lost earning power of those injured or killed, the social security payments to dependents of the deceased as well as public assistance and aid to dependent children—expenditures which must be maintained as the result of such accidents.

These data demonstrate that the excessive drinker is subject to significantly greater physical and social stress leading to higher injury and fatality rates than the general population. The greater vulnerability appears to be due to the general stress involved in the alcoholic's living conditions, the presence of an inadequate diet, the diseases connected with alcohol consumption itself, and the increased chance of death after injury with large quantities of alcohol in the blood (Brenner, 1967).

Specific Recommendations

Society at present pays a heavy price for the widespread availability of alcohol. The social costs of long-term, heavy use are much higher than any other drug "problem" we have.

The Commission does not believe that it is realistic to reconsider prohibition of availability for self-defined purposes. This country's earlier experiment with such controls amply demonstrated that they are ineffective and extremely costly. Impracticality of strict control, however, does not argue for a system of controls so lax and haphazard that heavy use is in no way discouraged and in some cases even encouraged. Without reviving Prohibition, society can demonstrate to users that alcohol is not an ordinary commodity but, rather, is a powerful psychoactive drug.

The Commission recommends that the National Institute on Alcohol Abuse and Alcoholism devote substantial effort to the development of better non-prohibitory means of controlling the availability of alcohol. In particular, society should alter availability controls to minimize the social costs of alcohol use.

Alcohol Industry

The manufacture and sale of alcoholic beverages is a major industry in the United States. In 1971, it had over 100 million customers and retail sales totaling $23.8 billion. This meant that Americans over 15 years of age averaged an annual per capita consumption of 2.62 gallons of spirits, 2.08 gallons of wine and 25.9 gallons of beer. Taxes from sales of alcoholic beverages totaled $3.2 billion at state and local level and $5.05 billion at the federal level (Deering, 1972).

The massive economic growth of the alcoholic beverage industry since the end of Prohibition leaves little doubt that alcohol is the drug of choice in America. Present regulation of the industry is largely a revenue control function, though state laws do prohibit distribution to minors and generally impose some restrictions on times and places of sale. Nonetheless, alcohol is freely available to adults almost everywhere. This widespread availability is not without serious costs. According to current estimates of the National Institute of Alcohol Abuse and Alcoholism, there are at least nine million alcohol-dependent persons in the United States (Brodie, 1973).

The Commission believes that the alcohol industry has an obligation to spearhead the private institutional response to that part of the drug problem with which it is directly involved. Specifically, the Commission recommends that the industry take the lead in funding research into the nature of compulsive alcohol-using behavior and the relation between alcohol use and traffic accidents, violent crimes, and domestic difficulties. We further urge manufacturers and distributors of alcoholic beverages to inform the public that compulsive use of alcohol is the most widespread and destructive drug-use pattern in this nation. Advertising should emphasize moderate, responsible use and point out the dangers of excessive consumption.

The Commission also recommends that the industry reorient its advertising to avoid making alcohol use attractive to populations especially susceptible to irresponsible use, particularly young people. By general agreement within the industry, hard liquor commercials do not appear on the broadcast media. The Commission urges the industry to pay special attention to the impact of advertising in the print media as well.

In addition, the Commission notes with approval that broadcasters and the industry have agreed voluntarily not to advertise beer and wine on television and radio programs whose probable audience are under 18. We further urge that the wine and beer industry consider eliminating their broadcast advertising altogether. While such action by governmental fiat would be inappropriate, the alcohol industry itself should revise its marketing methods to comport with an overall discouragement policy.

U.S. DEPARTMENT OF HEALTH, EDUCATION, AND WELFARE
Office of the Assistant Secretary for Health and Scientific Affairs

First Special Report to the U.S. Congress on

alcohol & health

from the Secretary of Health, Education, and Welfare
DECEMBER 1971

EDITORIAL STAFF

Mark Keller - Consulting Editor

Shirley Sirota Rosenberg - Editor

Terry C. Bellicha, Judith W. Katz, Lillian Light, Danielle L. Spiegler

DEPARTMENT OF HEALTH, EDUCATION, AND WELFARE

Office of the Assistant Secretary for Health and Scientific Affairs

Health Services and Mental Health Administration   National Institute of Mental Health

National Institute on Alcohol Abuse and Alcoholism

DHEW Publication No. (HSM) 72—9099

REVISED EDITION

For sale by the Superintendent of Documents, U.S. Government Printing Office
Washington, D.C. 20402 - Price $1.50
Stock Number 1724—0193
Library of Congress Card No. 73—189814

DECEMBER 1971

February 18, 1972

Honorable Carl Albert
Speaker of the House of Representatives
Washington, D. C.   20515

Dear Mr. Speaker:

It is my pleasure to submit to the United States Congress the first
special report on <u>Alcohol</u> <u>and</u> <u>Health</u>. As required by Title I,
Section 102(1), of Public Law 91-616, the "Comprehensive Alcohol Abuse
and Alcoholism Prevention, Treatment, and Rehabilitation Act of 1970,"
this report contains current information on the health consequences
of using alcoholic beverages.

No recommendations for legislative action are being submitted at the
present time. However, we are continuing to study the findings and
implications of this report. If appropriate, legislative recommendations
will be submitted at a later date.

Alcoholism is one of the most tragic, destructive, and costly illnesses
in the Nation today. Directly or indirectly, alcohol-related problems
affect the lives of tens of millions of our men, women, and children.

This report summarizes a substantial portion of current scientific
knowledge on the health consequences of using alcoholic beverages, and
represents the first part of a three-year comprehensive study being
undertaken by the National Institute on Alcohol Abuse and Alcoholism
to help the Nation combat alcohol-related problems.

In this initial fact-finding phase, NIAAA established a consultant task
force to gather and develop information, analyze existing literature,
and to identify those human health problems that are correlated with the
use and abuse of alcohol. This information is placed in the perspective
of how the United States assesses these problems, and the laws and
resources it has mustered to deal with them.

Subsequent phases will design and test methodologies for assessing precisely and completely the ways alcohol affects selected areas of well-
being, as well as identifying the most feasible methods for mounting
effective prevention and treatment programs in the field of alcohol
abuse and alcoholism. These studies will also be made available to both
the Congress and the people of the United States.

Sincerely,

Secretary

TABLE OF CONTENTS

Foreword

The past 5 years have witnessed a sharpened awareness and understanding about the problems of alcohol abuse and alcoholism unsurpassed in American history. We have emerged from an era when alcohol abuse and alcoholism were equated by the public with moral degeneration and despair . . . to the day in 1970 when President Nixon signed into law the landmark Public Law 91–616, the "Comprehensive Alcohol Abuse and Alcoholism Prevention, Treatment, and Rehabilitation Act of 1970." Passed unanimously by both Houses of Congress, this law followed a historical precedent of bringing together diverse and often divided interests in our society in support of a major public health measure.

Voluntary agencies in the field of alcoholism were frontrunners in the effort to develop a partnership between the public and private sectors of our Nation that would foster Federal alcoholism legislation. The National Council on Alcoholism was a leader in awakening Congress to the need to establish a Federal agency dedicated to providing visibility to the depth and scope of this public health program. The North American Association of Alcoholism Programs, representing directors of State alcoholism programs, assisted in preparing the legislation. And, of course, Alcoholics Anonymous, the pioneering demonstration that effective efforts can produce successful results, was instrumental in gathering support for the Comprehensive Act. Many other voluntary and professional organizations, as well as private groups, also joined the ranks of supporters of the Comprehensive Act.

Focus for Action

With the enactment of the Comprehensive Act, the new National Institute on Alcohol Abuse and Alcoholism was then established as the focal point for an augmented Federal effort. The broad and foresighted provisions also provided the Department of Health, Education, and Welfare, for the first time, with the tools and resources needed to begin reducing the prevalence of alcohol-related problems in the Nation. President Nixon emphasized the Federal commitment to this effort in his health message of February 1971. Calling for a national health strategy that "would marshal a variety of forces in a coordinated assault" on the health problems currently faced by the Nation, the President specifically directed the attention of Congress to the problems of alcohol abuse and alcoholism.

This First Special Report to the U.S. Congress on "Alcohol and Health" has grown out of the legislative requirement in the Comprehensive Act which mandated a special report from the Secretary of Health, Education, and Welfare on the health consequences of using alcoholic beverages. Assembled by a task force representing various disciplines concerned with alcohol abuse and alcoholism, "Alcohol and Health" brings together, in one document, a substantial portion of current knowledge on the health consequences of using these beverages. It is anticipated that this report will be of interest and value to the general public; to the members of the organizations, disciplines, and professions concerned with alcohol abuse and alcoholism; and to the industries engaged in the manufacture and distribution of alcoholic beverages. Subsequent reports representing two additional phases of a 3-year comprehensive study being undertaken by NIAAA will also be made available to the Congress and the people of the United States.

Another Step Forward

Meanwhile, the continuing nationwide effort to encourage a consistent pattern of alcoholism legislation throughout this country resulted last summer in the adoption of a Uniform Alcoholism and Intoxication Treatment Act by the National Conference on Uniform State Laws. As Secretary of Health, Education, and Welfare, I have publicly recommended that all States adopt this Uniform Act which regards the disease of alcoholism as a public health problem, and removes alcoholism from the criminal justice system, while in no way altering the provisions of the criminal law that protect public safety. Hopefully, the report on "Alcohol and Health" will speed the recognition throughout our land that alcoholism is an illness, with an inherent potential for prevention, control, and recovery. Only in this way can we put to work and develop the appropriate attitudes and resources that see the alcoholic individual as a person who wants help, will accept help, and can benefit from help.

ELLIOT L. RICHARDSON,
Secretary of Health, Education, and Welfare.

MEMBERS OF THE TASK FORCE

Preface

Man's desire to alter reality is one of the most ancient, persistent, and understandable of human needs. The many means used by people in diverse cultures reflect the universal necessity to transform oneself and one's world. In all times and places, people have enjoyed the mood-changing and pleasure-giving properties of alcoholic beverages. But, as is true with most pleasures, too much can be deleterious.

All individuals experience stress. In the face of stress, we all employ methods to maintain a dynamic equilibrium, both internally and externally. Most people, however, tend to believe that other people's coping mechanisms are not as good as their own. Thus while we are horrified by the abuse of such drugs as hallucinogens, narcotics, and stimulants by our youth, we pay little heed to the most abused drug of all: Alcohol.

Threat to Life

Alcohol abusers shorten their life spans by 10 to a dozen years. Although these early deaths often result from the deleterious effects of alcohol on major body organs, alcohol is also implicated in death-through-violence: One-half of all traffic fatalities and one-third of all homicide victims have significant amounts of alcohol in their bloodstreams at the time of autopsy. We may not be able to quantify the violated quality of life incurred by alcohol abuse and alcoholism, but we know that many tens of millions of individuals and families are directly and indirectly affected by the 9 million persons with alcohol-related problems. A poignant aspect of these problems is their relation to many other forms of unhappiness: illness; family problems; poverty; job problems; or general demoralization. Although it cannot be said how often excessive drinking is the cause, and how often the effect, it is dramatically evident that alcohol-related problems go hand in hand with other forms of unhappiness.

Prevalence of Problems

A Harris survey conducted in November 1971 for the National Institute on Alcohol Abuse and Alcoholism discloses that most people understand—even if imprecisely—that alcohol abuse and alcoholism can lead to tragedy. The same study reveals that the tragedy is not a distant one: Many people live daily with alcohol-related problems. Almost one-in-five persons reported that someone close to them—most often a family member—drinks too much. Moreover, persons close to someone with an alcohol-related problem usually endure it a long time—in over half the instances, for at least 10 years.

When this nation became concerned about drug use among the young, the public was finally forced to recognize that adult use of alcohol—a central nervous system drug which we use as a social beverage—is actually the major drug problem in this country . . . and that young people learn from imitation and identification with adults.

The Road Ahead

As a result, many of us are rightly concerned that the abuse of the drug, alcohol, will mire millions of Americans in a state of dependency, and maim or kill millions of others. Because of our extreme concern, we hunger for a "victory by vaccine" over this complex problem. Because life does not often offer simple solutions, however, we face several challenges.

The first is to dispel the many myths surrounding alcohol.

The second is for this nation to erase the needless hardships, particularly those imposed on members of disadvantaged groups, that sometimes make heavy drinking appear to be the only avenue of escape from unjust stresses and strains.

The third is to redirect unhealthy needs for alcohol into nondestructive and rewarding channels. We must develop alternatives to reliance on potions and pills that bring temporary surcease from the pains of living.

We live in a tense, anxious, and frightening time. New stresses arise before the old are resolved. By building programs based on understanding and caring, rather than fear and guilt, we can lessen the desire to use alcohol and other drugs to deal with life's problems.

MERLIN K. DuVAL, M.D.,
Assistant Secretary for Health and Scientific Affairs.

Findings

The Task Force Finds That:

- Alcohol is the most abused drug in the United States. The extent of problems related to alcohol abuse and alcoholism is increasing and has reached major proportions.

  An estimated 5 percent of the adult population in the United States manifest the behaviors of alcohol abuse and alcoholism. Among the more than 95 million drinkers in the nation, about 9 million men and women are alcohol abusers and alcoholic individuals.

  The most visible victims of alcoholism are inhabitants of skid rows across the nation. Yet they represent only from 3 to 5 percent of the alcoholic population in the United States. Most alcoholic individuals are in the nation's working and homemaking population. It has been estimated that as many as 5 percent of the nation's work force are alcoholic individuals and that almost another 5 percent are serious alcohol abusers.

  Alcohol plays a major role in half the highway fatalities in the United States, and cost 28,000 lives in one recent year. The ratio of alcohol-related traffic fatalities is even greater among youths age 16 to 24; among these young people, the proportion rises to six out of 10 highway deaths.

Alcohol abuse and alcoholism drain the economy of an estimated $15 billion a year. Of this total, $10 billion is attributable to lost work time in business, industry, civilian government, and the military . . . $2 billion is spent for health and welfare services provided to alcoholic persons and their families . . . and property damage, medical expenses, and other overhead costs account for another $3 billion or more.

Public intoxication alone accounts for one-third of all arrests reported annually. If such alcohol-related offenses as driving while under the influence of alcohol, disorderly conduct, and vagrancy are considered, the proportion would rise to between 40 and 49 percent.

Among American Indians, the incidence of alcoholism is at an epidemic level. The rate is estimated to be at least two times the national average. On some American Indian reservations, the rate of alcoholism is as high as 25 to 50 percent.

- Alcohol abuse can impair health and lead to alcoholism.

- Alcoholism is not a crime. It is an illness or disease which requires rehabilitation through a broad range of health and social services tailored to persons at different stages of alcohol abuse and alcoholism.

- The criminal law is not an appropriate device for preventing or controlling health problems. To deal with alcoholic persons as criminals because they appear in public when intoxicated is unproductive and wasteful of human resources.

- The causal factors of alcohol abuse and alcoholism are not yet established. Social, psychological, physiological, and cultural factors all play roles in their development and course. The full understanding of these factors and their interrelationships awaits further study.

- Many minority groups in our society have experienced exceptional deprivations. For these disadvantaged citizens, heavy drinking has accentuated or been a response to such hardships as limited access to job opportunities, unequal housing and schooling, and inadequate medical care.

- In addition to intoxication, the illnesses associated with alcohol abuse and alcoholism include emotional disorders and chronic progressive diseases of the central and peripheral nervous systems and of the liver, heart, muscles, gastrointestinal tract, and other bodily organs and tissues.

- Scientific research has made progress in understanding the metabolic course of alcohol through the body. Nevertheless, we still lack important knowledge of the complex and interactive role that alcohol plays in producing some of the biochemical changes and physiological damage seen in heavy drinkers.

- Present programs dealing with alcohol abuse and alcoholism are accorded a low priority and are unrelated to most of the health and social resources within communities. Existing research, as well as social, health, and rehabilitation laws and activities have not been effectively mobilized to solve the problems of alcohol abuse and alcoholism. These inadequacies have contributed to the inability of many private and public national, State, and local institutions, agencies, and organizations to recognize their responsibilities for meeting alcohol-related problems.

- Too often the only community health resource for acutely intoxicated individuals is an emergency facility commonly known as a detoxification center. When isolated from other human services, these centers duplicate the "revolving door" syndrome long associated with repeated incarceration, rather than providing for the rehabilitation of alcohol abusers and alcoholic persons.

- Establishment of modern public-health oriented facilities to deal with intoxicated persons will free police, courts, correctional institutions, and other law enforcement agencies from being over-burdened by a large population of ill people. It will also facilitate:
    Early detection and prevention of alcoholism.
    Effective treatment and rehabilitation of alcoholic persons.
    Early diagnosis and treatment of other diseases caused by, exacerbated by, or coexisting with alcohol abuse and alcoholism.

- Although many communities do provide some treatment facilities for persons with alcohol-related problems, these services are frequently fragmented and fail to take into account either changing life styles or the unique characteristics of various population groups. Thus, alcohol abusers and alcoholic individuals may be deterred from seeking or accepting help in the communities where treatment should be readily accessible and designed for their specific needs.

- Many public and private general hospitals have not yet implemented the position taken by the American Medical Association and the American Hospital Association that no patient can be excluded from hospital care because his illness is identified as alcoholism. As a result, many physicians are still forced to make subterfuge diagnoses so patients can gain hospital admittance for treatment of alcoholism. This situation reinforces society's denial that alcoholism is a significant health problem and thereby undermines attempts to develop effective methods of prevention and treatment.

- Minimal success has been achieved by our traditional, punitive methods of dealing with persons who drive while under the influence of alcohol. Research findings indicate that a therapeutic approach to the problem of drinking drivers holds a greater promise of reducing the incidence of alcohol-related traffic accidents.

- Employment-connected alcoholism programs have demonstrated their therapeutic value.

- Faced with shortages of professional personnel and increasing demands for service, many alcoholism programs have demonstrated that the ability to care for people is not built into any one profession. A variety of professional and trained paraprofessional persons, and trained members of such voluntary groups as Alcoholics Anonymous, can serve as effective providers of therapeutic and rehabilitative services.

- Historically, difficulties have been experienced in planning necessary long-range programs to provide training, services, and preventive activities because of the lack and uncertainty of adequate financial support for alcoholism programs.

- Test cases, Crime Commission reports, and even adoption of progressive new uniform legislation, do not guarantee the provision of adequate and appropriate treatment and rehabilitation services. They merely provide the statutory framework within which a State can undertake to handle the problems of intoxication and alcoholism according to the best current knowledge. Implementation is up to the will of the State, and can be demonstrated only by appropriate funding and the dedication of the health, welfare, and rehabilitation resources necessary to do the job.

- Alcohol abuse and alcoholism are recognized as major health problems in most developed and many developing nations. Despite the global nature of these problems, however, there has been little multinational cooperation aimed to develop more effective methods for combating alcohol abuse and alcoholism.

- No battle against a public health problem can gain a significant victory if it attends only to the casualties. Appropriate treatment of persons who are abusing alcohol—the primary condition that may lead to alcoholism—can intercept the development of many cases of alcoholism. Yet much of the work in the field of alcoholism has been focused on treating late-stage victims of the disorder. Programs that are exclusively therapeutic or rehabilitative will not result in long-term conquest of the problem unless ways of preventing new cases of alcoholism are developed.

Programs

In response to the findings of the Task Force, the Secretary of
  Health, Education, and Welfare Is Establishing Programs With-
  in the National Institute on Alcohol Abuse and Alcoholism,
  and Coordinating All Departmental Research, Prevention, and
  Treatment Programs, To Develop and Implement a Detailed,
  Comprehensive Federal Plan Designed to:

  (1) Evaluate the adequacy and appropriateness of any pro-
       visions relating to the prevention and treatment of alco-
       hol abuse and alcoholism in all State health, welfare, and
       rehabilitation plans submitted to the Government in
       accordance with Federal law.

  (2) Assist such Federal Departments as the Civil Service
       Commission, Department of Defense, Department of
       Housing and Urban Development, Department of Trans-
       portation, Department of Labor, Department of the
       Interior, Office of Economic Opportunity, and Veterans'
       Administration; and such DHEW agencies as the Social
       Security Administration, Indian Health Service, National
       Institute on Occupational Health and Safety, Social and
       Rehabilitative Services; and other Federal departments
       and agencies in developing and maintaining appropriate

prevention and treatment programs for alcohol abuse and alcoholism.

(3) Assist State and local governments in coordinating programs among themselves for the prevention and treatment of alcohol abuse and alcoholism, and provide assistance and consultation to local governments and private organizations with respect to prevention and treatment of alcohol abuse and alcoholism.

(4) Encourage States to adopt the Uniform Alcoholism and Intoxication Treatment Act, and provide technical assistance to help States implement this Uniform Act.

(5) Establish a clearinghouse of information to gather, systematize, maintain, and make widely available—in appropriate contexts and languages to all sectors of the population—the knowledge on alcohol abuse and alcoholism.

(6) Make available research facilities and resources to appropriate authorities, health officials, and individuals engaged in special studies related to the prevention, control, and treatment of alcohol abuse and alcoholism.

(7) Formulate and publish criteria of quality treatment for alcohol abuse and alcoholism, and require that all programs supported by the Comprehensive Alcohol Abuse and Alcoholism Prevention, Treatment, and Rehabilitation Act of 1970 meet such criteria.

(8) Issue regulations that establish State standards that require providers of services for alcohol abuse and alcoholism to offer a continuum of care ranging from emergency treatment for acute intoxication, to outpatient therapy, to residential centers for the small number of alcoholic individuals unable to return to unsupervised life in the community.

(9) Establish interdisciplinary training programs for professional and paraprofessional personnel with respect to alcohol abuse and alcoholism; develop guidelines and courses to educate health and social workers about the factors contributing to alcohol abuse and alcoholism; and provide training for health, education, and other professionals to help them become leaders, teachers, researchers, and program developers in this field of public health.

(10) Develop regulations for training grants that establish standards of education and experience for professional

and paraprofessional workers who provide treatment services to alcoholic persons.

(11) Recruit and train paraprofessional workers, including recovered alcoholic persons and other individuals whose life experiences enable them to bring special empathies to this work, to serve in community services for the prevention and treatment of alcohol abuse and alcoholism.

(12) Stimulate programs of research designed to understand the uses and abuses of alcohol, and the processes of alcohol addiction or dependence, particularly with respect to elucidating the mechanisms by which alcohol acts as a central nervous system intoxicant.

(13) Stimulate and support multinational cooperation and collaboration in undertaking basic and applied research concerning the causes of alcohol abuse and alcoholism, and the most effective methods of combating them. Such investigations should include international epidemiological studies as well as evaluations of the effectiveness and costs of different treatment modalities and delivery systems.

Introduction

THIS SPECIAL REPORT TO THE CONGRESS OF THE UNITED STATES brings together a substantial portion of the current scientific knowledge on the health consequences of using, and especially of abusing, alcoholic beverages. The information is presented within the perspective of the history and epidemiology of alcohol use, as well as its effects on both the central nervous system and other body organs, tissues, and systems. The causal theories, treatment methods, and legal status of alcohol-related problems are reviewed. In addition, directions for future action are charted in research, training, treatment, and prevention for the field of alcohol abuse and alcoholism.

In our concern over the depth and scope of alcohol-related problems, it is important to remember that drinking alcoholic beverages is typical behavior in the United States, and that most people who drink do not abuse alcohol or develop alcoholism. Some people reserve drinking for sanctification of religious ritual or celebration of special occasions. Some find the custom of a cocktail a convenient means for separating the demands of the workaday world from those of the home. One person takes a drink before lunch. Another may confine his liquor consumption to the evening—sometimes because he is without and sometimes because

1

he is with his family. Others find alcoholic beverages a help occasionally in relieving fatigue, tedium, depression, or anxiety, or to enhance their ease and promote festivity at social gatherings.

The medicinal value of alcohol is recognized by physicians to this day. It may be prescribed as a mild relaxant for geriatric and convalescent patients, and serve as a source of readily available caloric energy for them. For patients who enjoy alcoholic beverages, alcohol may be recommended to stimulate lagging appetite and digestion. Alcohol is also used as an occasional remedy for insomnia, as a solvent for many other drugs, and, in dehydrated form, can be injected near nerves or sympathetic ganglia for relief of pain.

Drinking does not become a problem until the repetitive use of, or preoccupation with, alcohol causes physical, psychological, or social difficulties to the drinker or to society.

Defining the Problem

Alcohol abuse, in one sense, is present any time a person becomes drunk. Repeated episodes of intoxication or heavy drinking which impairs health, or consistent use of alcohol as a coping mechanism in dealing with the problems of life to a degree of serious interference with an individual's effectiveness on the job, at home, in the community, or behind the wheel of a car, is alcohol abuse . . . and may raise a strong inference of alcoholism.

When a person develops increased adaptation to the effects of alcohol, so that he needs increasing doses to achieve and sustain a desired effect, and shows specific signs and symptoms of withdrawal upon suddenly stopping drinking, this is considered to be alcohol dependence or addiction. Under certain circumstances and for certain periods of time that are unique for him, an alcoholic person—one who manifests the behaviors of alcohol dependence, or alcoholism, *needs* to drink, even though he may know the potential destructive consequences of his behavior.

The most visible population and stereotype of alcoholism is seen on skid row. Yet these individuals represent only 3 to 5 percent of the persons with alcohol-related problems in the United States. This estimate is based on the best existing population studies. Hard numbers on the proportion of persons with alcohol-related problems are difficult to gather at the present time because public stigma and insufficient funds for study impede efforts to collect such data. The fixation upon the skid row individual as the model of an alcoholic person has led to an inappropriate view by

2

society of the problems of alcohol abuse and alcoholism. Having reached the point in life where he has few essential resources left, the skid row inebriate requires extensive efforts for rehabilitation. For many years we have identified this person—outcast, neglected, distained—as "the alcoholic," persisting in punishing him by arrest and rearrest, and denying him adequate medical, psychological, and social assistance. Largely to protect ourselves against our own confusion and conflicts about our own use of alcohol, we have focused on these unfortunate individuals in an attempt to minimize and isolate our own concerns.

Preventive Efforts

This stereotyping takes a toll. Identifying early alcohol-related problems, when intervention is most likely to be beneficial, is avoided and little help for persons with these problems has been available. With enlightened attitudes to alcohol-related problems, early casefinding results in improved therapeutic outcomes which are now strengthened by varieties of approaches tailored to individual needs. The new directions and approaches point up ways to lessen the emotional distress and impact of alcohol-related problems on the Nation.

Today's pressing need is for a massive and comprehensive program that puts to work and builds on the knowledge we already have. To initiate such a program, the National Institute on Alcohol Abuse and Alcoholism envisions new career personnel trained to make certain that no individual needing help is lost in the cracks. Such personnel would enhance the concept of continuity-of-care ... help identify and establish needed resources ... and serve as the link among new and established programs to assure that a span of services is truly available in the six priority areas of research and services:

- Providing help to alcoholic employees.

- Rehabilitating public inebriates.

- Reducing alcoholism among American Indians.

- Delivering comprehensive services to all alcoholic persons.

- Treating alcoholic individuals identified through traffic safety programs.

- Preventing alcohol abuse and alcoholism.

3

*Providing Help
to Alcoholic
Employees*

A price of $10 billion is paid each year by industry and workers as a result of lost work time, medical expenses, impaired job efficiency, and accidents incurred by employed persons suffering from alcoholism. About 4.5 million workers suffer from alcohol-related problems; 240,000 are jobholders for the largest employer of all, the U.S. Government.

A number of industrial corporations today have personnel policies consonant with the emerging view that alcoholism is a treatable illness. This approach generally calls for helping an alcoholic employee locate resources for help, rather than ignoring his needs and worth, and forcing him into job dismissal. Preliminary results are heartening. When faced with these alternatives and offered competent treatment programs, from six to seven out of 10 alcoholic employees achieve control of their condition. The Civil Service Commission is currently working with NIAAA to develop prevention, treatment, and rehabilitation programs and services for alcohol abuse and alcoholism among its civilian Federal employees. To keep in step with this trend, industries should be encouraged to establish similar programs among their own workers.

*Rehabilitating
Public
Inebriates*

Although public inebriates make up a small minority of the alcoholic population, they account for one-third of all arrests, excluding traffic violations. Handled primarily within the criminal justice system, their treatment is generally acknowledged to be inhumane and ineffective. Sleeping it off in jail may provide them with desperately needed food and shelter and sometimes with emergency medical services, but incarceration reinforces both their own and the public stigmatization of themselves, costs society more than $100 million a year in arrest and imprisonment proceedings, and has proved ineffective in changing modes of behavior of the alcoholic individual.

Short-term studies have shown that by providing these individuals with all the elements of a regular comprehensive treatment program, plus special cooperative outreach and court referral procedures, many public inebriates can be successfully recruited into rehabilitation programs. Even those who appear to have been

4

totally deprived of resources with little chance for recovery have shown a success rate of one-out-of-four.

Reducing Alcoholism Among American Indians

In December 1969, a special Health Service task force reported that among American Indians (including Alaskan natives), "the majority of suicides, murders, accidental deaths, and injuries are associated with drinking, as are many cases of infection, cirrhosis, and malnutrition." In addition, the report pointed out that 76 percent of all fines, arrests, and imprisonments incurred by these people resulted from drinking.

Given the parameters by which we measure emotional and physical wellbeing—morbidity and mortality, annual income, level of education, availability of preventive and curative health and social services, opportunities for employment—the first Americans stand out as one of the most deprived American groups. As resources for prevention and treatment are mustered on behalf of this group of people, whose overall alcoholism rate is twice the National average, attention will be given to helping them overcome basic economic and social disadvantages.

Delivering Comprehensive Services

Although alcoholism has been labeled an "iceberg problem"—primarily because many people with this illness are forced by societal attitudes to deny that they are suffering from it—many alcoholic individuals make contact with one or more of the persons and agencies providing helping services in their communities.

The general public pays a price for alcohol-related problems. A bill of at least $2 billion is run up each year for medical payments and for welfare benefits to alcoholic individuals who are physically or emotionally incapacitated. Thus many alcohol abusers and alcoholic persons are already known in their communities, where they could be referred to comprehensive resources enlisted in their behalf.

Identifying and Treating Drunken Drivers

More than half the individuals involved in fatal auto accidents each year have significant amounts of alcohol in their bloodstreams. This highway carnage has snuffed out 28,000 lives in 1 year. Alcohol-related accidents also cause injuries annually to half-a-million people, result in several hundred thousand arrests, and carry a pricetag of more than $1 billion for property damage, insurance costs, and medical services.

Punitive methods—fines, jailing, and license revocations—have not kept the alcoholic driver off the road very long. In some cities, conviction for driving while intoxicated may lead to referral for treatment. Working in concert, health workers and law enforcement officers can make a determined and feasible casefinding effort to reach alcoholic drivers in the early stages of their illnesses. Such coordinated efforts may prove to be the prototype of joint local safety and health planning programs that reduce the prevalence of both alcoholism and traffic fatalities.

Prevention of Alcoholism and Alcohol Abuse

As President Nixon made clear in his proposal for a national health strategy, people tend to utilize our present health system when they are troubled by acute disease. The President said: "We should build a true 'health' system—and not a 'sickness' system alone."

An essential aspect of a health system is a concerted effort at secondary prevention or early casefinding. Casefinding of those who are especially vulnerable to alcoholism can occur at various levels from the early school years to adulthood. This could also include identifying emotionally deprived and immature children in nursery and elementary schools, and referring their families to special developmental clinics provided by school systems and social agencies. Work with adolescents could also be an important mechanism for early casefinding. We know that most Americans have their first taste of alcohol during childhood or adolescence, and this usually takes place in the home. By high school age, the majority of teenagers drink occasionally, partly in a ritual of identification with the adult world. Intervention at this time of life among adolescents who are exhibiting delinquent behavior or personality traits of incipient alcohol abuse, might well reduce the rate of alcohol-related problems. Early casefinding could also include identification of early signs of unhealthy relationships in marriage, with couples directed to remedial programs conducted by private therapists, comprehensive mental health centers, or family agencies.

Physicians can be a prime source in identifying and treating persons with alcohol-related problems. Alcohol is implicated in numerous illnesses which combine to shorten the victim's life by

6

10 to 12 years. Since persons with alcohol-related problems run many times the average risk of being involved in an accident, hospital emergency rooms are obvious places of entry into an appropriate referral and treatment system. People arrested for drunken driving are another obvious example of an identifiable group presenting potential for therapy.

Despite the growing recognition of the symptoms of alcohol abuse and alcoholism, treating the casualties is no final solution. Primary prevention—or ways to prevent alcohol abuse and alcoholism before they start—is a crucial undertaking. As with so many problems, identification of the precursors of the condition has been retrospective: reconstructing the cause by the wisdom of hindsight. We now know enough to begin a commitment to prospective studies and preventive techniques. While identification of important early causative factors could not affect any genetic factors that may predispose an individual to alcohol abuse and alcoholism, it would allow the introduction of corrective measures which may reduce the receptivity of the person to development of alcoholism.

The ethnic diversity that enriches the American culture may well serve as a prototype for investigating differing predispositions to alcoholism. For, although researchers have thus far failed to identify a genetic, physiological, or environmental cause of alcoholism, cross-cultural studies have determined that the condition is widespread among certain cultural groups and virtually unknown among others.

The rate of alcoholism, for example, has been shown to be low in groups whose drinking-related customs, values, and sanctions are widely known, established, and congruent with other cultural values. On the other hand, alcoholism rates are higher in those populations where ambivalence about alcohol is marked. Apparently, in cultures which use alcohol but have a low incidence of alcoholism, people drink in a definite pattern. The beverage is sipped slowly, consumed with food, taken in the company of others—all in relaxing, comfortable circumstances. Drinking is taken for granted. No emotional rewards are reaped by the man who shows prowess of consumption. Intoxication is abhorred. Other cultures with a high incidence of alcohol-related problems usually assign a special significance to drinking. Alcohol use is surrounded with attitudes of ambivalence and guilt. Maladaptive drinking, drinking without food, and intoxication are common.

We all tend to learn patterns of behavior and preferred coping mechanisms from our parents and the "significant others" in our

7

lives. The guilt that so many families feel about their own drinking behavior is reflected in society's attitudes. Ours is a Nation that is ambivalent about its alcohol use. This confusion has deterred us from creating a National climate that encourages responsible attitudes toward drinking for those who choose to drink; that is, using alcohol in a way which does not harm oneself or society.

Too often, in our attempt to solve human problems, we gravitate toward simplistic answers to deal with complicated issues. Certainly most cultures that have tried, have failed to persuade all people to give up the consumption of alcoholic beverages.

Our goal recognizes the right of each individual to exercise his time on this planet as he sees fit, provided he does not harm others. At the same time, the National Institute on Alcohol Abuse and Alcoholism aims to help private nonprofit and public agencies reach out to offer the alcoholic individual the help we have every reason to believe that he wants . . . that he will accept . . . and that he will utilize. In addition, we seek to develop ways to identify the potential alcoholic person, and to devise ways to circumvent unhealthy use of alcohol.

MORRIS E. CHAFETZ, M.D.,
Chairman of the Task Force.

Chapter I

ETHANOL: THE BASIC SUBSTANCE IN ALCOHOLIC BEVERAGES

INVOLVED IN ALL ALCOHOL-RELATED PROBLEMS are the nature of man, his society, his experiences, and a chemical compound known as ethyl alcohol, or ethanol. This compound with the chemical formula CH_3CH_2OH has such remarkable and seemingly magical properties as the ability to induce euphoria, sedation, intoxication, and narcosis. Of the many known alcohols, it is the only one universally agreeable to man as a beverage ingredient. Other alcohols, including the well-known methyl and isopropyl, have immediate toxic effects that make them unsuitable for drinking. Thus, ethanol, the significant and desired ingredient in the three major classes of alcoholic beverages—distilled spirits, wines, and beers—is the only one called simply alcohol.

ORIGINS

Alcoholic beverages were presumably discovered, rather than invented, in prehistoric times. Their origin is buried in antiquity, though the presence of wine and beer is well attested in archaeological records of the oldest civilizations (18, 19, 29) and in the diets of most preliterate peoples.

The surmise that man discovered alcohol very early is based on the nature of the compound. Alcohol can be formed when fermentation is started in sugar-containing plants by yeasts from the environment; the sugar is thereby converted to alcohol. A

9

mismash of fruit or berries left exposed in a warm atmosphere and, thus, to the action of airborne yeasts, would normally be fermented into a crude wine. The early men who first consumed the product of this natural event must have felt an effect far more interesting than mere satiation of hunger and thirst.

Ample evidence exists that prehistoric man was technologically, as well as artistically, creative. A likely guess would be that, in many parts of the world, men quickly proceeded from accidental discovery to purposeful production of alcoholic beverages, and from merely gathering the raw materials to purposeful cultivation. Relatively primitive agriculturists, for example, devised simple ways of converting the starch in grains to fermentable sugar to produce beer; the enzyme necessary for this additional process was provided from their saliva by chewing some of the grain and spitting it out into the vessels of prepared mash. Men soon learned that besides fruits and grains, other plants such as flowers and cactuses, and many plant products, including the saps of trees and even milk and honey, could be fermented to become alcoholic beverages. The result must have been considered well worth the effort.

Religious Uses

The near-universality of alcoholic beverages imposes an irresistible inference: Man from earliest times appreciated the mood-changing effect of these fluids, regarding them as useful and beneficent. In his attempts to appease or manipulate the divine or magical powers that he perceived as determining his fate. . . in his early groping for relatedness to the mystical forces in nature . . . man offered up to these forces something precious. Water may have been the first sacrifice offered to the divinities, especially in the relatively arid lands where some of the earliest agricultural civilizations developed. Water was followed perhaps by milk and honey.

In many cultures, wine or beer eventually replaced other fluids in religious rituals, both as libation and as a sacred drink whereby man could incorporate the "divine" power of the alcohol (12). This is hardly surprising, for alcoholic beverages were obviously more suitable than any others for evoking those moods of release, mystification, and ecstasy that were sought as a way to communicate with and relate to powers that were invisible and beyond knowing. In particular, alcoholic beverages facilitated the rites of orgiastic communicants. Small wonder that Dionysos-Bacchus became the most popular of the gods among the Greeks and Romans.

Secular Uses

In the best-documented early civilizations, such as the Sumerian-Akkadian, the Babylonian-Chaldean, and the Egyptian (18, 19) as well as among the classical peoples (21, 22)—Greeks, Hebrews, and Romans—alcoholic beverages were secularized for common use. This may have been due, in part, to their being more satisfying as beverages than other available fluids. But the secularization of alcohol was undoubtedly related also to the fact that its traditional role in religion tended to impart a desired aura of sanctity or solemnity to its use on nonreligious but important occasions. Alcoholic beverages became mandatory not only in worship and in the practice of magic and medicine, but also to solemnify formal councils, to ratify compacts and crownings, to commemorate festivals, to display hospitality, to stimulate warmaking, and to celebrate peacemaking, as well as to confirm all rites of passage through life—births, initiations, marriages, and funerals.

Drunkenness or Alcoholism

If we assume that these public events are accompanied by conscious or unconscious anxiety, the ability of alcohol to assuage apprehension may have suggested the extension of its use not only from religious to public events, but also to personal occasions of unease. The advice of King Lemuel's mother to "Give. . . wine unto them that be of heavy hearts" (Prov. 31:6) is the summation of ancient experience and wisdom.

A widespread impression exists that the classical Hebrews and Greeks were moderate drinkers. This impression is erroneous (16, 22). The ancients knew that alcoholic beverages could do more than relieve heavy hearts; they also enhanced light-heartedness and light-headedness whenever gaiety or courage was desired. The everyday use of wine or beer, both as a beverage and for its immediate mood-altering qualities, led to private excesses and to personal and social troubles—quite a different matter from such fiestal drunkenness as at the Bacchanalia. Drunkenness, and undoubtedly what was to become known as alcoholism, were

11

problems among ancient Greeks and Jews, as well as among the peoples of Perso-Media, India, and China (19, 29). Teachers and governments made numerous formal and informal attempts to reform or control the drinking excesses among these nations. Government efforts included total prohibitions accompanied by harsh penal threats (25) which do not seem to have worked.

Among the Jews, temperate drinking became the established norm only when their national culture was reformed around 525 B.C. to 350 B.C. (16). But the cultures of the Greeks and Judaeans and, later, of the Romans all mingled in the centuries following 300 B.C. (38), and this mix powerfully influenced what was to become Western or European culture, including drinking customs and attitudes.

Thus, notions that drunkenness or alcoholism are modern phenomena, or associated exclusively or specifically with poverty or affluence or industrialization or advertising, are simplistic and ignore the facts of history. The Bible, the Graeco-Roman classics, the Russian *Collection of the Moral Sermons and Admonitions of the Twelfth Century (35)*, the German 13th century *Ocean Cruise of the Viennese (9)* and 16th-century *Horrible Vice of Drunkenness* (11), Nash's *Pierce Penilesse* (27), and, even more, Skelton's earlier *Tunnyng of Elynour Rummyng (33)* (both the latter in 15th–16th century England) all reveal that multitudes of the rich as well as poor in various cultures and times have resorted to intoxicating amounts of alcohol for what troubled them. Skelton's satire reveals that women too were given to drunkenness (to the extent that they showed florid signs of alcoholic diseases) and, moreover, that alcoholism could be achieved by drinking English ale as well as the gin of Dutch ancestry.

An historic exception must be entered for the Moslems, who abstained from wine in obedience to the injunction recorded in the Koran. Faithful attachment to religious teachings among the Brahmin caste in India, and the adherents of Buddhism more widely, also kept multitudes of devotees abstinent (6). Following the Protestant Reformation, members of large as well as smaller denominations in Western Europe, and later in America, adopted total abstinence as a religious tenet (20). Since the temperate drinking of the Jews seems also to be associated with a religious-cultural orientation (4, 16, 34) it appears that religion rather than government, moral rather than legal controls, proved capable of stemming the tide of drunkenness. In recent years, however, there are indications that abstinence is declining among members of

12

some Moslem and Christian groups (5, 8, 24, 30); this may be related to a change in the quality of their religious attachment.

CHARACTERISTICS OF BEVERAGES

From prehistoric times until about the 16th century, alcoholic beverages were derived from fermentation and consisted of wines and beers containing, at most, about 14 percent alcohol. This upper limit is fixed by the inability of the fermentative yeasts to survive in stronger solutions of alcohol. In the fermentation of any substance, moreover, the yield of alcohol is also limited by the amount of available sugar, and the willingness or patience of the producer to wait until the maximum possible yield of alcohol is obtained. As a result, to this day, many fermented beverages contain less than 14 percent alcohol. Sometimes the proportion is as little as 2 percent or less, as in the *koumiss* (fermented mare's milk) of nomadic tribes in Asia, the Russian *kvas*, or the deliberately mild beers of some Scandinavian countries.

Food Values

In addition to their mood-changing properties, the crude alcoholic beverages were undoubtedly valuable foods; this is still true of such brews as the beer of the African Bantu tribes. In many of these primitive beverages, the nutrients of the raw materials, including essential vitamins and minerals, are conserved (28). By comparison, little of these nutrients survive in the alcoholic beverages refined by modern technology for contemporary tastes, and none are left in the products of distillation. Yet one food value remains in the distillate: The alcohol itself is a rich source of calories usable for heat and energy.

Calories

Each gram of alcohol metabolized in the body yields seven calories; this adds up to approximately 200 calories per fluid ounce (about 30 milliliters) of absolute alcohol, or 100 calories per fluid ounce of 100-U.S.-proof distilled spirits. In beer, some additional calories, about four per ounce, remain from the surviving cereal content of the original grain. (These nonalcohol calories, however, are currently being eliminated by some manufacturers catering to weight-conscious consumers.)

13

DISTILLATION

The popularization of distillation in Europe, beginning in the 15th century, introduced a new and more potent alcoholic beverage—the spirit of wine—and very soon the spirit of any fermented fluid from any source—grains and tubers as well as other berries and fruits besides grapes (31). Now instead of beers and wines containing probably between 6 and 14 percent alcohol, beverages containing as much as 50 percent and more alcohol could be drunk.

Magic and Medicine

Distilled spirits gained immediate acceptance among those who wanted a quicker, easier, or more potent alcoholic effect. In addition, even more powerful magical-beneficent virtues were attributed to them than to the original alcoholic beverages. This is manifested in the glorified names the distilled spirits acquired—the "water of life"—*aqua vitae*, in scholastic Latin, and *eau-de-vie* and *uisge beatha* in popular French and Irish.

Aqua vitae quickly established itself in medicine and surgery (15) and easily crept into folkloristic healing, often replacing the relatively weak traditional wines. This beverage was not, as some early users had wishfully thought, the long-sought philosopher's stone. It did not really rejuvenate the body, as was at first claimed, or completely banish all worry and sadness. It did not cure many of the diseases for which it was prescribed and imbibed. But then, neither did anything else. Alcohol, at least, reduced the intensity of emotional distress and physical aches, and was the best anesthetic available to surgeons. Its medical use brought it into the lexicon of drugs, where it remains to this day.

ATTEMPTS AT CONTROL

The understanding of drunkenness or alcoholism was generally not more profound in those times than more recently. Drunkenness was looked on as a vice or sin—especially a vice in the lower classes. The attempts to cope with it were as naive as most later and modern measures. King Edgar had required taverns to have pegged cups in which the quantity was measured off, and those who drank beyond each gradation forfeited a penny for each peg. King James imposed fines in shillings for getting drunk. There was

14

no lack of suggestions in the oldest classical writings that drunkenness might be a disease, but the orientation to the concept of sin and vice prevailed (20). It was transplanted to the American Colonies, where fining those found drunk and shaming them, as by confinement in stocks, were the treatments of choice (3).

With the beginning of the Industrial Revolution in the 18th century, drunkenness may have become more widespread (36). The resulting displacement and alienation of populations, and the availability of cheap spirits, perhaps added incentive for disadvantaged people to resort to alcoholism (7). The increase in drunkenness, however, may not have been as great as has been supposed. The phenomenon may only have become more noticeable and less tolerable under the new, more complex, social conditions. Alcoholism had been rampant before industrialization and the upper classes, hardly disadvantaged by the Industrial Revolution, equally manifested the behaviors of alcoholism.

Young America

In the American Colonies, newer approaches to the problem of damaging drinking were attempted. A growth of inebriety here has been attributed to the development of the rum trade but, in fact, the colonists had brought their native drinking and carousing customs with them (20). Centuries passed before the Puritan settlers' "Good Creature of God" was metamorphosed by their descendants into the Demon Rum (17). Contemporary drinking ways are a mix imported by successive waves of immigrants from different geographic areas and ethnocultural backgrounds. In time, some indigenous customs developed in the particular American situation, notably the reckless frontier drinking in the 18th and 19th centuries (37) and, later, the cocktail hour.

The gross excesses of the frontier drinking style, as well as waxing industrialization, aroused the concern of leaders of public opinion, including Benjamin Franklin, over the growth of problems associated with the common copious intake of spirits. The Quaker, Anthony Benezet, campaigned in a private pamphlet against the use of spirits, emphasizing their harmful effects on health (2). He was soon followed by Dr. Benjamin Rush, a signer of the Declaration of Independence and a Surgeon-General in the Continental Army, who denied the value of spirits for preserving the health of soldiers. In 1785, Rush published his classic *Inquiry Into the Effects of Ardent Spirits on the Human Body and Mind*

15

(32). In it, Rush explicitly called the intemperate use of distilled spirits a "disease," referred to it as an "addiction," and was the first to estimate the rate of death by alcoholism in the United States: "Not less than 4,000 people" per year in a population then less than 6 million. Thus at the very formation of the United States of America, its foremost physician recognized the abuse of alcohol as a public health problem.

The Temperance Movement

Undoubtedly Benezet and Rush, followed by other leaders of public opinion early in the 19th century, laid the foundations for the organized temperance movement which, at first, opposed only the use of distilled spirits and advocated methods of moral suasion for achieving widespread temperance. The moderationist temperance movement proved effective in gaining a large and influential membership throughout the country over a period of about 40 years. By the middle of the 19th century, however, the movement had been taken over by those who advocated total abstinence and legislative repression of the trade in alcoholic beverages (2).

In the next 80 years, the teetotalist Temperance Movement proved itself politically effective. An anti-alcohol clause was included in the 1844 Constitution of the newly organized Oregon Territory. Statewide prohibition was first mandated in Maine in 1851. Four years later, statewide prohibition laws had been adopted in 13 of the 31 States. By 1863, however, all States except Maine had repealed or modified their prohibition laws. Then in 1880, a second wave of statewide prohibition began. It affected eight States but, again, most of these laws were repealed in the next two decades.

Prohibition

In the years before World War I, the third and most effective drive for prohibition developed. It was by the AntiSaloon League and the Woman's Christian Temperance Union, and was supported by a substantial block of Protestant churches. Their campaign culminated in the 18th amendment to the Constitution, adopted in 1919 and imposing nationwide prohibition in 1920.

Other Countries

The temperance movement inspired an echo crusade in many European countries; in some, notably Finland and Iceland, pro-

16

hibition was similarly tried. A substantial part of Canada also came under prohibition. But the attempt to suppress all use of alcoholic beverages by legislation collapsed in the face of defiant resistance on the part of substantial segments of the population in all these countries as well as in the United States. Indeed, prohibition produced its own evils, including contempt for law and corruption of law-enforcement personnel.

Repeal

After 13 years of frustrated trial, national prohibition was repealed in the United States by the 21st amendment to the Constitution. Statewide prohibition remained for a time in three States, but in 1966 Mississippi became the last State to repeal its law. In smaller political jurisdictions within many States, however, prohibition is still the rule by local option. The national prohibitions tried in all other Western countries have also been repealed.

The prohibition amendment was passed in the United States by the action of a sufficient number of State legislatures. Repeal, on the other hand, was effected by popular referendums in the States. The majorities in the States that ratified the 21st amendment may have consisted largely of people who preferred to drink, and wished to purchase their supplies legally. But they may well have included many people who, while preferring abstinence, did not think prohibition a wise or workable kind of law. About one in three of the adult American population are nondrinkers at the present time, but their proportion was undoubtedly greater at the time of repeal. The repeal movement may have owed its success, in part, to a growing antipathy among Americans toward legislated moralism, so that many people preferred to have the right to choose their own behavior; that is, whether to drink or not.

PROPORTIONS OF DRINKERS
AND ABSTAINERS

To appreciate the possible role of alcohol in health and social problems in contemporary America, it is necessary to know some basic numerical facts about the drinkers in the population and the kinds and amounts of alcoholic beverages they consume. It is useful also to make some comparisons with data from other countries. For, as will be evident from a consideration of these facts and the contents of subsequent chapters, enough alcohol in any form will insure trouble for any group or nation. Yet alcohol alone may cause no substantial trouble, even in a universally drinking population. And the type of alcoholic beverage may not matter so much as the patterns and purposes of drinking.

In the years since prohibition, the proportion of abstainers in the United States has declined and the proportion of drinkers has correspondingly increased. These proportions were indeterminate until 1940, when the first estimate was made of the size of these groups in the adult age bracket of 21 and over. This estimate, and the results of several national surveys during the next 25 years, are shown in figure 1. The largest increase in the proportion of adult drinkers is among women.

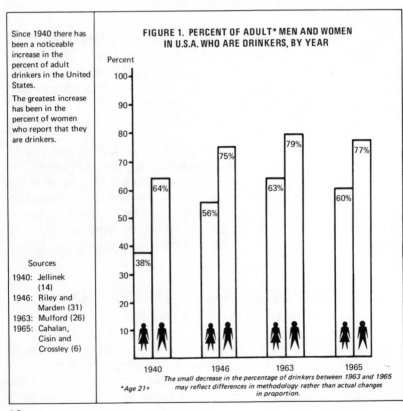

Since 1940 there has been a noticeable increase in the percent of adult drinkers in the United States.

The greatest increase has been in the percent of women who report that they are drinkers.

Sources

1940: Jellinek (14)
1946: Riley and Marden (31)
1963: Mulford (26)
1965: Cahalan, Cisin and Crossley (6)

FIGURE 1. PERCENT OF ADULT* MEN AND WOMEN IN U.S.A. WHO ARE DRINKERS, BY YEAR

Percent

1940: 38%, 64%
1946: 56%, 75%
1963: 63%, 79%
1965: 60%, 77%

*Age 21+

The small decrease in the percentage of drinkers between 1963 and 1965 may reflect differences in methodology rather than actual changes in proportion.

Surveys of adults, however, leave out a sizable portion of the drinkers. Numerous studies of younger populations, mostly in high schools, reveal that a substantial proportion of teenagers are drinkers (1, 23). Estimates based on an aggregation of such surveys show that, in recent years, about 57 percent of boys and 43 percent of girls aged 15 through 20 years are drinkers. For the year 1970, the projected total number of drinkers 15 years of age and over is 95,648,000—nearly 44 million women and girls, and over 52 million men and boys (10).

ALCOHOL CONSUMPTION

The amounts of tax-paid alcoholic beverages—distilled spirits, wines, and beers—apparently consumed in the United States in 1970 by the average person in the drinking-age population (which includes all those aged 15 years and more), are shown in table I for each State, for the District of Columbia, and for the whole country. The quantities are given in terms of both U.S. gallons of each class of beverage apparently consumed by the average person, and in terms of the absolute alcohol derived from each class. The last column totals the absolute alcohol derived from all the beverages.

The anomalously high amounts attributed to the District of Columbia can be due to several factors: The consumption in this and all subsequent tables and figures actually represents the tax-paid quantities that enter—not even those that leave—consumer outlets. Temporary stocking up or inventory overloads can distort the apparent consumption in any one year.

The District is not a State, with urban and rural areas counterbalancing high and low purchase and consumption rates, but a large metropolis where a high rate of both is expected. It is a foremost tourist and convention center, where a high drinking rate is expected. And it is a low-price center attracting purchases from a vast suburban and transient population. (The amount of nontax-paid alcohol that may be consumed in the District of Columbia because of the presence of numerous foreign embassies, however, has been left out of account.)

Another caution applies to comparisons among States. Some States attract multitudes of vacationers and tourists from others where prices of spirits are as much as 35 percent to 40 percent higher. These mostly automobile-borne transients stock up while in the low-price States, thus artificially inflating the "consump-

19

TABLE I

APPARENT CONSUMPTION,* BY STATES,
OF EACH MAJOR BEVERAGE CLASS,
AND OF ABSOLUTE ALCOHOL FROM EACH CLASS,
IN U.S. GALLONS PER PERSON
IN THE DRINKING-AGE POPULATION,** U.S.A. 1970

State	Distilled Spirits	Absolute Alcohol	Wine	Absolute Alcohol	Beer	Absolute Alcohol	TOTAL Absolute Alcohol
Alabama	1.59	0.72	0.58	0.09	13.66	0.61	1.42
Alaska	4.79	2.16	2.36	0.38	27.22	1.22	3.76
Arizona	2.41	1.08	2.03	0.32	31.30	1.41	2.81
Arkansas	1.35	0.61	0.86	0.13	16.20	0.73	1.47
California	3.12	1.40	4.06	0.65	25.20	1.13	3.18
Colorado	2.72	1.22	2.00	0.32	26.96	1.21	2.75
Connecticut	3.34	1.50	2.17	0.35	22.81	1.03	2.88
Delaware	4.14	1.86	1.38	0.22	26.82	1.21	3.29
Florida	3.58	1.61	1.89	0.30	24.86	1.12	3.03
Georgia	2.32	1.04	0.89	0.14	18.06	0.81	1.99
Hawaii	2.58	1.16	1.61	0.26	25.35	1.14	2.56
Idaho	1.72	0.77	0.63	0.10	27.48	1.24	2.11
Illinois	3.05	1.37	1.74	0.28	27.72	1.25	2.90
Indiana	1.68	0.76	0.77	0.12	22.94	1.03	1.91
Iowa	1.56	0.70	0.39	0.06	24.93	1.12	1.88
Kansas	1.48	0.67	0.59	0.09	19.52	0.88	1.64
Kentucky	1.94	0.87	0.53	0.08	21.38	0.96	1.91
Louisiana	2.13	0.96	1.85	0.30	27.60	1.24	2.50
Maine	2.36	1.06	0.62	0.10	28.30	1.27	2.43
Maryland	3.17	1.43	1.63	0.26	29.89	1.35	3.04
Massachusetts	3.09	1.39	1.92	0.31	26.12	1.18	2.88
Michigan	2.44	1.10	1.54	0.25	31.45	1.42	2.77
Minnesota	2.65	1.19	1.01	0.16	26.09	1.17	2.52
Mississippi	1.62	0.73	0.53	0.08	18.88	0.85	1.66
Missouri	2.28	1.03	1.25	0.20	25.68	1.16	2.39
Montana	2.35	1.06	0.86	0.14	35.31	1.59	2.79
Nebraska	2.33	1.05	0.85	0.14	29.33	1.32	2.51
Nevada	7.25	3.26	4.30	0.69	39.51	1.78	5.73
New Hampshire	6.44	2.90	2.02	0.32	38.36	1.73	4.95
New Jersey	3.15	1.42	2.44	0.39	26.72	1.20	3.01
New Mexico	2.26	1.02	2.36	0.38	27.56	1.24	2.64
New York	3.26	1.47	2.55	0.41	26.84	1.21	3.09
North Carolina	2.09	0.94	1.02	0.16	16.37	0.74	1.84
North Dakota	2.39	1.08	0.69	0.11	27.87	1.25	2.44
Ohio	1.86	0.84	1.20	0.19	27.81	1.25	2.28
Oklahoma	1.91	0.86	0.94	0.15	17.76	0.80	1.81
Oregon	2.06	0.93	2.52	0.40	26.81	1.21	2.54
Pennsylvania	1.88	0.85	1.24	0.20	28.82	1.30	2.35
Rhode Island	2.68	1.21	2.42	0.39	29.23	1.32	2.92
South Carolina	2.88	1.30	1.07	0.17	18.25	0.82	2.29
South Dakota	2.08	0.94	0.86	0.14	21.35	0.96	2.04
Tennessee	1.33	0.60	0.41	0.07	19.91	0.90	1.57
Texas	1.74	0.78	1.12	0.18	30.02	1.35	2.31
Utah	1.31	0.59	0.79	0.13	17.28	0.78	1.50
Vermont	3.96	1.73	2.48	0.40	31.64	1.42	3.60
Virginia	2.32	1.04	1.32	0.21	25.44	1.14	2.39
Washington	2.46	1.11	2.51	0.40	27.26	1.23	2.74
West Virginia	1.57	0.71	0.57	0.09	19.79	0.89	1.69
Wisconsin	2.86	1.29	1.40	0.22	39.19	1.76	3.27
Wyoming	2.64	1.19	1.01	0.16	29.39	1.32	2.67
D.C.	10.39	4.68	5.24	0.84	31.48	1.42	6.94
U.S.A.	2.56	1.15	1.84	0.29	25.95	1.17	2.61

* For comparative purposes only. Amounts calculated according to tax paid withdrawals.
** Age 15+

tion" in the latter. Similarly, many residents of areas dry by local option buy their supplies in contiguous States, thus artificially inflating the consumption of their neighbors and masking the consumption in their own States.

Somewhat more realistic indices of apparent consumption are shown in figure 2a and figure 2b. Here the apparent consumption is divided among the populations of larger geographic units—the Bureau of Census regions—rather than State by State. These data show the consumption, per person in the drinking-age population, in terms only of the absolute alcohol contained in the various beverages, and the proportion of the total absolute alcohol contributed by each major class of beverage. Interesting and possibly important differences appear. Thus, at one extreme, inhabitants of the South Central regions consume the least alcohol while the Pacific and New England regions consume the most. In contrast, the distribution among different classes of beverages reveals that the inhabitants of the West South Central region apparently consume only 37 percent of their alcohol in the form of distilled spirits, obtaining 54 percent from beer; those in the South Atlantic region get 51 percent from distilled spirits and 40 percent from beer. And while the national average of absolute alcohol consumption from wine is 11 percent, the Pacific region—dominated by California—stands out by taking 19 percent of its alcohol in the form of wine.

The Trend over Time

The brief historical perspective on American drinking practices presented earlier in this chapter invites examination of actual alcohol consumption over time; this is shown in table II and figure 3. Disregarding the artificially low values of 1934–1935 and the immediately following years, when the relegalized trade was only beginning to replace the bootleg supplies of the prohibition era, no great swings are evident in the average consumption of total absolute alcohol, per person in the drinking-age population, until recently.

Shifts in Beverage Preferences

A noteworthy change occurred, however, in the relative consumption of spirits and beer during the latter half of the 19th

21

FIGURE 2a. APPARENT CONSUMPTION* OF ABSOLUTE ALCOHOL, IN U.S. GALLONS PER PERSON IN THE DRINKING-AGE POPULATION, BY REGION, U.S.A. 1970**

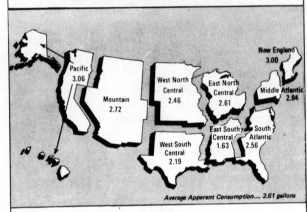

Note: The regions are the standard regions of the U.S. Census Bureau.

*For comparative purposes only. Amounts calculated according to tax-paid withdrawals.

**Age 15+

century. Only about 10 percent of the national consumption of alcohol at mid-19th century was in the form of beer; 85 percent came from distilled spirits. About 50 years later, more than half the alcohol was being taken in the form of beer, and less than half from distilled spirits, with no substantial change in the contribution of wine.

The remarkable shift from distilled spirits to beer can hardly be credited to the propaganda of the temperance movement; in that campaign, all alcoholic beverages were equally condemned. Rather, it may be accounted for by the large immigration of populations from traditionally beer-drinking countries that is reflected, to this day, in the relatively high consumption of beer in such a State as Wisconsin.

In the preceding tables and figures, the apparent consumption of absolute alcohol has been divided up among the Census population aged 15 years of age and over. This yields a truer picture than using the entire U.S. population, first because children under 15 drink only a tiny fraction of the total and, second, because the size of this youngest nondrinking part of the population tends to change from time to time (13).

22

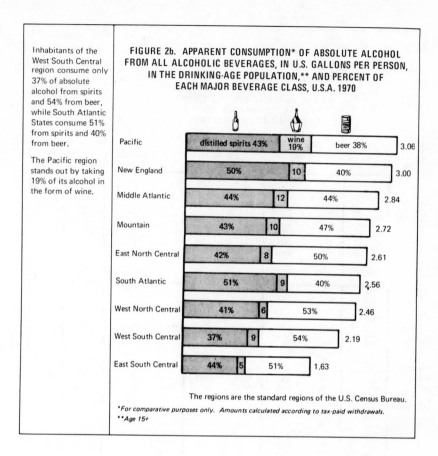

Inhabitants of the West South Central region consume only 37% of absolute alcohol from spirits and 54% from beer, while South Atlantic States consume 51% from spirits and 40% from beer.

The Pacific region stands out by taking 19% of its alcohol in the form of wine.

FIGURE 2b. APPARENT CONSUMPTION* OF ABSOLUTE ALCOHOL FROM ALL ALCOHOLIC BEVERAGES, IN U.S. GALLONS PER PERSON, IN THE DRINKING-AGE POPULATION,** AND PERCENT OF EACH MAJOR BEVERAGE CLASS, U.S.A. 1970

Region	distilled spirits	wine	beer	Total
Pacific	distilled spirits 43%	wine 19%	beer 38%	3.06
New England	50%	10	40%	3.00
Middle Atlantic	44%	12	44%	2.84
Mountain	43%	10	47%	2.72
East North Central	42%	8	50%	2.61
South Atlantic	51%	9	40%	2.56
West North Central	41%	6	53%	2.46
West South Central	37%	9	54%	2.19
East South Central	44%	5	51%	1.63

The regions are the standard regions of the U.S. Census Bureau.

*For comparative purposes only. Amounts calculated according to tax-paid withdrawals.

**Age 15+

The Average Drinker

The latter consideration makes it obvious that the truest picture of alcohol consumption requires a division among the drinkers themselves, leaving out the abstainers. It is not possible to do that for the entire period in U.S. history, when alcohol and population statistics became available, because the proportions of drinkers and abstainers remained unknown until 1940.

Figure 4, however, compares the average consumption of absolute alcohol in terms of total population, drinking-age population, and actual drinkers in 1946–1947 (the first postwar year) and in 1969–1970. By this most realistic comparison, the average drinker in the latter year consumed 3.93 U.S. gallons of absolute

23

TABLE II
APPARENT ANNUAL CONSUMPTION,* OVER TIME,
OF EACH MAJOR BEVERAGE CLASS,
AND OF ABSOLUTE ALCOHOL FROM EACH CLASS,
IN U.S. GALLONS PER PERSON
IN THE DRINKING-AGE POPULATION,** U.S.A. 1850-1970

Year	Distilled Spirits	Absolute Alcohol	Wine	Absolute Alcohol	Beer	Absolute Alcohol	Total
1850	4.17	1.88	0.46	0.08	2.70	0.14	2.10
1860	4.79	2.16	0.57	0.10	5.39	0.27	2.53
1870	3.40	1.53	0.53	0.10	8.73	0.44	2.07
1871-80	2.27	1.02	0.77	0.14	11.26	0.56	1.72
1881-90	2.12	0.95	0.76	0.14	17.94	0.90	1.99
1891-95	2.12	0.95	0.60	0.11	23.42	1.17	2.23
1896-1900	1.72	0.77	0.55	0.10	23.72	1.19	2.06
1901-05	2.11	0.95	0.71	0.13	26.20	1.31	2.39
1906-10	2.14	0.96	0.92	0.17	29.27	1.47	2.60
1911-15	2.09	0.94	0.79	0.14	29.53	1.48	2.56
1916-19	1.68	0.76	0.69	0.12	21.63	1.08	1.96
PROHIBITION*							
1934	0.64	0.29	0.36	0 07	13.58	0.61	0.97
1935	0.96	0.43	0.50	0.09	15.13	0.68	1.20
1936	1.20	0.59	0.64	0.12	17.53	0.79	1.50
1937	1.43	0.64	0.71	0.13	18.21	0.82	1.59
1938	1.32	0.59	0.70	0.13	16.58	0.75	1.47
1939	1.38	0.62	0.79	0.14	16.77	0.75	1.51
1940	1.43	0.67	0.01	0.16	16.29	0.73	1.56
1941	1.58	0.71	1.02	0.18	17.97	0.81	1.70
1942	1.89	0.85	1.11	0.20	20.00	0.90	1.95
1943	1.46	0.66	0.94	0.17	22.26	1.00	1.83
1944	1.00	0.76	0.02	0.17	25.22	1.13	2.06
1945	1.95	0.88	1.13	0.20	25.97	1.17	2.25
1946	2.20	0.99	1.34	0.24	23.75	1.07	2.30
1947	1.69	0.76	0.90	0.16	24.56	1.11	2.03
1948	1.56	0.70	1.11	0.20	23.77	1.07	1.97
1949	1.55	0.70	1.21	0.22	23.48	1.06	1.98
1950	1.72	0.77	1.27	0.23	23.21	1.04	2.04
1951	1.73	0.78	1.13	0.20	22.92	1.03	2.01
1952	1.63	0.73	1.22	0.21	23.20	1.04	1.98
1953	1.70	0.77	1.19	0.20	23.04	1.04	2.01
1954	1.66	0.74	1.21	0.21	22.41	1.01	1.96
1955	1.71	0.77	1.25	0.22	22 39	1.01	2.00
1956	1.31	0.81	1.27	0.22	22.18	1.00	2.03
1957	1.77	0.80	1.26	0.22	21.44	0.97	1.99
1958	1.77	0.80	1.27	0.22	21.35	0.96	1.98
1959	1.86	0.84	1.28	0.22	22.15	1.00	2.06
1960	1.90	0.86	1.32	0.22	21.95	0.99	2.07
1961	1.91	0.86	1.36	0.23	21.47	0.97	2.06
1962	1.99	0.90	1.32	0.22	21.98	0.99	2.11
1963	2.02	0.91	1.37	0.23	22.51	1.01	2.15
1964	2.01	0.95	1.41	0.24	23.08	1.04	2.23
1965	2.21	0.99	1.42	0.24	23.07	1.04	2.27
1966	2.26	1.02	1.40	0.24	23.52	1.06	2.32
1967	2.34	1.05	1.46	0.25	23.81	1.07	2.37
1968	2.44	1.10	1.51	0.26	24.33	1.09	2.45
1969	2.51	1.13	1.62	0.26	24.90	1.12	2.51
1970	2.56	1.15	1.84	0.29	26.95	1.17	2.61

*For comparative purposes only. Amounts calculated according to tax-paid withdrawals.
** Age 15+
***Figures unavailable

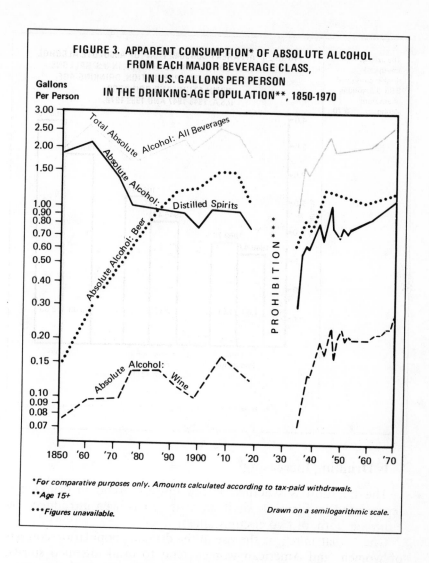

FIGURE 3. APPARENT CONSUMPTION* OF ABSOLUTE ALCOHOL FROM EACH MAJOR BEVERAGE CLASS, IN U.S. GALLONS PER PERSON IN THE DRINKING-AGE POPULATION**, 1850-1970

Gallons Per Person

Total Absolute Alcohol: All Beverages

Absolute Alcohol: Distilled Spirits

Absolute Alcohol: Beer

Absolute Alcohol: Wine

PROHIBITION***

3.00 2.50 2.00 1.50 1.00 0.90 0.80 0.70 0.60 0.50 0.40 0.30 0.20 0.15 0.10 0.09 0.08 0.07

1850 '60 '70 '80 '90 1900 '10 '20 '30 '40 '50 '60 '70

*For comparative purposes only. Amounts calculated according to tax-paid withdrawals.

**Age 15+

***Figures unavailable.   Drawn on a semilogarithmic scale.

alcohol. This allows, for one drinker, about 44 fifths of whiskey; or 98 bottles of fortified wine; or 157 bottles of table wine; or 928 bottles of beer . . . or, for a drinker with eclectic tastes, about 12 fifths of whiskey plus 15 bottles of sherry plus 30 bottles of table wines plus 350 bottles of beer. The average may also be calculated as a little over 3 ounces of whiskey a day, or the equivalent in other beverages—for example, one cocktail, one glass of wine, and a bottle of beer a day.

25

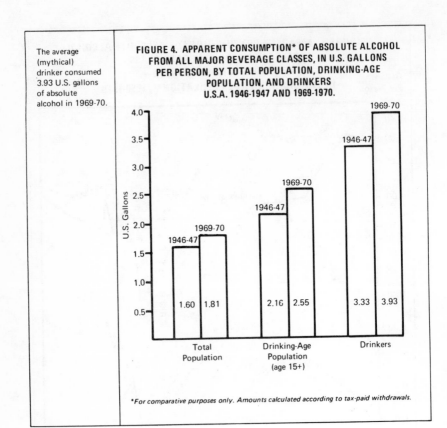

The average (mythical) drinker consumed 3.93 U.S. gallons of absolute alcohol in 1969-70.

FIGURE 4. APPARENT CONSUMPTION* OF ABSOLUTE ALCOHOL FROM ALL MAJOR BEVERAGE CLASSES, IN U.S. GALLONS PER PERSON, BY TOTAL POPULATION, DRINKING-AGE POPULATION, AND DRINKERS U.S.A. 1946-1947 AND 1969-1970.

*For comparative purposes only. Amounts calculated according to tax-paid withdrawals.

Is Drinking Increasing?

The question is whether a true upward trend in drinking is represented in figure 4, or if an artifact has been introduced by either, or both, of two circumstances:

One is that much of the rise in the drinking population consists of women, and American women tend to drink distilled spirits, especially in cocktails, while beer remains the drink of men. (The consumption of beer rose by less than 11 percent since 1947, while the consumption of distilled spirits rose by 50 percent.) The greater proportion of women drinkers, however, can account for only some of the proportionately greater increase in distilled spirits, especially as women drink much less than men.

The second relevant circumstance is that the post-war rise in consumption of distilled spirits may represent, in part, not additional drinking but the replacement of nontax-paid distilled

26

spirits; the latter are the only source of data in these tabulations. Certain socioeconomic changes in the United States suggest this possibility. The United States has proportionately fewer farmers than ever today and fewer of them are "making their own"; in addition, the traditional moonshine industry has probably declined.

The possibility of a real increase in alcohol consumption, however, particularly in the form of distilled spirits, cannot be ruled out. The fact cannot be determined from tax-paid trends alone; direct study of the moonshine industry and of home production is required.

All the preceding calculations have ascribed the alcoholic beverages to an "average" drinker. The average drinker, however, is a myth. The United States probably does not have a single man or woman who consumed exactly 3.93 U.S. gallons of absolute alcohol during 1969 or 1970. Even less likely is the existence of an individual who divided this quantity evenly over all the days of the year. Inhabitants of different regions and States drink different average quantities each year. In addition, the average man drinker consumes three times as much as the average woman drinker, and the average alcoholic person ingests about 11 times as much as the average nonalcoholic person who drinks (14). Assuming that about 5 million people in this country suffer from alcoholism, and that perhaps another 4 million abuse alcohol, then the average drinker with no alcohol-related problems actually drinks much less than the national average of 3.93 U.S. gallons of absolute alcohol. Thus, as surveys show, this nation has millions of occasional and very moderate drinkers (5).

INTERNATIONAL COMPARISONS

Table III compares the drinking in the United States with that in 19 other countries. Included are only those countries from which adequate statistics on both alcohol consumption and population are available for recent years.

France heads the list, with a consumption of 6.53 U.S. gallons of absolute alcohol per person aged 15 years or older. Not only do the French drink more wine than any of the other people, but they also get more alcohol from distilled spirits.

Italy is next in consumption of total alcohol. As with the French, the main Italian alcoholic beverage is wine. Its wine consumption, however, is only about three-fourths the French

27

TABLE III

**APPARENT CONSUMPTION, IN 20 COUNTRIES, OF EACH MAJOR
BEVERAGE CLASS, AND OF ABSOLUTE ALCOHOL FROM EACH CLASS,
IN U.S. GALLONS PER PERSON IN THE DRINKING-AGE POPULATION***

(listed in descending order of total)

Country	Year**	Distilled Spirits	Absolute Alcohol	Wine	Absolute Alcohol	Beer	Absolute Alcohol	TOTAL Absolute Alcohol
1. France	1966	2.35	1.18	43.03	4.52	20.10^a	0.83	6.53
2. Italy	1968	[1.11]	0.55	41.29	3.30	3.54	0.16	4.01
3. Switzerland	1966	1.53	0.61	13.61	1.43	29.73^a	1.35	3.39
4. West Germany	1968	[2.35]	0.89	4.04	0.40	44.65	1.97	3.26
5. Australia	1966	0.54	0.31	2.58	0.44	42.86	2.14	2.89
6. Belgium	1967	0.67	0.33	3.14	0.44	42.07^a	2.10	2.87
7. U.S.A.	1970	2.56	1.15	1.84	0.29	25.95	1.17	2.61
8. New Zealand	1964	0.79	0.45	0.98	0.17	39.28	1.96	2.58
9. Czechoslovakia	1968	[0.83]	[0.42]	[3.51]	[0.49]	[30.91]	[1.54]	2.45
10. Canada	1967	[1.86]	0.75	[1.12]	0.18	[25.47]	1.27	2.20
11. Denmark	1968	0.78	0.34	1.53	0.22	29.03	1.38	1.94
12. United Kingdom	1966	0.51	0.29	1.08	0.18	31.77	1.43	1.90
13. Sweden	1968	2.13	0.85	1.77	0.24	15.57	0.65	1.74
14. Japan	1968	[1.10]	0.35	[5.10]^b	0.81	8.22	0.37	1.53
15. The Netherlands	1968	[1.38]	[0.69]	[0.86]	[0.15]	[15.38]	[0.69]	1.53
16. Ireland	1966	0.70	0.40	0.56	0.09	22.26	1.00	1.49
17. Norway	1968	1.20	0.52	0.70	0.10	10.82	0.51	1.13
18. Finland	1968	1.33	0.52	1.06	0.17	6.85	0.34	1.03
19. Iceland	1966	2.11	0.73	0.62	0.08	4.26	0.15	0.96
20. Israel	1968	0.89	0.44	1.66	0.20	3.58	0.18	0.82

NOTES: (a) Includes cider.   *(b) Includes saké.*   *[ ] Bracketed data converted from source terms.*

* *Age 15+*

** *Latest available year for each country.*

level, while the consumption of distilled spirits is less than half; beer is consumed at a rate less than one-sixth that in France.

The United States ranks seventh among the countries in total alcohol, but of the 20 on the list, it is the only country that comes close to France in drinking hard liquor. Wine consumption in the United States is comparatively low, however, and beer consumption is at a medium level.

At the bottom of the list is Israel, with an average annual consumption of only four-fifths of a U.S. gallon of absolute alcohol. Israel's position may come as no surprise, but the distribution of absolute alcohol among beverage types may be unexpected: More than half the Israeli consumption (0.44 U.S. gallon of absolute alcohol) is in the form of distilled spirits, not wine, as might have been anticipated; the remaining sources of absolute alcohol are almost equally divided between wine (0.20 gallon) and beer (0.18 gallon).

Also surprising may be the low rank of Ireland, in view of the high rate of alcoholism attributed to the Irish in America.* Yet that country is in 16th place in per person consumption of alcohol. Moreover, the average Irish consumption of distilled spirits is one-tenth lower than in Israel; of wine, it is one-half less. But the average Irishman consumes five times more beer than the average Israeli.

Some caution is necessary in evaluating these data: The time period is not the same for all the countries; the assignment of a uniform drinking age of 15 years is surely inaccurate; in some cases, the information about average alcohol content of beverages is not too certain. If the numbers are not treated as absolute but looked on as approximations, however, they are of reasonable use. The more regrettable feature of this table is the absence of many countries from which adequate information could not be obtained.

Nevertheless, the data reinforce cautions against simplistic explanations of alcohol problems. A people that drinks most of its alcohol in the form of distilled spirits may have a low rate of alcohol consumption and a low rate of problems. Yet another people with an almost equally low total alcohol consumption may have a high rate of problems; here the drinking is apparently being telescoped in few but extreme bouts.

France, the country ranking the highest in alcohol consumption, appears to have the highest rate of problems. Italy, the next ranking country, has an alcohol consumption more than fivefold that of Israel, the lowest and most trouble-free nation. Yet Italy appears to be relatively low on the problems scale and, in any case, has a much lower rate of alcohol problems than several countries with substantially lower alcohol consumptions.

SUMMARY AND CONCLUSION

The basic desired substance in alcoholic beverages is the chemical compound ethyl alcohol. The discovery of wine and beer and their purposeful production are prehistoric, and they were presumably adopted for their euphoriant as well as nutrient qualities. Ancient religious-ceremonial-medicinal uses of wine and beer became secularized and popular before classical times: Drunkenness, and apparently alcoholism, were reported as serious prob-

*See fig. 4, ch. II.

lems in the classical literatures. The historic attempts to cope with this problem by prohibitions and punitive laws were unsuccessful, but religious influence inculcated moderation or abstinence among some peoples, both long ago as well as relatively recently.

Beers and wines owed their historic popularity to their nutrient and medicinal properties as well as the euphoriant quality which made them useful in social intercourse and ceremonial solemnification. Distillation was popularized in Europe in the 16th century. The process removed all but the caloric nutrient values, but enhanced the much-desired pharmacological effects and the ease of achieving intoxication. In the 18th century, colonial America saw the start of a temperance movement, which had a public health as well as moralistic orientation aimed at reducing the common use of distilled spirits. By mid-19th century the movement had shifted its aims to opposing all drinking and outlawing the trade in alcoholic beverages. After numerous statewide prohibitions, national prohibition was instituted (1920), but repealed as a failure after 13 years.

In the United States, the proportion of drinkers (among adults aged 21 and over) rose from about 40 percent of women and 65 percent of men before World War II to over 60 percent of women and near 80 percent of men in recent years. Including youths (aged 15 and over) the number of drinkers in 1970 is estimated at 95,648,000. These drinkers consumed an average of 3.93 gallons of absolute alcohol per year in 1969–1970; about 45 percent was obtained from distilled spirits, 45 percent from beer, and 10 percent from wine. Total alcohol consumption, divided among the drinking-age population (15 and over), did not change greatly during the century before 1960 (although prohibition-time consumption is unknown). But a huge shift occurred—from a slight to a substantial proportion of beer rather than whiskey—during the latter half of the 19th century. In the past decade, a rise of nearly 20 percent in consumption of absolute alcohol has apparently occurred. The consumption data are incomplete because the contributions of nontax-paid sources are unknown, and the rise may reflect only substitution for declining moonshine and home production.

Division of the national alcohol consumption among a mythical average in the drinking-age or actual-drinker population, however, tends to mask certain facts: Men drink three times as much as women; alcoholic persons drink 11 times as much as others; there are huge differences between States and regions both in quantities consumed and preferences for beer, wine, or spirits. Finally, alcohol consumption compared in 20 countries shows France highest in consumption—and highest in spirits as well as wine, and medium in beer; Italy next but high only in wine; the United States in seventh position, second highest in spirits but medium in beer and low in wine.

From the differences in proportions of drinkers and abstainers both in age groups and over time, differences in consumption of alcohol from various beverage classes by different groups in different countries and in regions and States in the United States, and reported differences in rates of alcohol-related troubles, it is inferred that sufficient alcohol can produce troubles anywhere, but neither the proportions of drinkers nor the kinds of beverages are as important as the patterns and purposes of drinking. The patterns and purposes, as well as the actual consumption by various demographic groups, need to be studied in other countries as well as across the United States, including the contributions of moonshine and homemade beverages. These facts need to be compared with appropriate measures of relevant problems.

The ethnic diversity that enriches the American culture may well serve as a prototype for investigating differing predispositions to alcoholism. For, although researchers have thus far failed to identify a genetic, physiological, or environmental cause of alcoholism, cross-cultural studies have determined that the condition is widespread among certain cultural groups and virtually unknown among others.

The rate of alcoholism, for example, has been shown to be low in groups whose drinking-related customs, values, and sanctions are widely known, established, and congruent with other cultural values. On the other hand, alcoholism rates are higher in those populations where ambivalence about alcohol is marked. Apparently, in cultures which use alcohol but have a low incidence of alcoholism, people drink in a definite pattern. The beverage is sipped slowly, consumed with food, taken in the company of others—all in relaxing, comfortable circumstances. Drinking is taken for granted. No emotional rewards are reaped by the man who shows prowess of consumption. Intoxication is abhorred. Other cultures with a high incidence of alcohol-related problems usually assign a special significance to drinking. Alcohol use is surrounded with attitudes of ambivalence and guilt. Maladaptive drinking, drinking without food, and intoxication are common.

31

We all tend to learn patterns of behavior and preferred coping mechanisms from our parents and the "significant others" in our lives. The guilt that so many families feel about their own drinking behavior is reflected in society's attitudes. Ours is a Nation that is ambivalent about its alcohol use. This confusion has deterred us from creating a National climate that encourages responsible attitudes toward drinking for those who choose to drink; that is, using alcohol in a way which does not harm oneself or society.

Too often, in our attempt to solve human problems, we gravitate toward simplistic answers to deal with complicated issues. Certainly most cultures that have tried, have failed to persuade all people to give up the consumption of alcoholic beverages.

Our goal recognizes the right of each individual to exercise his time on this planet as he sees fit, provided he does not harm others. At the same time, the National Institute on Alcohol Abuse and Alcoholism aims to help private nonprofit and public agencies reach out to offer the alcoholic individual the help we have every reason to believe that he wants . . . that he will accept . . . and that he will utilize. In addition, we seek to develop ways to identify the potential alcoholic person, and to devise ways to circumvent unhealthy use of alcohol.

REFERENCES

(1) Bacon, M. and Jones, M.B. Teen-age Drinking. New York: Crowell, 1968.

(2) Bacon, S.D. The classic temperance movement of the U.S.A.; Impact today on attitudes, action and research. Brit. J. Addict. 62:5–18, 1967.

(3) Baird, E.G. The alcohol problem and the law. Quart. J. Stud. Alc. 4:535–556, 1944; 5:126–161, 1944; 6:335–383, 1945; 7:110–162, 271–296, 1946; 9:80–118, 1948.

(4) Bales, R.F. Cultural differences in rates of alcoholism. Quart. J. Stud. Alc. 6:480–499, 1946.

(5) Cahalan, D., Cisin, I.H., and Crossley, H.M. American Drinking Practices; A National Study of Drinking Behavior and Attitudes. Monograph No. 6. New Brunswick, N.J.: Rutgers Center of Alcohol Studies, 1969.

(6) Carstairs, G.M. Daru and bhang; Cultural factors in the choice of intoxicant. Quart. J. Stud. Alc. 15:220–237, 1954.

(7) Coffey, T.G. Beer Street: Gin Lane; Some views of 18th-century drinking. Quart. J. Stud. Alc. 27:669–692, 1966.

(8) Dajani, R.M., Ghandour-Mnaymneh, L. and Saadeh, F. Effect of the congeners in

araq on the incidence of alcoholic fatty liver in the rat. Quart. J. Stud. Alc., Suppl. No. 5, 1970, pp. 34–49.

(9) Der Freudenleere (pseud.; before 1284). Der Wiener Mervart. (The ocean cruise of the Viennese.) In: von der Hagen, F.H., ed., Gesammtabenteuer. (Global adventure.) Stuttgart: 1850.

(10) Efron, V. and Keller, M. Selected Statistics on Consumption of Alcohol (1850–1968) and on Alcoholism (1930–1968) New Brunswick, N.J.: Publications Division, Rutgers Center of Alcohol Studies, 1970.

(11) Franck, S. Von dem grewlichen laster der trunckenheyt. (On the horrible vice of drunkenness.) Ulm; 1531.

(12) Goodenough, E.R. Jewish Symbols in the Greco-Roman Period. Vol. 5, Fish, Bread and Wine. New York: Pantheon, 1956.

(13) Jellinek, E.M. Recent trends in alcoholism and in alcohol consumption. Quart. J. Stud. Alc. 8:1–42, 1947.

(14) Jellinek, E.M. Distributions of alcohol consumption and of calories derived from alcohol in various selected populations. Proc. Nutr. Soc. 14:93–97, 1955.

(15) Keller, M. Alcohol in health and disease: Some historical perspectives. Ann. N.Y. Acad. Sci. 133:820–827, 1966.

(16) Keller, M. The great Jewish drink mystery. Brit. J. Addict. 64:287–296, 1970.

(17) Keller, M. and McCormick, M. A Dictionary of Words about Alcohol. (Introduction.) New Brunswick, N.J.: Publications Division, Rutgers Center of Alcohol Studies, 1968.

(18) Kramer, S.N. From the tablets of Sumer. In: Medicine: The First Pharmacopoeia. Indian Hills, Colo.: Falcon's Wing Press, 1956, pp. 56–60.

(19) Loeb, E.M. Primitive intoxicants. Quart. J. Stud. Alc. 4:387–398, 1943.

(20) McCarthy, R.G. and Douglass, E.M. Alcohol and Social Responsibility––A New Educational Approach. New York: Crowell, 1949.

(21) McKinlay, A.P. Bacchus as health-giver. Quart. J. Stud. Alc. 11:230–246, 1950.

(22) McKinlay, A.P. New light on the question of Homeric temperance. Quart. J. Stud. Alc. 14:78–93, 1953.

(23) Maddox, G.L. and McCall, B.C. Drinking among Teenagers; A Sociological Interpretation of Alcohol Use by High-School Students. Monograph No. 4. New Brunswick, N.J.: Rutgers Center of Alcohol Studies, 1964.

(24) Midgley, J. Drinking and attitudes toward drinking in a Muslim community. Quart. J. Stud. Alc. 32:148–158, 1971.

(25) Moore, M. Chinese wine; Some notes on its social use. Quart. J. Stud. Alc. 9:270–279, 1948.

(26) Mulford, H.A. Drinking and deviant drinking, U.S.A., 1963. Quart. J. Stud. Alc. 25:634–650, 1964.

(27) Nashe, T. (1567–1601) Pierce Penilesse. In: McKerrow, R.B., ed., The Works of Thomas Nashe, London: Bullen, 1904–1910.

33

(28) Platt, B.S. Some traditional alcoholic beverages and their importance in indigenous African communities. Proc. Nutr. Soc. 14:115–124, 1955.

(29) Ravi Varma, L.A. Alcoholism in Ayurveda. Quart. J. Stud. Alc. 11:484–491, 1950.

(30) Riley, J.W., Jr. and Marden, C.R. The social pattern of alcoholic drinking. Quart. J. Stud. Alc. 8:265–273, 1947.

(31) Roueche, B. The Neutral Spirit. A Portrait of Alcohol. Boston: Little, Brown, 1960.

(32) Rush, B. An Inquiry into the Effects of Ardent Spirits upon the Human Body and Mind; With an Account of the Means of Preventing and of the Remedies for Curing Them. (1785) Brookfield: Merriam, 8th ed., 1814.

(33) Skelton, J. (1460?–1529) The Tunnying of Elynour Rummyng. In: Dyce, A., ed., The Poetical works of John Skelton. London: Rodd, 1843.

(34) Snyder, C.R. Alcohol and the Jews; A Cultural Study of Drinking and Sobriety. Monograph No. 1. New Brunswick, N.J.: Rutgers Center of Alcohol Studies, 1958.

(35) St. Basil the Great. Slovo Svyatogo velikogo Vassiliya o tom, kak podobayet vzderzhatsya ot p'yanstva. (The sermon of St. Basil the Great on how it is seemly to abstain from drunkenness.) From the Collection of the Moral Sermons and Admonitions of the Twelfth Century of the Trinity-St. Sergius Monastery. Reprinted in: Ponomareff, A.I. Pamyatniki drevne-russkoi tzerkovno-uchitel'noi literatury. (Monumenta of the Ancient Russian Instructional Church Literature.) St. Petersburg: Strannik, 1897.

(36) Webb, S. and Webb, B. The History of Liquor Licensing in England, Principally from 1700 to 1830. London: Longmans, Green, 1903.

(37) Winkler, A.M. Drinking on the American frontier. Quart. J. Stud. Alc. 29:413–445, 1968.

(38) Zeitlin, S. The Rise and Fall of the Jewish State. Philadelphia: Jewish Publication Society of America, 1962–1969.

34

Chapter II

EXTENT AND PATTERNS
OF USE AND ABUSE
OF ALCOHOL

ALCOHOLISM IS CONSIDERED by many drug experts to be a more significant problem than all other forms of drug abuse combined (21). Yet alcohol differs from most other drugs because of its accepted uses in so many different contexts—as a thirst-quencher, as an adjunct to gracious living, as a social lubricant, as a food, as a medicine, as an intoxicant, as a psychedelic agent, or as a symbol of defying authority.

Two-thirds of American adults drink, so adult drinking is normal behavior in most circles. Whether a person drinks at all, how much, and why are closely tied in with sociocultural factors. Heavy drinking, and the alcohol-related problems usually associated with heavy drinking, also frequently bring into play certain social and personality variables.

For these reasons, the correlates of both the mere use of alcohol, and the use of alcohol to the point where it produces problems, were considered separately in three national surveys of drinking behavior of U.S. adults, aged 21 and over, conducted by the social research group of the George Washington University. The final analyses of these surveys are now being completed at the School of Public Health at the University of California at Berkeley. Most of the findings in this chapter are drawn from these three surveys:

- A 1964–65 survey, published in "American Drinking Practices" and hereafter referred to as ADP, measured drinking practices and attitudes among 2,746 persons representing the adult household population of the United States (8).

  Two additional surveys measured and analyzed the prevalence of various types of alcohol-related problems among adults:
- A 1967 followup of the ADP survey studied a subsample of 1,359 adult men and women (9).
- A 1969 survey studied a subsample of men aged 21 to 59 (10).

These latter two surveys also provided a total of 1,561 interviews for analysis of the group—men aged 21 to 59—who stand the greatest risk of incurring problems related to heavy drinking.

Some additional information is available from a Harris survey (20) made as recently as November 1971 on behalf of the National Institute on Alcohol Abuse and Alcoholism. Although the results of this last survey are as yet only incompletely analyzed, the preliminary data for the most part appear to confirm those in the earlier surveys, thus filling out the picture of the drinking practices of American adults. They also suggest some new areas of interest and understanding. Comparisons between the Harris and other surveys must be treated as tentative, however, especially since Harris included the population aged 18 and over, while the others studied only those aged 21 and over.

DRINKING PRACTICES
AND ATTITUDES

As figure 1 shows, the ADP survey found that 68 percent of the adult population drink at least once a year: 77 percent of the men and 60 percent of the women, but not all of these people are regular drinkers. When the infrequent drinkers and abstainers are added together, the adult population is rather evenly divided between the 47 percent who drink less than once a month, and the 53 percent who drink once a month or more.

The survey found that of the 32 percent abstainers, one-third used to drink but had stopped, while two-thirds never had any alcoholic beverages at all. Heavy drinkers made up 12 percent of the sample studied; one-fifth of the adult men and one-twentieth of the adult women in the sample were heavy drinkers.

32% of the total adult population are abstainers. The remaining 68% drink at least once a year, with 12% of all adults classified as heavy drinkers.

77% of adult men and 60% of adult women drink at least once a year, with 21% of all men and 5% of all women classified as heavy drinkers.

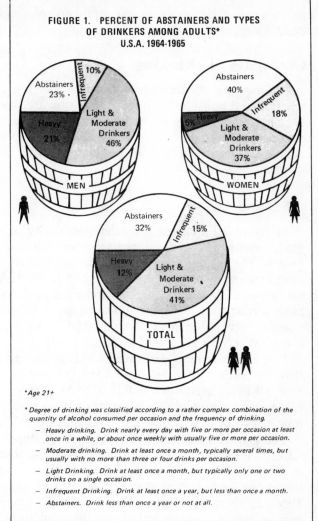

FIGURE 1.   PERCENT OF ABSTAINERS AND TYPES
OF DRINKERS AMONG ADULTS*
U.S.A. 1964-1965

*Age 21+

* Degree of drinking was classified according to a rather complex combination of the
quantity of alcohol consumed per occasion and the frequency of drinking.

  – Heavy drinking. Drink nearly every day with five or more per occasion at least
     once in a while, or about once weekly with usually five or more per occasion.

  – Moderate drinking. Drink at least once a month, typically several times, but
     usually with no more than three or four drinks per occasion.

  – Light Drinking. Drink at least once a month, but typically only one or two
     drinks on a single occasion.

  – Infrequent Drinking. Drink at least once a year, but less than once a month.

  – Abstainers. Drink less than once a year or not at all.

Mulford, 1964, and Gallup, 1966, reported similar proportions of drinkers and nondrinkers (1, 31).

The ADP and Gallup surveys found that a much larger proportion of younger women drank than was true of women over 50. The ADP findings also parallel Gallup data indicating that the proportion of drinkers in the adult population has increased somewhat since World War II, particularly among women. Further studies are needed to clarify the circumstances that bring about

37

increases and decreases in the numbers of drinkers and heavy drinkers in the United States.

Correlates of Drinking

Among the sociocultural factors that are associated with whether and how much a person will drink are: sex and age; ethnic background; religious affiliation; socioeconomic level; education; occupation; degree of urbanization; and behavioral factors such as childhood experiences and association with drinkers or nondrinkers.

Sex and Age

In figure 2, it can be seen that a majority of men in each age group up to 65 years of age reported drinking at least once a month. The highest proportion of heavy drinkers (30 percent) was found among men aged 30 to 34 and 45 to 49. Half or more of the women in each group either did not drink at all, or drank less than once a month. The highest proportion of heavy drinkers among women occurred at ages 21 to 24 and 45 to 49, and constituted about 10 percent in each of these age groups.

The Harris survey data are in substantial agreement showing that 76 percent of those aged 18 to 29 and 71 percent of those aged 30 to 49 are drinkers. But only 58 percent of those aged 50 to 64 and a minority (45 percent) of those aged 65 and over were reported to be drinkers (20).

The greater proportion of drinkers in younger age groups may reflect the recent decline in attitudes favoring abstinence, as noted in chapter I. But, in part, it may also reflect a trend observed by Glenn and Zody (19) in their analysis of Gallup data from 1945 to 1960. In these studies, it was consistently found that, in all age groups over a 15-year period, people tend to quit drinking with advancing age.

Ethnic Background

The United States no longer is a melting pot of recent immigrants. Fathers of three-fourths of the adults interviewed in the survey were born in this country. Nevertheless, ethnic background is still important in determining patterns of American life, including drinking habits.

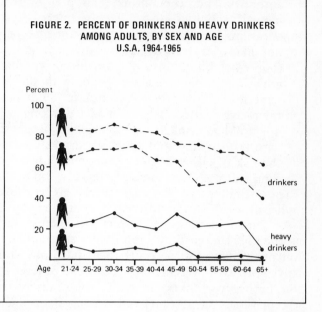

Among both men and women, the percent of drinkers tends to decline with age.

The highest percent of heavy drinkers (30%) was found among men aged 30 to 34 and 45 to 49. In contrast, the highest percent of heavy drinkers among women came to only about 10% and occurred at ages 21 to 24 and 45 to 49.

FIGURE 2. PERCENT OF DRINKERS AND HEAVY DRINKERS AMONG ADULTS, BY SEX AND AGE U.S.A. 1964-1965

ADP survey findings are generally congruent with the hypothesis that the rate of alcoholism will tend to be low among groups whose drinking customs, values, and sanctions are well-established, known, and agreed upon by all the group members, and integrated with the rest of the culture. The rate of alcoholism, on the other hand, will tend to be high in groups with marked ambivalence toward alcohol.

Lolli and associates (28) found that first-generation Italians in the United States, just as natives in Italy, drink frequently but have low rates of alcohol-related problems. Subsequent generations of Italian Americans have higher rates of heavier drinking (23).

There are many reports of high rates of alcoholism among Irish Americans (4, 18) although, as noted in chapter I, Ireland rates 16th in apparent consumption of alcohol among the 20 countries reported.

Thus no correlation necessarily exists between widespread drinking and a high incidence of alcohol-related problems. As Blum (7) puts it:

When drinking is part of an institutionalized set of behaviors which includes important other people in roles of

39

authority and when drinking is part of ritualized or ceremonial activities (e.g., family meals, festivals, religious occasions, etc.) as opposed to leisure time or private use, it is not likely to be associated with high individual variability (unpredictability, loss of control) in conduct nor with the growth of drug dependency nor with the judgment by observers of "abuse" or "alcoholism." Further, when parents themselves reflect safe or model drinking behavior (i.e., are not problem drinkers), when drinking occurs shortly before or with food taking, and when the drinks used are wine or beer, the risk of either long- or short-term adverse effects are quite slim. Adverse effects nevertheless can still occur.

These findings of the ADP survey are consistent with earlier studies of sociocultural differences in drinking behavior.

As shown in figure 3, respondents whose fathers were born outside the United States reported a substantially higher proportion of drinkers (80 percent) than did those whose fathers were native-born (64 percent). However, the difference in the proportion of heavy drinkers in each group was relatively small (15 percent versus 11 percent) and, among all drinkers, the difference was negligible.

Figure 4 shows that, when standardized for age level, those whose fathers were born in Ireland had the highest proportion of drinkers (93 percent) as well as the highest proportion of heavy drinkers (33 percent) within the drinking population. Those whose fathers came from Latin America or the Caribbean had the lowest

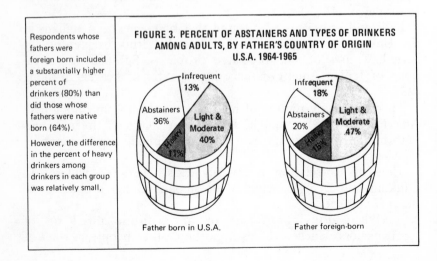

Respondents whose fathers were foreign born included a substantially higher percent of drinkers (80%) than did those whose fathers were native born (64%).

However, the difference in the percent of heavy drinkers among drinkers in each group was relatively small,

FIGURE 3. PERCENT OF ABSTAINERS AND TYPES OF DRINKERS AMONG ADULTS, BY FATHER'S COUNTRY OF ORIGIN U.S.A. 1964-1965

Infrequent 13%
Abstainers 36%
Light & Moderate 40%
Heavy 11%
Father born in U.S.A.

Infrequent 18%
Abstainers 20%
Light & Moderate 47%
Heavy 15%
Father foreign-born

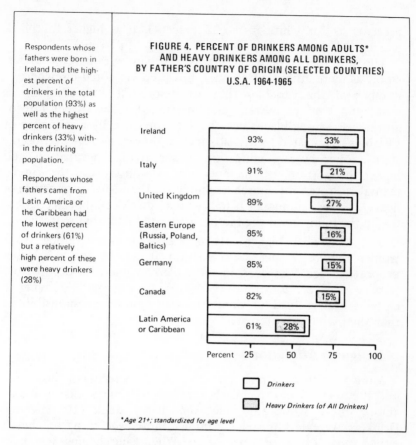

Respondents whose fathers were born in Ireland had the highest percent of drinkers in the total population (93%) as well as the highest percent of heavy drinkers (33%) within the drinking population.

Respondents whose fathers came from Latin America or the Caribbean had the lowest percent of drinkers (61%) but a relatively high percent of these were heavy drinkers (28%)

FIGURE 4. PERCENT OF DRINKERS AMONG ADULTS*
AND HEAVY DRINKERS AMONG ALL DRINKERS,
BY FATHER'S COUNTRY OF ORIGIN (SELECTED COUNTRIES)
U.S.A. 1964-1965

Ireland 93% 33%

Italy 91% 21%

United Kingdom 89% 27%

Eastern Europe (Russia, Poland, Baltics) 85% 16%

Germany 85% 15%

Canada 82% 15%

Latin America or Caribbean 61% 28%

Percent 25 50 75 100

☐ Drinkers

▢ Heavy Drinkers (of All Drinkers)

*Age 21+; standardized for age level

proportion of drinkers (61 percent), but a relatively large proportion of those who drank were heavy drinkers (28 percent).

National surveys have not found great differences in rates of drinking between whites and blacks, in the aggregate. The ADP survey found a higher proportion of black abstainers (38 percent) compared to whites (31 percent), but a slightly higher proportion of heavy drinkers among those blacks who drink. The Harris survey also found a higher proportion of abstainers (42 percent) among the blacks, taken as a group.

A sharper ethnic difference emerges if the sexes are analyzed separately. More white than black men are abstainers, but the difference is slight: 23 percent versus 21 percent. On the other hand, more black than white women are abstainers, but here the difference is considerable—51 percent versus 39 percent. While the proportion of heavy drinkers is about the same for black men (19

41

percent) as for white men (22 percent), it is higher for black women (11 percent) than for white women (4 percent).

The differences between blacks and whites cannot be understood as mere ethnic differences, however. As noted elsewhere, a number of the variables that are associated with drinking or abstaining tend to overlap and intermingle. The higher rate of abstinence among blacks may be accounted for by a piling up of variables associated with abstinence—lower average economic status, lower average education, lower average occupation, and higher proportion of membership in conservative or fundamentalist Protestant churches. Similarly, the higher proportion of heavy drinkers among all blacks who do drink could be accounted for by the piling up of the factors associated with that pattern.

The somewhat higher rate of heavy drinkers among black women requires a special explanation. It may be due to a higher proportion being engaged in particularly vulnerable occupations (service jobs) or, as some investigators have suggested, having to carry a heavier load of domestic and economic responsibilities than their white counterparts.

Religious Affiliation

More than twice as high a proportion (22 percent) of those who said they never went to church were heavy drinkers, than was true among those who said they went every week (10 percent). Drinkers were less prevalent among those who went to church either most often or least often. When churchgoing was held constant, however, the proportion of heavy drinkers was higher among Catholics than among liberal Protestants, and higher among the latter than among conservative or fundamentalist Protestants.

Catholics had above-average proportions of both drinkers (83 percent) and heavy drinkers (19 percent). Among those who drank, slightly less than one-fourth were heavy drinkers.

Compared to other religious groups, the more conservative or fundamentalist Protestant denominations had relatively low proportions of drinkers (52 percent) and heavy drinkers (7 percent).

Jews and Episcopalians had higher proportions of drinkers (slightly more than 90 percent) than any other religious groups. They also had relatively low proportions of heavy drinkers (slightly more than 10 percent), both within the total population and among drinkers themselves.

Socioeconomic Status

As shown in figure 5, when considered in terms of age, sex, and socioeconomic level, the proportion of drinkers was highest (88 percent) among young men aged 21 to 39 in the highest socioeconomic group. It was lowest (34 percent) among women over 60 years of age in the lowest socioeconomic level. The lower level groups, in both sexes, had smaller proportions of light and moderate drinkers than did the higher level groups, but the proportion of heavy drinkers among all adults was about the same at all levels.

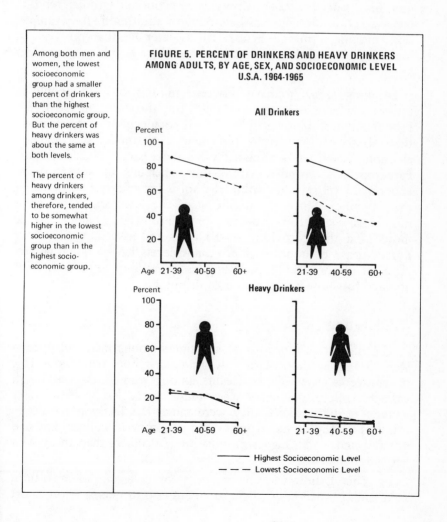

Among both men and women, the lowest socioeconomic group had a smaller percent of drinkers than the highest socioeconomic group. But the percent of heavy drinkers was about the same at both levels.

The percent of heavy drinkers among drinkers, therefore, tended to be somewhat higher in the lowest socioeconomic group than in the highest socioeconomic group.

FIGURE 5. PERCENT OF DRINKERS AND HEAVY DRINKERS AMONG ADULTS, BY AGE, SEX, AND SOCIOECONOMIC LEVEL U.S.A. 1964-1965

All Drinkers

Percent

Age 21-39   40-59   60+

Percent   Heavy Drinkers

Age 21-39   40-59   60+

——— Highest Socioeconomic Level
— — — Lowest Socioeconomic Level

Among the drinkers themselves, the proportion of heavy drinkers tended to be somewhat higher at the lower socioeconomic levels. Relatively more well-to-do and middle-class people reported drinking at least occasionally, but few of those who did drink were heavy drinkers.

A larger proportion of those of higher socioeconomic levels started drinking later in life, and also continued drinking to a more advanced age, than was true among those at lower levels. This finding is consistent with the general age differential in the phasing of various activities among socioeconomic groups noted by Kinsey and his associates (24). Upper socioeconomic groups tend to initiate certain activities associated with adulthood—for example, sex, smoking, drinking—at a relatively later age than do those of lower status, and then tend to continue these activities to an older age.

Drinking seems to have different implications for people in lower socioeconomic groups than for those in higher levels. Proportionately more people of high socioeconomic levels drink than those of low levels, but they drink moderately and see alcoholic beverages as a relatively harmless part of their lifestyles. Paradoxically, proportionately more persons of lower socioeconomic level say they think alcohol is harmful to themselves or their families. Since the wellbeing of the lower-status person is more easily jeopardized by any untoward event, alcohol may be more of a threat to him. As Knupfer and associates (25) have noted, those of upper socioeconomic levels have a much greater range of options in life, including less possibility of being fired or arrested for showing the effects of drinking.

Education

The highest proportions of abstainers among men and women were found in those with only grammar-school education. This difference is especially noticeable among women. And although women college graduates were much more likely than other women to be drinkers, they were much less likely to be heavy drinkers if they drank. Women who had gone to college, but had not finished, had a higher proportion of drinkers than those who had graduated.

In general, however, the majority of college graduates—both men and women—were light or moderate drinkers. Those most likely to be heavy drinkers were men who had completed high school and men who did not finish college.

Occupation

Figure 6 shows that farm owners had the lowest proportion of drinkers (60 percent of men and 26 percent of women); they also showed the lowest proportion of heavy drinkers (20 percent of men and practically no women). About 80 percent of men whose main occupations were in the professional and business fields reported they were drinkers, with the businessmen having a higher proportion of heavy drinkers among drinkers (30 percent) than the professionals (18 percent). Of the men who drank, semiprofessionals had the highest proportion of heavy drinkers (38 percent). Of the women who drank, service workers had the highest proportion of heavy drinkers (17 percent).

Residence

Geographical differences in drinking were considerable. The highest proportion of both drinkers and heavy drinkers were found in the Middle Atlantic, New England, Pacific, and East North Central areas—all relatively more urban in population than the rest of the Nation. The lowest proportion of drinkers were in the East South Central States, followed by other southern areas and the Mountain States. Factors which affect the high rate of abstinence in the South include its less urban character and its higher proportion of members of conservative Protestant denominations whose tenets forbid drinking.

Large cities had the highest proportion of drinkers, a finding also noted by Riley and Marden (35) and Mulford (31). The proportion of drinkers ranged from only 43 percent among farm residents to 87 percent among those living in large suburbs of 50,000 to 1 million population in metropolitan areas. Among drinkers, the highest rate of heavy drinkers was found among residents of the largest inner cities.

These regional findings are consistent with Malzberg's (30) analysis of admission rates to hospitals for alcoholic psychosis.

Behavioral Variables

Parental approval of drinking was generally correlated with the proportion of drinkers. Younger persons and those of higher

Farm owners had the lowest percent of drinkers (60% of men and 26% of women) and also the lowest percent of heavy drinkers (20% of men and practically no women) among those who drank.

FIGURE 6. PERCENT OF DRINKERS AMONG ADULTS* AND HEAVY DRINKERS AMONG ALL DRINKERS, BY OCCUPATION AND SEX U.S.A. 1964-1965**

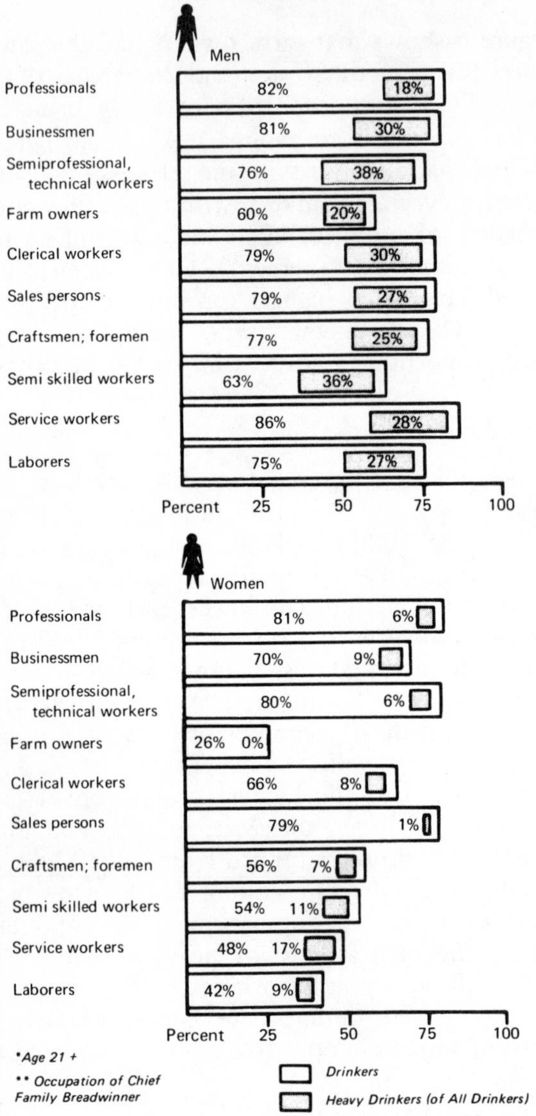

Men
Professionals 82% 18%
Businessmen 81% 30%
Semiprofessional, technical workers 76% 38%
Farm owners 60% 20%
Clerical workers 79% 30%
Sales persons 79% 27%
Craftsmen; foremen 77% 25%
Semi skilled workers 63% 36%
Service workers 86% 28%
Laborers 75% 27%
Percent 25 50 75 100
Women
Professionals 81% 6%
Businessmen 70% 9%
Semiprofessional, technical workers 80% 6%
Farm owners 26% 0%
Clerical workers 66% 8%
Sales persons 79% 1%
Craftsmen; foremen 56% 7%
Semi skilled workers 54% 11%
Service workers 48% 17%
Laborers 42% 9%
Percent 25 50 75 100
Drinkers
Heavy Drinkers (of All Drinkers)

*Age 21 +

** Occupation of Chief Family Breadwinner

socioeconomic levels tended to have greater proportions of parents who drank frequently and who approved of drinking than did older people and people in the lower socioeconomic levels. Heavy drinking by women was closely correlated with heavy drinking by their husbands, and vice versa.

People drank most often with friends (including those from work), next most often with family members, and least often by themselves. In general, alcoholic beverages were served more often when people met socially with co-workers than when they were with their close friends. Although heavy drinkers were more likely than other drinkers to say that they drank alone, less than one-fourth said they drank alone fairly often. Thus even heavy drinking tends to be social drinking, and self-reports of solitary heavy drinking are relatively rare.

What Do People Drink?

Wine was consumed at least once a year by four out of 10 persons, but only 1 percent of the total adult population were heavy drinkers of wine. Half of the respondents drank beer at least once a year; 7 percent were heavy beer drinkers. Distilled spirits (either straight or in mixed drinks) were consumed by 57 percent of the respondents at least once a year; 6 percent were heavy drinkers of distilled spirits. One-fourth said they drank all three classes of beverages at least once a year.

Compared with the other two classes of beverages, wine was consumed relatively more often by women, by moderate than by heavy drinkers, by persons of upper socioeconomic level, by residents of the wine-producing Pacific and Middle Atlantic States, and by people living in the larger suburbs. Beer was consumed more often by men, by an above-average proportion of the heavier drinkers, and by younger persons. Distilled spirits were consumed by men in their thirties and forties, and women in their twenties, by relatively more of the heavier drinkers, and by persons of upper socioeconomic status.

Attitudes toward Drinking

About equal proportions of respondents mentioned favorable and unfavorable effects of drinking. Two-thirds, however, said they did not recall any particular effects from their own drinking during the last year. This implies that many drinkers do not think

PROFILE ANALYSIS
OF TYPES OF
DRINKERS

Comparisons among the four types of drinkers' practices that were analyzed in the ADP survey, reveal:

—Compared with both light and heavy drinkers, abstainers were more likely to be older people and lower than average in socioeconomic level. Relatively more abstainers lived in the South and in rural areas, had native-born parents, belonged to conservative or fundamentalist Protestant denominations, and took part in religious activities frequently.

—Compared with other groups, heavy drinkers reported more drinking by parents and friends. Heavy drinkers also found drinking helpful to relieve depression.

—Compared with other groups, heavy drinkers restainers and heavy drinkers tended to be somewhat more alienated from society and more unhappy with their lot in life.

of themselves as drinking primarily for the effect of alcohol. Nevertheless 9 percent of all drinkers in the ADP survey reported that they worried about their own drinking. This is matched by the finding of the Harris survey that 10 percent worry they drink too much.

Ambivalent attitudes toward alcohol may be discerned in two ADP findings:

- Three-fourths of the sample (including a majority of male heavy drinkers) said they thought drinking "does more harm than good."
- Three-fourths of the sample regarded alcoholism as a serious public health problem in the United States.

Of possible great significance for the measurement of serious alcohol abuse and alcoholism is the Harris finding that 6 percent of drinkers said they sometimes have trouble stopping drinking, or drink more than they had intended. These are classical Jellinek indicators of loss of control over drinking and, hence, possible signs of alcoholism (22). This finding correlates with currently accepted estimates of the rate of alcohol addiction in the United States (16).

ALCOHOL-RELATED PROBLEMS

Until recent years, most of the research on the consequences of excessive drinking focused on the characteristics of institutionalized persons or those labeled as "alcoholics." The primary usefulness of such research has been to document the fact that heavy use of alcohol tends to shorten life and to lead to medical complications and alcoholic psychoses (14, 29, 33).

But the study of institutionalized persons cannot provide conclusive evidence regarding either the sociocultural or personality characteristics of drinkers in the broader population, or dependable information on the processes through which moderate drinking may evolve into heavy drinking. In his analysis of five groups of alcoholic persons or clinic patients Room (37) found "remarkably wide and somewhat consistent variations in purported prevalences (of symptoms) from one sample to another." He also cites the conclusions of other investigators that the number and kind of symptoms are dependent upon the nature of the institution or clinic serving the patient, as well as on the motives of the alcoholic persons when responding to questions about their backgrounds and symptoms (22, 41).

Another factor in the reliability of generalizing from institutionalized or officially labeled alcoholic persons is the tendency for physicians to be more willing to recognize lower class patients as "alcoholics" (5, 43). In addition, while the problems in recognized alcoholic persons are easily seen and well-known, the general population of alcoholic individuals has less visible problems of a health, social, and psychological nature. But the chief reason that data on institutionalized alcoholic patients cannot be generalized to the total population is the fact that the downhill process toward institutionalization ordinarily takes many years. For these reasons, it is impossible to use piecemeal statistics based on institutionalized alcoholic patients or on the skid row population to arrive at valid estimates of people with alcohol-related problems within the population as a whole.

A number of epidemiological studies and clinical observations have focused on identifying persons with potential, subtle, and actual alcohol-related problems (3, 11, 12, 26, 32). The 1967 and 1969 studies described in this chapter built on a number of these studies, focusing on measuring the degree of severity of 11 problems—all compatible with the Knupfer definition of "a problem—any problem—connected fairly closely with drinking . . ." (26).

The studies took into account the following variables:

- Severity of problems, where relevant, in terms of the frequency and degree of the problem as, for example, the number of times the person has had trouble with police over his drinking.
- Certainty or reliability of measurement in terms of the number of items or indicators of a problem. Thus a person who was scored as having drinking problems vis-a-vis his wife on five items was given a higher score than if the problem were reflected in positive responses on only two items.
- Immediacy of problems in terms of whether the problem had occurred during the last 3 years or before.

The following is a description of the 11 problem categories used:

Frequent intoxication was measured by the amount respondents drank on an occasion, the frequency with which they drank fairly large amounts, and their reports of how often they got "high" or "tight." A high score on this potential problem was attained by drinking a minimum of five or more drinks at least once a week, and eight or more drinks on one of the most recent two drinking occasions and twice in the last 2 months, or 12 or more drinks on one of the last two occasions and twice in the last year, or currently getting high or tight at least once a week. While fairly heavy drinking may not by itself constitute a problem, a high level of alcohol intake was included as a potential problem so that later analyses could be made of the extent to which heavy intake leads to demonstrable health or interpersonal problems.

Binge drinking consisted of being intoxicated for at least several days at a time, or for 2 days on more than one occasion. (Binge drinking is one manifestation of Jellinek's "loss of control over drinking" concept, and indicative of alcoholism.)

Symptomatic drinking refers to signs of Jellinek's gamma alcoholism. It includes exhibition of signs attributed to physical dependence and loss of control—for example, drinking to get rid of a hangover, having difficulty in stopping drinking, blackouts or lapses of memory, skipping meals while drinking, tossing down drinks for quicker effect, or sneaking drinks.

Psychological dependence on alcohol included drinking to alleviate depression or nervousness or to escape from the problems of everyday living.

50

Problems with spouse or relatives included the spouse leaving, threatening to leave, or becoming concerned over the person's drinking; or the spouse or relative asking the drinker to cut down; or the person himself judging his drinking as having had a harmful effect on his home life. Trouble with spouse or relatives was usually accompanied by other drinking problems, and persons with a high score on spouse-or-relatives trouble had an average of 2.4 additional problems related to drinking.

Problems with friends or neighbors included the report that friends or neighbors had suggested the drinker cut down, or that he himself felt his drinking had been harmful to his friendships and social life.

Job problems consisted of losing or nearly losing a job because of drinking, having coworkers suggest that one cut down on drinking, or rating oneself as having harmed one's work opportunities through drinking.

Problems with law, police, accidents included reporting trouble with the law over drinking after driving, overdrinking, or drinking contributing to an accident in which there was personal injury.

Health problems were based on reports that drinking had been harmful to health and also that a physician had advised the person to cut down.

Financial problems were based on reports that drinking had harmed the respondent's finances during the prior 3 years.

Belligerence associated with drinking included either feeling aggressive or cross, or getting into a fight or heated argument after drinking.

Association of Alcohol-Related Problems With Demographic Variables

Both the 1967 and 1969 surveys analyzed a variety of demographic variables assumed to have existed, for the most part, before the development of adult drinking habits. These variables included: Family status; geographic region and urbanization; ethnicity; religion; and socioeconomic status. While some persons do change their religion or social class, particularly in societies characterized as "open," changes in status on most of these variables are less common than the maintenance of stability. Only longitudinal studies can determine which came first—changes in the demographic variables or changes in drinking behavior. Until such longitudinal studies have been concluded, the demographic

51

PROFILE ANALYSIS
OF PERSONS WITH
HIGH PROBLEM RATES

The highest rates of alcohol-related problems in the aggregate for men aged 21 to 59 were found among:
—Men under 25.
—Men of lower socioeconomic levels.
—Residents of cities.
—Those who had moved from rural areas or small towns to large cities.
—Those with childhood disjunctions (for example, from broken homes).
—Catholics and liberal Protestants.
—Those who did not attend church.
—Single and divorced men.

variables in the 1967 and 1969 surveys may be taken as useful predictors of drinking behavior and alcohol-related problems.

Within some of these subgroups, there were some differences in rates of specific types of problems. In addition, some of these groups overlap. For example, city residence, moving to larger cities, childhood disjunction, and marital status tend to be correlated.

Besides being scored on individual problems, each respondent was also given an overall combined score of "moderate" or "severe" that took into account all of the reported problems and noted their severity. A current-problems score of seven points or more (7+) out of a possible 58 was the point at which a person was deemed to have a fairly high index of alcohol-related problems. This score could usually be attained only by having problems in two or more areas, with at least one being rated in severe form . . . or problems in three or more areas, with at least one being moderately severe . . . or problems in five or more areas with at least one being moderate or severe . . . or slight problems in seven or more of the 11 problem areas.

Sex and Age

Figure 7 reveals that in the 1967 survey, the major alcohol-related problems of men were psychological dependence (39 percent), frequent intoxication (17 percent), problems with spouse or relatives (16 percent), and symptomatic drinking (16 percent). The major problems of women were psychological dependence (15 percent), belligerence (8 percent), health (8 percent), and symptomatic drinking (7 percent). The largest proportion of women with severe alcohol-related problems never rose above the 4 percent who reported it in the area of health. Men, however, experienced severe problems in substantially large proportions in several areas: frequent intoxication (14 percent),

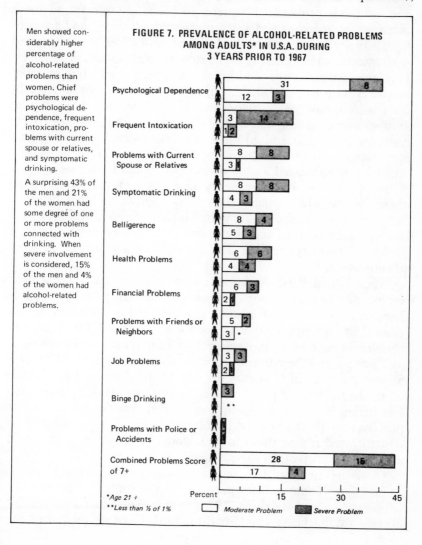

Men showed considerably higher percentage of alcohol-related problems than women. Chief problems were psychological dependence, frequent intoxication, problems with current spouse or relatives, and symptomatic drinking.

A surprising 43% of the men and 21% of the women had some degree of one or more problems connected with drinking. When severe involvement is considered, 15% of the men and 4% of the women had alcohol-related problems.

FIGURE 7. PREVALENCE OF ALCOHOL-RELATED PROBLEMS AMONG ADULTS* IN U.S.A. DURING 3 YEARS PRIOR TO 1967

Psychological Dependence — 31 / 8 ; 12 / 3

Frequent Intoxication — 3 / 14 ; 1 2

Problems with Current Spouse or Relatives — 8 / 8 ; 3

Symptomatic Drinking — 8 / 8 ; 4 / 3

Belligerence — 8 / 4 ; 5 / 3

Health Problems — 6 / 6 ; 4 / 4

Financial Problems — 6 / 3 ; 2

Problems with Friends or Neighbors — 5 / 2 ; 3 / *

Job Problems — 3 / 3 ; 2

Binge Drinking — 3 ; **

Problems with Police or Accidents

Combined Problems Score of 7+ — 28 / 15 ; 17 / 4

Percent — 15 — 30 — 45

*Age 21 +
**Less than ½ of 1%

☐ Moderate Problem   ▨ Severe Problem

53

psychological dependence, problems with spouse or relatives, and symptomatic drinking (each 8 percent).

A surprising 31 percent of the total sample had experienced some degree of one or more problems connected with drinking during the 3 years preceding the survey—43 percent of the men and 21 percent of the women. When more severe involvement (a high score) is considered alone, 15 percent of the men and 4 percent of the women could be said to have problems or potential problems connected with drinking. Many people had more than one drinking problem. Frequent intoxication was found most often to be accompanied by symptomatic drinking and psychological dependence, and binge drinking most often was associated with symptomatic drinking and problems with spouse or relatives. Problems with friends and neighbors were associated in most instances with frequent intoxication, symptomatic drinking, problems with spouse or relatives, and health problems. This may be another way of saying that by the time friends and neighbors (who have no clear responsibility for the respondent) get around to remonstrating with him about his drinking, the individual usually will have accumulated a host of alcohol-related problems in other areas of his life. Further, heavy drinkers may gravitate toward those people who initially do not disapprove of their drinking behavior. Since half of those with a high score on health problems did not achieve high scores on any other potential problems, a health problem related to drinking may be a relatively isolated phenomenon.

When findings are examined separately for men and women within different age groups, somewhat different patterns of problems emerge. Figure 8 shows age trends for problems in the combined high-risk sample of men aged 21 to 59. Every type of problem is seen to be most prevalent among men in the youngest age groups, and the current-problems score among men 21 to 24 is almost twice as high as it is for any of the older groups. Among men, alcohol-related problems generally taper off sharply by their late fifties. However, relatively few women in their twenties report problems, with the bulk of problems for women appearing to be concentrated among those in their thirties and forties, with, again, a very sharp drop-off in their fifties.

These age findings are congruent with those of recent studies reviewed by Tremper (40), particularly the studies of Drew (15), Gibbins (17), and Malzberg (29). The evidence is that a substantial portion of the heavy drinkers do indeed moderate their drinking

54

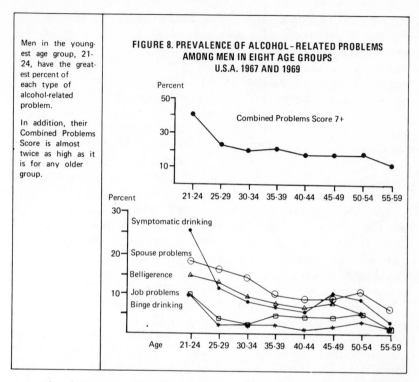

Men in the youngest age group, 21-24, have the greatest percent of each type of alcohol-related problem.

In addition, their Combined Problems Score is almost twice as high as it is for any older group.

FIGURE 8. PREVALENCE OF ALCOHOL-RELATED PROBLEMS AMONG MEN IN EIGHT AGE GROUPS U.S.A. 1967 AND 1969

Percent

50

30

Combined Problems Score 7+

10

Percent   21-24 25-29 30-34 35-39 40-44 45-49 50-54 55-59

30

Symptomatic drinking

20   Spouse problems

Belligerence

10   Job problems

Binge drinking

Age   21-24 25-29 30-34 35-39 40-44 45-49 50-54 55-59

over the long run. Another part of the reduced proportion of heavy drinkers in the older age groups may be accounted for by a higher mortality among them. Alcohol-related problems (particularly for men) probably had their beginnings at a relatively early age. Studies of college students with alcohol-related problems have shown they are similar to alcoholic adults in their self-concepts of being neurotic, cynical, impulsive, and having a low self-evaluation. The implication is that these personality characteristics may predispose some people to later development of alcoholism (42). Thus the available evidence indicates the need for more intensive inquiry into the acquisition of drinking habits and attitudes at an early age.

Socioeconomic Level

Although drinking is more prevalent among those of higher socioeconomic level, most studies of alcohol-related problems or alcoholism have found the conditions more prevalent among the poor than among the remainder of the population (3, 9, 26, 31,

55

36). Figure 9 shows that both alcohol-related problems and abstinence are positively associated with lower socioeconomic levels among men aged 21 to 59. On the other hand, drinkers without even minimal problems are over twice as common in the highest groups as in the lowest. The proportion of tangible consequences of heavy intake or binge drinking is relatively high in the two lower groups, and particularly high within the very lowest group. Thus, consistent with their more insecure existence, the poor tend to have a higher ratio of consequences of heavy drinking than the well-to-do. Adjusting for socioeconomic level, highest prevalences of tangible consequences were consistently found in the youngest adults (aged 21 to 29). The youngest men at the highest socioeconomic level had a lower ratio of consequences in relation to heavy or binge drinking than the older men at the same level. This may imply that our society particularly protects young men of high socioeconomic level, allowing them their youthful "wild-oats" sowing.

Geographic region. When regions were classified as to their "dryness" or "wetness" (on the basis of temperance sentiments and drinking patterns), those living in the drier areas (primarily Southern, Mountain, and Plains areas) had a lower rate of alcohol-related problems, but also a relatively high ratio of interpersonal problems to heavy or binge drinking.

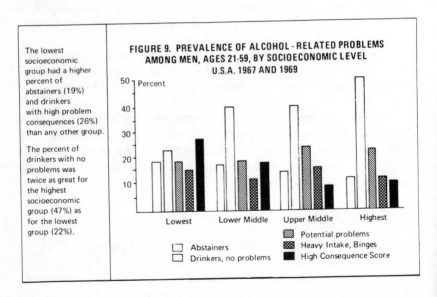

The lowest socioeconomic group had a higher percent of abstainers (19%) and drinkers with high problem consequences (26%) than any other group.

The percent of drinkers with no problems was twice as great for the highest socioeconomic group (47%) as for the lowest group (22%).

FIGURE 9. PREVALENCE OF ALCOHOL - RELATED PROBLEMS AMONG MEN, AGES 21-59, BY SOCIOECONOMIC LEVEL U.S.A. 1967 AND 1969

Percent

Lowest   Lower Middle   Upper Middle   Highest

Abstainers
Drinkers, no problems
Potential problems
Heavy Intake, Binges
High Consequence Score

Other Factors Influencing
Alcohol-Related Problems

Many environmental and personality variables have been found to be associated with drinking and alcohol-related problems (9). Plaut (34) summarizes the role of such variables:

> A tentative model may be developed for understanding the causes of problem drinking, even though the precise roles of the various factors have not yet been determined. An individual who: (1) Responds to beverage alcohol in a certain way, perhaps physiologically determined, by experiencing intense relief and relaxation; and who (2) has certain personality characteristics, such as difficulty in dealing with and overcoming depression, frustration, and anxiety; and who (3) is a member of a culture in which there is both pressure to drink and culturally induced guilt and confusion regarding what kinds of drinking behavior are appropriate, is more likely to develop trouble than will most other persons. An intermingling of certain factors may be necessary for the development of problem drinking, and the relative importance of the differential causal factors no doubt varies from one individual to another.

In the 1969 survey, the variables found to be most strongly associated with alcohol-related problems were those involving favorable attitudes toward drinking and environmental support for heavy drinking, impulsivity and nonconformity, and several indicators of alienation and maladjustment (childhood disjunctions, adult disjunction, somatic complaints, affective anxiety or irritability, and alienation and paranoia). The concepts used in analyzing the correlates of alcohol-related problems in the survey were partly derived from preceding studies of social structure and problems (13, 23).

Correlating all intervening and demographic variables for men aged 21 to 59 against overall problem-drinking scores, the principal finding is that those intervening variables which are involved specifically with drinking behavior and attitudes are correlated most highly with alcohol-related problems. It may be argued that the association between a person's attitudes and the drinking behavior and attitudes of his associates toward his own alcohol-related problems may be as much a consequence of his heavy drinking as an antecedent of it. However, support for the hypothesis that drinking attitudes may "cause" later alcohol-related problems is found in the earlier two-stage study in the same series, in which favorable attitudes toward drinking were found to precede alcohol-related problems more often than the problems preceded the favorable attitude.

It was also found that environmental factors predominate among the correlates of alcohol-related problems although certain personality characteristics—notably impulsivity, alienation, maladjustment—are important in determining the level and character of alcohol-related problems (6). Such correlations alone do not prove the existence or the direction of causal relationships. However, the fact that environmental factors such as the permissiveness of one's family, one's socioeconomic status, ethnic background, and size of city have high correlations with alcohol-related problems should serve as a stimulus for preventive and remedial programs designed to take into account these background characteristics. These findings are also consistent with findings that the alcohol abuser or alcoholic individual does not represent a unique personality or psychiatric type (2, 38, 39).

The 1967 and 1969 national surveys that are primarily concerned with correlations between certain types of drinking practices and specific types of problems represent an early stage in the investigation of alcohol-related problems. To establish more clearly whether the drinking caused the problem or the problem caused the drinking, two subsequent stages of research are needed. The first would be to carry out longitudinal studies in which changes in people's lives between two points in time are related to subsequent changes in drinking behavior, health, or interpersonal relations. A subsequent stage would be controlled experimental studies in which various remedial measures for persons with alcohol-related problems are implemented over a period of time, and their effects evaluated on problems relating to drinking.

PATTERNS OF CHANGE IN DRINKING BEHAVIOR

The magnitude and character of change in drinking habits over time are especially crucial issues in planning preventive and remedial programs to control alcohol abuse and alcoholism. Available evidence clearly indicates that many people who drink at a given time either quit drinking or reduce their drinking. Even one-third of the abstainers said they once used to drink (8). The 1967 survey found that as many persons had fairly severe drinking problems prior to 3 years ago as had drinking problems within the last 3 years. The retrospective data on past changes in drinking behavior are borne out by separate measurements. During the short period between the 1964—65 and 1967 surveys, 15 percent of the persons interviewed had either moved into or out of the group reporting they drank five or more drinks on one occasion at least some of the time.

The findings that those with severe alcohol-related problems show considerable fluctuation in drinking implies that many persons with these problems have occasions when it is easier to bring their drinking under better control. The process of cutting down appears to be most successful among men in their forties and fifties in upper socioeconomic levels, and among people in smaller towns and rural areas. In the combined national surveys, an analysis of men aged 21 to 59 also found that those who matured out of alcohol-related problems fastest (on the basis of retrospective reports) were more secure in their jobs, less impulsive, and lived in an environment that was less permissive of heavy drinking than was true for persons with alcohol-related problems. A 1964 San Francisco study also found that those retaining alcohol-related problems tended to show more signs of childhood stress, drinking problems in the home while growing up, anxiety, depression, maladjustment, guilt, and need for approval (27).

SUMMARY AND CONCLUSION

(1) In most areas of the United States, drinking is typical behavior. Both abstinence and alcohol-related problems are atypical.

(2) The proportion of drinkers, especially among women, appears to have increased since World War II. Evidence about change in the rates of alcohol-related problems is tentative, however.

(3) Whether a person drinks at all, and how much, depends primarily on sociocultural variables, as shown in the great differences in drinker status by such factors as sex, age, social status, region, degree of urbanization, and religion. Certain personality measures are found useful in explaining some of the variations in drinking and heavy drinking within subgroups. These include such indicators as alienation, neurotic tendencies, and impulsivity.

(4) The factors which determine who will become an alcohol abuser or alcoholic individual are probably established at an early age.

(5) There is a one-third turnover in alcohol-related problems of many individuals, as well as a general tendency for older persons to drop out of the drinking and alcohol-related problem classes. The implications are that a person with alcohol-related problems may present a number of opportunities to help him mobilize his resources to bring his drinking under better control.

Alcohol abuse and alcoholism may not be as intractable as is commonly supposed. Attitudes and behavior can be changed. These studies reveal an encouraging amount of change in the drinking behavior of many individuals over a relatively short time. Such findings lend added confidence that effective preventive and treatment programs can be devised which will mobilize the recuperative resources of the individual and his environment to redirect problem behavior associated with heavy drinking into more constructive and rewarding channels.

REFERENCES

(1) American Institute of Public Opinion. Gallup political index; political, social and economic trends. Report, 1966, Princeton, N.J.

(2) Armstrong, J.D. The search for the alcoholic personality. Ann. Amer. Acad. Polit. Soc. Sci. 315:40–47, 1958.

(3) Bailey, M.B., Haberman, P.W., and Alksne, H. The epidemiology of alcoholism in an urban residential area. Quart. J. Stud. Alc. 26:19–40, 1965.

(4) Bales, R.F. Attitudes toward drinking in the Irish culture. In: Pittman, D.J. and Snyder, C.R., eds., Society, Culture and Drinking Patterns. Chapter 10. New York: Wiley, 1962.

(5) Blane, H.T., Overton, W.F., and Chafetz, M.E. Social factors in the diagnosis of alcoholics; characteristics of the patient. Quart. J. Stud. Alc. 24:640–663, 1963.

(6) Block, J. The Challenge of Response Sets: Unconfounding Meaning, Acquiescence, and Social Desirability in the MMPI. New York: Appleton-Century-Crofts, 1965.

(7) Blum, R.H. Mind-altering drugs and dangerous behavior: Alcohol. In: President's Commission on Law Enforcement and Administration of Justice. Task Force Report: Drunkenness. Appendix B. Washington, D.C.: U.S. Govt. Printing Office, 1967.

(8) Cahalan, D., Cisin, I.H., and Crossley, H.M. American Drinking Practices: A National Survey of Drinking Behavior and Attitudes. New Brunswick: Rutgers Center of Alcohol Studies, 1969.

(9) Cahalan, D. Problem Drinkers. San Francisco: Jossey-Bass, 1970.

(10) Cahalan, D. and Room, R. Problem drinking among American men. Monographs of the Rutgers Center of Alcohol Studies, No. 7. New Brunswick, N.J.: Rutgers Center of Alcohol Studies, in press, 1972.

(11) Chafetz, M.E. Alcohol prevention and reality. Proceedings of the IV World Congress of Psychiatry, Madrid, 1966. Also in Excerpta Med. Internat. Cong., Ser. No. 150.

(12) Clark, W. Operational definitions of drinking problems and associated prevalence rates. Quart. J. Stud. Alc. 27:648–688, 1966.

(13) Cloward, R. and Ohlin, L.E. Delinquency and Opportunity. New York: Free Press, 1960.

(14) Davies, K.M. The influence of alcohol on mortality. Proceedings, Home Office Life Underwriters Assn., 46:159–177, 1965.

(15) Drew, L.R.H. Alcoholism as a self-limiting disease. Quart. J. Stud. Alc. 29:956–967, 1968.

(16) Efron, V. and Keller, M. Selected Statistics on Consumption of Alcohol (1850–1968) and on Alcoholism (1930–1968). New Brunswick, N.J.: Rutgers Center of Alcohol Studies, 1970.

(17) Gibbins, R.J. The fate of a natural alcoholic population over a ten-year period. Paper presented at the 28th International Congress on Alcohol and Alcoholism. Washington, D.C.: September 15–20, 1968.

(18) Glad, D.D. Attitudes and experiences of American-Jewish and American-Irish male youth as related to differences in adult rates of inebriety. Quart. J. Stud. Alc. 8:406–472, 1947.

(19) Glenn, N.D. and Zody, R.E. Cohort analysis with national survey data. Gerontologist 10:233–240, 1970.

(20) Harris, L. and Associates, Inc. American attitudes toward alcohol and alcoholics. Study No. 2138. Report prepared for the National Institute on Alcohol Abuse and Alcoholism, 1971.

(21) Jaffe, J.H. Drug addiction and drug abuse. In: Goodman, L.S. and Gilman, A., eds., The Pharmacological Basis of Therapeutics. Chapter 16. New York: Macmillan, 1965, p. 294.

(22) Jellinek, E.M. The Disease Concept of Alcoholism. Highland Park, N.J.: Hillhouse Press, 1960.

(23) Jessor, R., Young, H.B., Young, E.B. and Tesi, G. Perceived opportunity, alienation, and drinking behavior among Italian and American youth. Paper presented at the 28th International Congress on Alcohol and Alcoholism, Washington, D.C., September 19, 1968.

(24) Kinsey,A.C., Pomeroy, W.B. and Martin, C.E. Sexual Behavior in the Human Male. Philadelphia: Saunders, 1948.

(25) Knupfer, G., Fink, R., Clark, W.B. and Goffman, A.S. Factors Related to Amount of Drinking in an Urban Community. California Drinking Practices Study,

61

Report No. 6. Berkeley: Division of Alcoholic Rehabilitation, California State Department of Public Health, 1963.

(26) Knupfer, G. The epidemiology of problem drinking. Amer. J. Public Health 57: 973–986, 1967.

(27) Knupfer, G. Ex-problem drinkers. Paper delivered at the Fourth Conference on Life History and Psychopathology, St. Louis, November 1970.

(28) Lolli, G., Serianni, E., Golder, G.M. and Luzzatto-Fegiz, P. Alcohol in Italian Culture: Food and Wine in Relation to Sobriety Among Italians and Italian Americans. Monographs of the Rutgers Center of Alcohol Studies, No. 3. New Brunswick, N.J.: Rutgers Center of Alcohol Studies, 1958.

(29) Malzberg, B. Rates of discharge and rates of mortality among first admissions to the New York State civil state hospitals. Ment. Hyg. 37:619–654, 1953.

(30) Malzberg, B. The Alcoholic Psychoses: Demographic Aspects at Midcentury in New York State. New Brunswick, N.J.: Rutgers Center of Alcohol Studies, 1960.

(31) Mulford, H.A. Drinking and deviant drinking, U.S.A., 1963. Quart. J. Stud. Alc. 25:634–650, 1964.

(32) Mulford, H.A. and Miller, D.E. Drinking in Iowa. IV. Preoccupation with alcohol and definitions of alcohol, heavy drinking, and trouble due to drinking. Quart. J. Stud. Alc. 21:279–291, 1960.

(33) Pell, S. and Alonzo, C.A. The prevalence of chronic disease among problem drinkers. Arch. Environ. Health 16:678–684, 1968.

(34) Plaut, T.F.A. Alcohol Problems: A Report to the Nation by the Cooperative Commission on the Study on Alcoholism. New York: Oxford University Press, 1967.

(35) Riley, J.W. and Marden, C.F. The social pattern of alcoholic drinking. Quart. J. Stud. Alc. 8:265–273, 1947.

(36) Room, R. Cultural contingencies of alcoholism: Variations between and within nineteenth-century urban ethnic groups in alcohol-related death rates. J. Health Soc. Behav. 9:99–113, 1968.

(37) Room, R. Assumptions and implications of disease concepts of alcoholism. Paper delivered at the 29th International Congress on Alcoholism and Drug Dependence, Sydney, February, 1970.

(38) Rosen, A.C. A comparative study of alcoholic and psychiatric patients with the MMPI. Quart. J. Stud. Alc. 21:253–266, 1960.

(39) Syme, L. Personality characteristics of the alcoholic. Quart. J. Stud. Alc. 18:288–301, 1957.

(40) Tremper, M. What happens to alcoholics. Unpublished manuscript, 1969.

(41) Trice, H.M. and Wahl, J.R. A rank order analysis of the symptoms of alcoholism. Quart. J. Stud. Alc. 19:636–648, 1958.

(42) Williams, A.F. Self-concepts of college problem drinkers. 1. A comparison with alcoholics. Quart. J. Stud. Alc. 26:586–594, 1965.

(43) Wolf, I., Chafetz, M.E., Blane, H.T., and Hill, M.J. Social factors in the diagnosis of alcoholism. II. Attitudes of physicians. Quart. J. Stud. Alc. 26:72–79, 1965.

Chapter III

ALCOHOL
AND THE CENTRAL
NERVOUS SYSTEM

MOST PEOPLE DRINK ALCOHOLIC BEVERAGES to obtain feelings of pleasure as well as relief from fears and tensions. Undoubtedly this is the basic reason for the widespread popularity of alcohol as a social beverage. This typical response is not universal, however. For some people, the same small amounts of alcohol result not in relaxation but in increased anxiety, not in happiness but in suspicion and distrust. These atypical responses may lead to belligerent feelings or actions, or episodes of confusion and disorientation. With the drinking of larger amounts, however, individual differences in behavior tend to decrease, and the pharmacological depressant effects of alcohol begin to predominate. As this occurs, a typical sequence of tiredness, sleepiness, and ultimately stupor occurs, although feelings of tiredness may nevertheless be accompanied by irritability on the one hand, or by mellowness and warmth on the other, depending on the individual and the circumstances.

Intoxicating
Effects of
Alcohol

These varied and complex effects of alcohol are due partly to changes in the function of the central nervous system; that is, to the effect of alcohol on the brain. Ingested alcohol is absorbed from

63

the alimentary tract and carried by the circulating blood to the brain and other organs. The concentration of alcohol in the blood which affects the functioning of the brain is lower than that which would significantly affect other tissues. The observable effects of alcohol intoxication, such as slurred speech and unsteady gait, are not due to the direct action of alcohol on the tongue or legs, but are caused by its effect on the parts of the brain which integrate and control their activities.

While the exact pharmacological mechanisms of the action of alcohol are unknown, we do know that the behavioral and depressant effects are dependent on dosage (5, 6, 11, 33, 39). The rapidity with which alcohol induces intoxication, and the behavioral expression of intoxication in altered function of the central nervous system, are related to the speed of its absorption from the stomach and small intestine, and to the drinking history of the individual.

Alcohol is metabolized, or burned and broken down, in the body at a fairly constant rate. As a person drinks at a rate faster than the alcohol can be metabolized, the drug accumulates in his body, resulting in higher and higher concentrations of alcohol in the blood. The larger the person, the greater the amount required to attain a given concentration of alcohol. In a 150-pound man, alcohol is metabolized at approximately the rate of one drink per hour. The typical drink—three-fourths ounce of alcohol—is provided by:

- a "shot" of spirits (1.5 oz. of 40 to 50 percent alcohol),
- a glass of wine (5 oz. of 12 percent alcohol),
- a pint of beer (16 oz. of 5 percent alcohol).

Consumption at this rate will result in little, if any, accumulation of alcohol in the blood.

Even the first few sips of an alcoholic beverage may cause changes in mood and behavior; these may be due to a conditioned or learned response based on previous drinking experiences. However, the first consistent sizable changes in mood and behavior which are attributable to the effects of alcohol on the central nervous system, appear at blood alcohol levels of about 0.05 percent. Thought, judgment, and restraint are loosened and sometimes disrupted at this level which would result from a 150-pound man consuming two drinks within an hour. The individual feels carefree, released from many of his ordinary anxieties and inhibitions; he may take small personal and social liberties as the impulse prompts. It is mainly to achieve this subjectively pleasant state that people drink alcoholic beverages in moderation.

As greater amounts of alcohol are consumed and correspondingly higher levels of alcohol are attained in the blood, the depressant action of alcohol progressively involves more functions of the brain. At a concentration of 0.10 percent alcohol in the blood, voluntary motor actions usually become perceptibly clumsy. At 0.20 percent, the function of the entire motor area of the brain is measurably depressed; that part of the brain which mediates emotional behavior is also affected. The individual staggers or he may tend to assume a horizontal posture; he may easily be angered, or shout, or weep. At a concentration of 0.30 percent, the more primitive perceptive areas of the brain are dulled. At this level a person is commonly confused, or may begin to be stuporous. Although aware, he has poor comprehension of what he hears or sees. With 0.40 or 0.50 percent alcohol in the blood, he is unaware of his environment; he is in coma. Higher levels of alcohol in the blood block the centers in the medulla of the lower brain which control breathing, and death rapidly ensues (48). The direct effects of extreme intoxication are estimated to account for about 1,000 deaths each year in the United States. This progression of effects is not unique to alcohol. It can be produced by many other hypnotic-sedative drugs, such as barbiturates, ether, and chloral hydrate.

Chronic Heavy
Alcohol Consumption

Chronic consumption of large amounts of alcohol over long periods of time seems to alter the sensitivity of the central nervous system to the effects of alcohol. As a result, larger amounts of alcohol are required to reproduce the same effect. This adaptation or reduced sensitivity of the central nervous system to the effects of alcohol is termed "tolerance" by pharmacologists. It is a phenomenon common to the chronic use of all addictive drugs (46) and is believed to be a basis of "addiction" or, in more recently adopted terminology, "dependence" (60).

The effects of alcohol on the moderate or heavy drinker, and on the person who is alcohol-dependent, are in some respects very different. In contrast to the pleasant, euphoric aspects of intoxication usually experienced by the normal drinker, alcoholic persons

65

may become progressively more tense and anxious while drinking (29, 30, 31, 32, 37, 40). One study has suggested, however, that the alcohol-dependent person selectively forgets the profound dysphoria and remembers only the positive aspects when sober (50).

Some of the other differences between the moderate or heavy drinker and the alcohol-dependent person are due, at least in part, to the latter's extraordinary adaptation to alcohol. The alcohol-dependent person must ingest relatively huge amounts through time to produce the changes in feelings and behavior which he had previously attained with smaller quantities. Moreover, the alcohol-dependent person's capacity to drink very large quantities without obvious behavioral impairment also distinguishes him from the moderate or heavy drinker. The alcohol-dependent person can consume between a fifth and a quart of whisky a day without signs of gross inebriation (35, 36). He can perform accurately on a series of complex behavioral tasks at blood alcohol levels several times as great as those that would lead to behavioral impairments in moderate to heavy drinkers. At present, it is not known what accounts for the dramatic "behavioral tolerance" of the alcohol-dependent person to alcohol. It was once thought that "tolerance" could be accounted for by differences in the rate of alcohol metabolism. It has been shown, however, that normal drinkers and alcoholic persons do not differ substantially in their overall rate of alcohol metabolism (3, 38, 41). This finding argues that the adaptive processes (subserving "behavioral tolerance") must occur in the central nervous system rather than at a metabolic level (34).

Another way in which the moderate or heavy drinker differs from the alcoholic person is that the abrupt removal of alcohol can produce dramatic alterations in behavior and perceptions in the alcoholic person. Whereas the normal drinker may experience the brief discomfort of the congeries of symptoms collectively referred to as the "hangover," the alcohol-dependent person may experience severe tremulousness, hallucinations and, in some instances, disorientation, confusion, delirium, and convulsions— the alcohol withdrawal syndrome. The time of onset of the alcohol withdrawal syndrome is usually within 12 to 48 hours following cessation of drinking (45), and may even occur when some alcohol is still present in the organism (15). The common alcohol withdrawal syndrome involving tremulousness, hyper-reflexia, profuse sweating, nausea, and anxiety should be distinguished from the severe and potentially lethal condition known as

66

delirium tremens. Delirium tremens is characterized by severe psychomotor agitation, confusion, disorientation, hallucinations, and autonomic and metabolic dysfunction. The critical determinants of the severity and duration of alcohol withdrawal symptoms are unknown, and do not appear to be directly related either to the volume of alcohol consumed or the duration of a drinking spree (34). Since alcohol withdrawal appears to reflect a state of heightened central nervous system excitability, it has been suggested that the removal of the depressant drug results in a rebound hyperactivity which is expressed in such behaviors as tremulousness and hyperreflexia. This general explanatory concept of drug withdrawal states has been described by Jaffee and Sharpless (18) as the "denervation supersensitivity model."

Although most people drink in social, convivial, informal settings, the effects of alcohol on behavior have usually been studied by brief tests under formal laboratory conditions. Measurements of performance in such tests may underestimate the detrimental effects of intoxication because the subjects under these conditions are able and often feel motivated to "pull themselves together," counteracting the depressant effects of alcohol on central nervous system functions which regulate sensory and motor performance, motivations, and emotions. Nevertheless, substantial detrimental effects on some measures of performance have been found in the laboratory, even with fairly low alcohol doses. Studies dealing with these effects, as detailed below, have been thoroughly reviewed in the literature (4, 19, 22, 56).

EFFECTS OF ALCOHOL
ON SENSATION AND PERCEPTION

Visual acuity seems to be relatively insensitive to the effects of alcohol. At high doses of alcohol, however, the eye responds in much the same way as it adapts to the dark. While perception of dim lights may be slightly improved by alcohol, there is a decrease in ability to discriminate accurately between lights of different intensities. Resistance to glare is also impaired, so that the eye requires a longer period of time to readjust after being exposed to a very bright light. In addition, sensitivity to certain colors, especially red, appears to decrease at high doses.

The ability to hear faint sounds remains intact but, as with vision, the ability to discriminate among different sounds is affected by moderate and high doses of alcohol. As is well-known, even low doses of alcohol impair sensitivity to odors and taste. And while alcohol has very little effect on the sense of touch, it definitely diminishes sensitivity to pain.

In general, sensory capabilities are rather resistant to alcohol, but the changes that do occur are predominately depressant or detrimental effects. Some studies also suggest that alcohol may alter perception of time and space. For example, individuals who have had a few drinks tend to underestimate the speed of objects and also underestimate the distance they have traveled over a period of time. These findings suggest that alcohol tends to make time appear to pass more quickly.

EFFECTS OF ALCOHOL
ON MOTOR PERFORMANCE

Tests of motor control or coordination show greater detrimental effects than sensory capabilities. Intoxicating doses of alcohol impair most types of performance, partly depending on familiarity with the task, but some skills are more susceptible than others to the negative effects of alcohol. A sensitive indicator of alcohol effect is the "standing steadiness" test. Alcohol increases swaying, especially if the eyes are closed and the stabilizing effect of visual cues is blocked. Sensorimotor coordination is also adversely affected by alcohol, as in tracking a moving object, especially if the task requires attention to multiple, concurrent events.

People differ from one another in their susceptibility to the effects of alcohol on motor performance, especially at blood alcohol levels of 0.10 percent and below. Although sufficient alcohol impairs everybody's performance, some people are better able than others to overcome the effects of small doses of alcohol and bring their performance up to its normal level. This ability seems to be related to the level of emotional arousal of the individual, so that more "highly anxious" persons are apparently more resistant to these effects of alcohol. In studies of how alcohol affects the performance of various types of individuals in a simulated driving test, "extroverts" did not alter their speed but made more errors. "Introverts" tended to change their speed, some in either direction; they made fewer errors, but there was more variation among them in the extent to which errors increased (8). In subjects whose sober performance was inferior from the start, there was a suggestion of greater detrimental effect of alcohol on neuromuscular control. On tests of very difficult problems in logic, however, highly intelligent young men performed better after small amounts of alcohol, but their performance deteriorated after drinking larger amounts (5).

EFFECTS OF ALCOHOL
ON EMOTIONS

The direct physiological action of alcohol, coupled with its apparent ability to relax feelings of self-criticism and inhibition, may give rise to the "high" associated with alcohol use. This in turn may be of special psychological utility in social situations as individuals interact with one another, each recognizing that the others are less responsible for what they say and do. Based on data from a number of cultures, MacAndrew and Edgerton (26) have suggested that "the way in which people comport themselves when they are drunk is determined . . . by what their society makes of and imparts to them concerning the state of drunkenness" rather than by "toxically disinhibited brains operating in impulse-driven bodies."

Some studies have shown that alcohol tends to decrease fear and increase the likelihood that an individual will accept risks. When a group of bus drivers were given several drinks, for example, they were more likely to try to drive their buses through spaces that were too narrow—and seemingly more likely to risk failure—than when they were sober (7). Studies with rats, mice, and cats tend to confirm this fear- and anxiety-reducing property of alcohol (1, 56). For example, cats that became afraid to eat after receiving several electric shocks lost their fear after they had been given alcohol (28).

Reaction time can be measured in the laboratory by the rapidity with which a subject makes a simple motor movement, such as pressing a button in response to an auditory or visual stimulus. If the dose is high enough, this performance is adversely affected by alcohol. Below a blood alcohol level of 0.07 percent, reaction time seems inconsistently affected. Between 0.08 and 0.10 percent, reaction time is increased slightly. Higher blood alcohol levels consistently produce large performance decrements. A much greater effect of alcohol is found on reaction time when attention is divided, as when the subject is simultaneously engaged in another task.

69

Other tests measuring both speed and accuracy suggest that alcohol has a greater effect on accuracy and consistency than on speed. In other words, an individual who has had several drinks tends to "breeze through" a complex test but makes more errors than he normally would and is more erratic in his responses. In many of these tasks, subjects feel that their performance has improved and show incredulity when shown the poor results.

Effects of alcohol on the powerful but poorly understood emotional response of humor were measured by Hetherington and Wray (15). A series of cartoons were rated more humorous by young men after drinking a small amount of alcohol than after drinking a placebo beverage. There was more appreciation of cartoons depicting aggressive humor than of those showing non-sense humor.

Projective tests, such as the Rorschach inkblots, are designed to study the feelings and emotions which remain hidden from conscious knowledge because of more overt, competing responses, or because the hidden feelings contain threatening or forbidden components which are repressed from memory. The few studies of alcohol effects with projective tests have generally shown an increase in impulsive, superficial, or disorganized responses, corresponding to the impairments found in tests of sensorimotor and intellectual functioning.

The Thematic Apperception Test (TAT) has been widely used for assessing alcohol effects on fantasy production. The subject is shown a representational picture and instructed to tell a story which includes the scene and the characters portrayed in the picture. Using the TAT, Takala and his co-workers (49) found that, when given alcohol, his Finnish subjects showed increases in general types of uninhibited expression, including themes of sexual behavior, aggression, and self-assertion. The stories generated under the influence of alcohol appeared to be more poorly organized and superficial than those reported in the sober state. Kalin and his co-workers (20) found in an American group that high blood alcohol levels were associated with increases in themes of physical aggression and sex, and decreases in themes of time concern, fear, and anxiety. Using the Draw-A-Person Test, Irgens-Jensen (16) found that young Norwegians with alcohol-related problems draw more incomplete and more sexually suggestive figures than control subjects, thus supporting findings of other studies using projective tests.

EFFECTS OF ALCOHOL ON SEXUALITY

The well-known capacity of alcohol to release inhibitions is connected in the public mind with the observation that after drinking, people tend to exhibit an increased amorousness. Moreover, some people seem to be able to engage in sexual activity only after drinking. These observations have given rise to an assumption that alcohol promotes or improves sexual activity. A subtle truth, however, was perceived and expressed by Shakespeare: Drink "provokes the desire, but it takes away the performance" (47).

Extensive studies in animals and man have revealed consistently that large doses of alcohol deteriorated sexual performance (14, 51). Studies of alcoholic persons have revealed that their sex life was markedly disturbed, deficient, and ineffectual (24). In persons with a long history of alcoholism, a tendency toward premature senility includes signs of dysfunction and degeneration of the sex glands (42, 58) and increased sex problems in both men and women (25).

It appears then that in nonalcoholic persons, a few drinks dull the sense of restraint and by helping to overcome lack of confidence or feelings of guilt about sex, facilitate sexual activity. Larger amounts of alcohol, however, may spoil the capacity to perform.

EFFECTS OF ALCOHOL ON SLEEP

The effects of alcohol on sleep are well known to anyone who has gone to bed after having had too much to drink at a party, only to toss and turn fitfully and awaken the following morning feeling headachy and fatigued. Taking several drinks before bedtime decreases the amount of REM or dreaming sleep (23). After drinking before bedtime for several nights and then stopping, there is usually a mild amount of increased REM, a sort of "rebound" phenomenon. The amount of REM sleep then returns to normal over the next several nights. There are indications, however, that the greater the dose of alcohol, the more prolonged is the block in REM sleep. The usual consequences of being deprived of REM sleep are impaired concentration and memory, as well as anxiety, tiredness, and irritability.

The effects of alcohol on REM and other aspects of sleep are currently under investigation, particularly since disorders of sleep may relate to the withdrawal reaction (12).

CORRELATIONS OF ALCOHOL WITH ACCIDENTS AND VIOLENCE

It has been seen that the depressive effects of alcohol on the central nervous system result in altered sensation, perception, motor performance, and emotions. It is not surprising, therefore, that a strong relationship exists between the abuse of alcohol and the occurrence of accidents, as well as acts of violence. Excessive alcohol intake is associated with a substantial portion of auto accidents and fatalities; other accidents on the streets, on the job, on vacation, and at home; and assaults, homicides, and suicides.

Highway Accidents

Tests of simple sensory or motor capabilities show little or no effects of alcohol on these abilities except at very high doses. More complex tasks, however, such as performance on driving simulators and in actual driving tests, are more susceptible to the detrimental effects of alcohol. These tasks require control of speed and, simultaneously, sensorimotor coordination in keeping a moving object on its course and braking. Thus, in actual driving tests, as in tests of complex reaction time, performance is impaired by amounts of alcohol as small as 0.05 percent (one-third to one-half the level required in most States for a conviction of driving while "under the influence").

The adaptive response to these alcohol effects would be to drive more slowly and cautiously. Alcohol, however, often has the opposite emotional effect, increasing boldness and impulsiveness, and resulting in a tendency to underestimate speed. Intoxicated people, therefore, tend to drive faster and more erratically, showing less caution. Excessive alcohol intake was reported to have been associated with approximately one-half of all auto fatalities in one year. Police estimates have suggested that fatally-injured drinking drivers were traveling at higher speeds than nondrinking drivers (9, 43).

A number of studies have shown that drivers who have been drinking heavily are much more likely to be involved in automobile accidents than nondrinking drivers. The more serious the automobile accident, the more likely that alcohol will have been involved. There is also evidence that driving fatalities are more closely associated with alcoholism or chronic alcohol abuse than they are with normal drinking. In fatal automobile accidents, a large proportion of the drivers had blood alcohol levels high enough to suggest that they had chronic alcohol-related problems and were not just "social drinkers" (2). Epidemiologic studies of fatal automobile accidents also show that they tend to occur at night, especially between 10 p.m. and 6 a.m., on weekends, and in the form of single-car accidents. These are times and circumstances under which chronically heavy drinkers are likely to be driving home after a long evening of drinking.

In addition, many single-car driving fatalities are suspected to be overt or unconsciously motivated acts of suicide. Excessive alcohol intake, generally of a chronic, long-continued nature, is associated with one-third of all reported suicides (45).

Other Accidents

A similar conclusion may be drawn from studies on the relationship between alcohol and home accidents. One study (55) of over 300 consecutive fatalities resulting from nonhighway accidents that were seen by the coroner of Sacramento County, Calif., reveals that alcohol plays a major role in deaths from unintentional injuries. Among all these cases, 58 percent of the fatalities had at least one indication of being an alcohol abuser or alcoholic individual; 30 percent were known to be heavy drinkers or alcoholic persons. The study also showed that death from alcohol-related injuries occurs more often at home or during recreational events, than at work. Only 18 percent had taken place at work while 50 percent had taken place at home.

The role of alcohol in nonfatal accidents has been investigated by Wechsler and associates (57). The Breathalyzer test was used to measure alcohol levels in patients admitted to the emergency service of a general hospital. Comparisons were made between the alcohol levels of patients in home accident injuries, and those admitted for injury resulting from transportation accidents, occupational accidents, fights, or assaults, as well as patients with medical conditions unrelated to accidental injuries.

Among accident victims, patients with injuries incurred in transportation had the highest frequency of positive blood alcohol levels (30 percent), and patients involved in accidents at home had the next highest (22 percent). Occupational accident cases had the lowest proportion with positive readings (16 percent).

Accidents and injuries result from a complex pattern of antecedent conditions. The role of alcohol as a causitive agent in many accidents may be suggestive but cannot be proved from statistical studies showing the association of drinking with accidents. The same conditions or personality characteristics which give rise to heavy drinking may also contribute to accident proneness, for example.

Violence

The disinhibitory effects of alcohol may be expected to release suppressed feelings of aggression and hostility and recent studies do, indeed, show an association of alcohol intoxication and violent behavior. In the Wechsler study on home accidents (57), patients injured in fights or assaults constituted by far the highest proportion with positive blood alcohol levels. Fifty-six percent had positive readings, and 39 percent had readings at or above the 0.05 percent level of blood alcohol. Alcohol levels in these patients were significantly higher than among accident cases and other cases. Analysis of some characteristics of male patients injured in fights or assaults revealed that 64 percent of those involved in accidents with unknown or unspecified persons had positive blood alcohol readings, compared with only 33 percent of the men injured by known persons. This suggests that persons under the influence of alcohol may be especially vulnerable to assault in the street, perhaps because they are out at times or places when the risk is greater, or because they may be readily identified as easy targets. Or else they may have "blanked out" the fact that they had "picked a fight."

A comprehensive investigation of 588 criminal homicides showed that 55 percent of the offenders had been drinking (59). Nine studies on the role of alcohol in murders have revealed that the median percent of people who had taken alcohol prior to committing murder was 54 percent (27). Three more recent investigations have associated alcohol with about 50 percent of the homicides studied (10, 13, 54). Similarly, alcohol has been strongly linked to assaultive behavior which did not involve death (48). These and a number of other studies have been thoroughly reviewed by Tinklenberg (52).

74

Thus, statistical studies show that violence is often associated with immediate intake of rather large amounts of alcohol. Chronic heavy drinking is more likely to be associated with feelings of self-destruction such as depression, suicide, and immature and irresponsible behavior (44). In this as in many other cases, it is helpful to keep in mind the distinction between acute and chronic effects of alcohol. Expressions of aggression and hostility in response to alcohol are partly determined by psychosocial factors such as the expectation of the drinkers and others about how alcohol will affect behavior. When people expect that aggression and loss of control will increase with the use of alcohol, the blame for a violent outcome can be shifted to alcohol away from the individuals involved. This signifies an implicit permission of violence.

SUMMARY AND CONCLUSION

In summary, the effects of alcohol consumption are modulated by a variety of factors having to do with rate of absorption, learned expectation, and differential central nervous system adaptation to drug effects. In the normal drinker, intoxication may be accompanied by feelings of exhilaration, loss of restraint, enhanced sociability, increased emotional lability, and impairment of performance on certain cognitive and perceptual tasks. Among the physical signs of intoxication are slurring of speech, abnormal gait, impaired motor performance, and, in some instances, disturbances of sensory perception. In the normal drinker, brief periods of intoxication leave no discernible behavioral or neurological residue, and therefore do not constitute a persistent health hazard. However, extreme intoxication may lead to a depression of the central nervous system, and to a state of stupor with an attendant risk of death.

REFERENCES

(1) Barry, H., III and Miller, N.E. Effects of drugs on approach-avoidance conflict tested repeatedly by means of a "telescope alley." J. Comp. Physiol. Psychol. 55:201–210, 1962.

(2) Bacon, S.D., ed. Studies of Driving and Drinking, Suppl. No. 4, Quarterly Journal of Studies on Alcohol, 1968.

(3) Bernhard, C.G. and Goldberg, L. Aufnahme und Verbrennung des alkohols bei alkoholisten. Acta Med. Scand. 86:152–215, 1935.

(4) Carpenter, J.A. Effects of alcohol on some psychological processes. Quart. J. Stud. Alc. 23:274–314, 1962.

(5) Carpenter, J.A., Moore, O.K., Snyder, C.R., and Lisansky, E.S. Alcohol and higher-order problem solving. Quart. J. Stud. Alc. 22:183–222, 1961.

(6) Carpenter, J.A. and Ross, B.M. Effect of alcohol on short-term memory. Quart. J. Stud. Alc. 26:561, 1965.

(7) Cohen, J., Dearnaley, E.J. and Hansel, C.E.M. The risk taken in driving under the influence of alcohol. Brit. Med. J. 1:1438–1442, 1958.

(8) Drew, G.C., Colquhoun, W.P., and Long, H.A. Effects of small doses of alcohol on a skill resembling driving. Great Britain Medical Research Council Memorandum No. 38. London: H.M. Stationery Office, 1959.

(9) Filkins, L.D., Clark, C.D., Rosenblatt, C.A., Carlson, W.L., Kerlan, M.W., and Manson, H. Alcohol Abuse and Traffic Safety: A Study of Fatalities, DWI Offenders, Alcoholics, and Court-Related Treatment Approaches. Report of Michigan's Highway Safety Research Institute to the U.S. Department of Transportation, National Highway Safety Bureau, June 26, 1970.

(10) Gillies, H. Murder in West Scotland. Brit. J. Psychiat. 111:1087, 1965.

(11) Grenell, R.G. Alcohols and activity of central neurons. Quart. J. Stud. Alc. 20:421–427, 1959.

(12) Gross, M.M. and Goodenough, D.R. Sleep disturbances in acute alcoholic psychoses. Psychiat. Rev. Rep. 24:132–147, 1968.

(13) Guttmacher, M. The normal and the sociopathic murderer. In: Wolfgang, M. ed., Studies in Homicide. New York: Harper & Row, 1967.

(14) Hart, B.L. Effects of alcohol on sexual reflexes and mating behavior in male dog. Quart. J. Stud. Alc. 29:839–844, 1968.

(15) Hetherington, E.M., and Wray, N.P. Aggression, need for social approval, and humor preferences. J. Abn. Soc. Psychol. 68:685–689, 1964.

(16) Irgens-Jensen, O. Problem Drinking and Personality; a Study based on the Draw-a-person Test. Publication No. 9. Oslo, Norway: National Institute for Alcohol Research, 1971.

(17) Isbell, H., Fraser, H., Wikler, A., Belleville, R., and Eisenman, A. An experimental study of the etiology of "rum fits" and delirium tremens. Quart. J. Stud. 16:1–33, 1955.

(18) Jaffee, J.H. and Sharpless, S.K. Pharmacological denervation supersensitivity in the central nervous system: A theory of physical dependence. In: Wikler, A., ed., The Addictive States. Baltimore: Williams and Wilkins, 1968, pp. 226–243.

(19) Jellinek, E.M. and McFarland, R.A. Analysis of psychological experiments on the effects of alcohol. Quart. J. Stud. Alc. 1:272–371, 1940.

(20) Kalin, R., McClelland, D.C., and Kahn, M. Effects of male social drinking on fantasy. J. Pers. Soc. Psychol. 1:441–452, 1965.

(21) Keller, M. Introduction. In: Keller, M. and McCormick, M. A Dictionary of Words about Alcohol. New Brunswick, N.J.: Rutgers Center of Alcohol Studies, 1968.

76

(22) Kissin, B. and Begleiter, H., eds. The Biology of Alcoholism. Vol. 2: Neurophysiology and Behavior. New York: Plenum Press, 1972.

(23) Knowles, J.B., Laverty, S.G., and Kuechler, N.A. Effects of alcohol on REM sleep. Quart. J. Stud. Alc. 29:342–349, 1968.

(24) Levine, J. The sexual adjustment of alcoholics: A clinical study of a selected sample. Quart. J. Stud. Alc. 16:675–680, 1955.

(25) Lisansky, E.E. Alcoholism in women: social and psychological concomitants. I. Social history data. Quart. J. Stud. Alc. 18:588–623, 1957.

(26) MacAndrew, C. and Edgerton, R.B. Drunken Comportment. Chicago: Aldine, 1969.

(27) MacDonald, J.M. The Murderer and His Victim. Springfield, Ill.: Thomas, 1961.

(28) Masserman, J.H., Jacques, M.G., and Nicholson, M.R. Alcohol as a preventive of experimental neuroses. Quart. J. Stud. Alc. 6:281–299, 1945.

(29) Mayfield, D. Psychopharmacology of alcohol. I. Affective change with intoxication, drinking behavior and affective state. J. Nerv. Ment. Dis. 146:314–321, 1968.

(30) Mayfield, D. Psychopharmacology of alcohol. II. Affective tolerance in alcohol intoxication. J. Nerv. Ment. Dis. 146:322–327, 1968.

(31) Mayfield, D. and Allen, D. Alcohol and affect: A psychopharmacological study. Amer. J. Psychiat. 123:1346–1351, 1967.

(32) McNamee, H.B., Mello, N.K., and Mendelson, J.H. Experimental analysis of drinking patterns of alcoholics: Concurrent psychiatric observations. Amer. J. Psychiat. 124:1063–1069, 1968.

(33) Mello, N.K. Some aspects of the behavioral pharmacology of alcohol. In: Efron, D.H., et al., eds.: Psychopharmacology. A Review of Progress. PHS Publ. No. 1836, Washington, D.C.: U.S. Government Printing Office, 1968, pp. 787–809.

(34) Mello, N.K. and Mendelson, J.H. Alterations in states of consciousness associated with chronic ingestion of alcohol. In: Zubin, J. and Shagass, C., eds., Neurobiological Aspects of Psychopathology. New York: Grune & Stratton, pp. 183–218, 1969.

(35) Mello, N.K. and Mendelson, J.H. Experimentally induced intoxication in alcoholics: A comparison between programmed and spontaneous drinking. J. Pharmacol. Exper. Ther., 173:101–116, 1970.

(36) Mello, N.K. and Mendelson, J.H. Drinking patterns during work-contingent and non-contingent alcohol acquisition. In: Mello, N.K. and Mendelson, J.H., eds., Recent Advances in Studies of Alcoholism. Washington, D.C.: U.S. Government Printing Office, 1971, in press.

(37) Mendelson, J.H., ed. Experimentally Induced Chronic Intoxication and Withdrawal in Alcoholics. Quart. J. Stud. Alc., Supplement No. 2, 1964.

(38) Mendelson, J.H. Ethanol–1–C^{14} metabolism in alcoholics and nonalcoholics. Science, 159:319–320, 1968.

(39) Mendelson, J.H. Biochemical pharmacology of alcohol. In: Efron, D.H., et al., eds.

Phychopharmacology. A Review of Progress. PHS Publ. No. 1836, Washington, D.C.: U.S. Government Printing Office, 1968, pp. 769–785.

(40) Mendelson, J.H., La Dou, J., and Solomon, P. Experimentally induced chronic intoxification and withdrawal in alcoholics. Pt. 3. Psychiatric Findings. Quart. J. Stud. Alc., Suppl. No. 2, pp. 40–52, 1964.

(41) Mendelson, J.H., Stein, S., and Mello, N.K. Effects of experimentally induced intoxication on metabolism of ethanol–1–C^{14} in alcoholic subjects. Metabolism 14:1255–1266, 1965.

(42) Neshkov, N.S. Sostoyaniye spermatogeneza i polovoi funktsii u zloupotreblyayushchikh alkogolem. (The state of spermatogenesis and sexual function in those who abuse alcohol.) Vrach. Delo, No. 2, pp. 130–131, 1969.

(43) Pollack, S. Drinking Driver and Traffic Safety Project. Vol. II. Report of University of Southern California Public Systems Research Institute to the U.S. Department of Transportation, National Highway Safety Bureau, July, 1969.

(44) Pitman, D.J., and Gordon, C.W. Revolving Door; a Study of the Chronic Police Case Inebriate. Monograph No. 2. New Brunswick, N.J.: Rutgers Center of Alcohol Studies, 1958.

(45) Robbins, E., Murphy, G., Wilkinson, R., Gasner, S., and Kayes, J. Some clinical considerations in the prevention of suicide based on a study of 134 successful suicides. Amer. J. Pub. Health 49:888, 1959.

(46) Seevers, M.H. and Deneau, G.A. Physiological aspects of tolerance and physical dependence. In: Root, W.S. and Hofmann, F.G., eds., Physiological Pharmacology. New York: Academic Press, 1963, pp. 565–640.

(47) Shakespeare, W. Macbeth, Act II, Sc. 3.

(48) Shupe, L.M. Alcohol and crime. A study of the urine alcohol concentration found in 882 persons arrested during or immediately after the commission of a felony. Journal of Criminal Law and Criminology 44:661, 1954.

(49) Takala, M., Pihkanen, T.A., and Markkanen, T. The Effects of Distilled and Brewed Beverages. A Psysiological, Neurological, and Psychological Study. Helsinki: The Finnish Foundation for Alcohol Studies, Publ. No. 4, 1957.

(50) Tamerin, J.S., Weiner, S., and Mendelson, J.H. Alcoholics' expectancies and recall of experiences during intoxication. Amer. J. Psychiat. 126:1697–1704, 1970.

(51) Teitelbaum, H.A. and Gantt, W.H. The effect of alcohol on sexual reflexes and sperm count in the dog. Quart. J. Stud. Alc. 19:394–398, 1958.

(52) Tinklenberg, J.R. Alcohol and Violence. In: Fox, R. and Bourne, P., eds., Alcoholism: Progress in Research and Treatment. New York: Academic Press, in press.

(53) Victor, M. and Adams, R.D. The effect of alcohol on the nervous system. Res. Publ. Ass. Nerv. Men. Dis. 32:526–573, 1953.

(54) Voss, H.L. and Hepburn, J.R. Patterns in criminal homicide in Chicago. Journal of Criminal Law, Criminology and Police Science 59:499, 1968.

(55) Waller, J.A. The Roles of Alcohol and Problem Drinking, Drugs and Medical Impairment. Report to the Department of Health, Education and Welfare, Environmental Control Administration, 1972.

(56) Wallgren, H. and Barry, H., III. Actions of Alcohol. Volume 1: Biochemical, Physiological and Psychological Aspects. Volume 2: Chronic and Clinical Aspects. New York: Elsevier, 1970.

(57) Wechsler, H., Kasey, E.H., Thum, D., and Demone, H.W. Alcohol level and home accidents. Public Health Reports 84:1043–1050, 1969.

(58) Weller, C.V. Degenerative changes in male geminal epithelium in acute alcoholism and their possible relationship to blastophthoria. Amer. J. Path. 6:1–18, 1930.

(59) Wolfgang, M.E. Patterns in Criminal Homicide. Philadelphia: University of Pennsylvania Press, 1958.

(60) World Health Organization. Expert Committee on Addiction-Producing Drugs; 13th Report. WHO Techn. Rep. No. 273, 1964.

Chapter IV

ALCOHOL-RELATED ILLNESSES

HEAVY DRINKING, ALCOHOL ABUSE, AND ALCOHOLISM have been implicated as primary or related causal factors in a large number of pathological conditions, although the exact frequency of most of these conditions is not known. (See table I for a partial listing of alcohol-related disorders.) For example, alcoholism is often associated with nutritional disorders, especially of vitamins such as folate, niacin, and thiamin. Deficiencies of these vitamins may be responsible for diseases of the neurological, digestive, and other body systems. Diseases of the heart and muscles, of the blood and other tissues, as well as mental disorders, are common in the course of prolonged alcohol abuse and alcoholism. Moreover, alcoholic persons whose alcohol dependency is not successfully treated are subject to an exceptionally high rate of morbidity and mortality. They more frequently fall victim to all sorts of illness not directly connected with alcoholism (9, 125), and their lifespan is reduced by as much as 10 to 12 years.

ENCEPHALOPATHIES

Among the most serious diseases associated with alcoholism are the encephalopathies: Wernicke's syndrome, Korsakoff's

TABLE I
ALCOHOL-RELATED DISORDERS

Gastrointestinal

Esophagitis
Esophageal carcinoma
Gastritis
Malabsorption
Chronic diarrhea
Pancreatitis
Fatty liver
Alcoholic hepatitis
Cirrhosis (may lead to cancer of liver)

Cardiac

Alcoholic cardiomyopathy
Beriberi

Skin

Rosacea
Telangiectasia
Rhinophyma
Cutaneous ulcers

Neurologic and psychiatric

Peripheral neuropathy
Convulsive disorders
Alcoholic hallucinosis
Delirium tremens
Wernicke's syndrome
Korsakoff's psychosis
Marchiafava's syndrome

Muscle

Alcoholic myopathy

Hematologic

Megaloblastic anemia

Vitamin deficiency disease

Beriberi
Pellagra
Scurvy

Metabolic

Alcoholic hypoglycemia
Alcoholic hyperlipemia

82

psychosis, niacin-deficiency (Jolliffe's) encephalopathy, and Marchiafava's disease.

The Wernicke's syndrome, characterized by clouding of consciousness and paralysis of eye nerves, is definitely associated with an acute severe deficiency of vitamin B_1, and responds well to prompt treatment with thiamin (2, 72, 73, 172). Korsakoff's psychosis is characterized by disorientation, failure of memory, and a curious tendency to make up for the defect by substituting imagined occurrences. Because it is often, though not always, accompanied by peripheral neuropathy and sometimes follows on the symptoms of Wernicke's syndrome, thiamin deficiency has been suspected of being implicated in the causation of Korsakoff's psychosis. In patients who do not recover from the acute form of this mental disorder within weeks, it may continue as a chronic condition requiring prolonged hospitalization (15, 72, 73, 171). Niacin-deficiency (Jolliffe's) encephalopathy is marked by clouding of consciousness, cogwheel rigidities of the arms and legs, and uncontrollable sucking and grasping reflexes. It is due to an acute total deficiency of niacin, and responds to massive doses of this vitamin together with other elements of the vitamin B complex. It is fatal if treatment is delayed (72, 73). Marchiafava's disease is a relatively uncommon degeneration of a specific part of the brain—the corpus callosum—causing severe mental malfunction. Because the behavioral symptoms are not specific, the diagnosis is rarely made except at autopsy (101, 172).

Many of the severe, chronic diseases closely associated with alcoholism result in serious damage to brain, liver, and other vital tissues. Most of these progressive pathological changes are largely due to the nutritional defects which almost inevitably accompany chronic heavy alcohol consumption (2, 72, 73, 175). Some recent evidence implicates alcohol more directly.

ALCOHOL AND THE LIVER

The liver is the organ which is most significantly involved with processing alcohol in the body and, at the same time, is most often seriously affected by heavy drinking and alcohol abuse.

Alcohol Metabolism

Alcohol is primarily a foreign compound. It does not require digestion like other foods. It passes directly into the bloodstream

83

and is distributed throughout the body by the circulating blood. A small portion is diffused into the blood directly through the stomach walls. The rest of the alcohol passes through the pylorus, the sphincter muscle separating the stomach from the intestines, and most of it is absorbed into the bloodstream through the walls of the small intestine. As the circulating alcohol—now enormously diluted in the body fluids—passes through the liver, it is subjected to the action of the enzyme ADH (alcohol dehydrogenase), as well as the coenzyme NAD (nicotinamide-adenine dinucleotide); this begins the process of metabolizing the alcohol by converting it into acetaldehyde. The latter, in turn, rapidly undergoes further metabolic change, producing acetate which is utilizable for energy and, finally, carbon dioxide and water. A small part (about 10% of the absorbed alcohol) is eliminated in an unmetabolized form through the kidneys, lungs, and sweat glands, The rest is oxidized mostly in the liver, since this organ contains the bulk of the necessary ADH.

This "organ specificity," plus the limited availability of NAD and the absence of a "feedback" mechanism that could adjust the rate of alcohol metabolism in the liver, probably explains why alcohol oxidation can produce striking imbalances in that organ. One of the effects of the metabolism of large amounts of alcohol is that blood lactic acid is increased. This slows the excretion of uric acid by the kidneys (89). Since high levels of uric acid in the blood are associated with gout, this may explain the common clinical observation that heavy consumption of alcoholic beverages is a frequent aggravating or precipitating factor in gouty attacks.

It has recently been reported that red blood cells in the capillaries of persons who have been drinking, tend to clump. It has been suggested that this clumping may result in sludging of blood cells and consequent interference with efficient oxygen transport to body cells (118).

Fat Metabolism

The process of alcohol oxidation releases excess hydrogen in the liver, an event which has a number of deleterious effects when very large amounts of alcohol are involved. The release of excess hydrogen is associated with an accumulation of increased fat in the liver (84). The increase in hydrogen also inhibits certain metabolic functions important in the production of energy from several sources (the citric acid cycle) (90). Under these conditions, the mitochondria (particles in the cell responsible for the production of energy) will utilize the hydrogen from the alcohol rather than oxidize fatty acids. In other words, alcohol becomes the "preferred fuel" and, instead of burning fat, the liver burns alcohol. The decreased oxidation of fat results in the deposition in the liver of dietary fat, when available or, in its absence, increased fat in the liver is derived from adipose tissue and from new internal formation (87).

The liver can dispose of excess fat (lipids) by increasing its secretion of lipoproteins into the blood (7). This contributes to the mildly elevated fat content in the blood (hyperlipemia) which is commonly associated with chronic heavy drinking (88). When potentiated by diabetes, pancreatitis, or underlying abnormalities in lipid metabolism, the alcohol-induced hyperlipemia can be strikingly exaggerated. The eponym "Zieve's syndrome" (185) is often used to characterize the simultaneous occurrence of fatty liver, hemolytic anemia, and jaundice in association with hyperlipemia. With severe liver disease, however, blood lipids may be normal or even subnormal.

Fatty Liver

If alcohol abuse is gross and prolonged, the hyperlipemia mechanism is insufficient to prevent lipid accumulation in the liver, and extensive fatty liver will develop. This may be exacerbated through continuous damage to liver function.

The accumulation of fat is the initial lesion produced in the liver by heavy consumption of alcohol. The frequency of fatty liver in alcoholic persons was reported 120 years ago (173). This disorder has little accompanying inflammation and few functional consequences, although in some cases minor derangements have been reported (87, 88). Cholestasis may develop. Rarely, an individual may develop jaundice and die in hepatic coma (142). Both moderate and massive fatty liver are usually entirely reversible when alcohol abuse is terminated.

Alcoholic Hepatitis

After a variable period of alcohol abuse—usually years—alcoholic hepatitis may supervene. This inflammatory liver disorder may or may not be associated with fat or cirrhosis (129), but usually there is fever, with an elevated white blood cell count, pain in the right upper abdominal quadrant, and jaundice. Frequently the clinical picture is similar to that produced by gallstones. The most characteristic feature seen under the microscope is the so-called alcoholic hyalin of Mallory (107), a form of cellular degeneration which, with few exceptions, is peculiar to alcoholic liver injury. Although alcoholic hepatitis usually subsides if drinking is stopped, it is a potentially lethal condition, and some patients may die in hepatic failure despite discontinued alcohol intake. If alcohol consumption continues, the hepatitis often progresses to cirrhosis, but in some cases it may do so even if alcohol abuse ceases.

Alcoholic Cirrhosis

The association of alcoholism and cirrhosis of the liver was noted long ago by the famous English clinician William Heberden (60). Some statistics of the present century indicate that liver cirrhosis is directly correlated with per capita consumption of alcohol (161). The incidence of alcoholic cirrhosis is increasing, and the extent of the problem can be inferred from statistics in New York City where cirrhosis of the liver, most of which is probably alcohol-related, ranks as the third leading cause of death between the ages of 25 and 65.

It has been estimated that about 10 percent of alcoholic persons develop cirrhosis, a disease characterized by diffuse scarring of the liver. This disabling and potentially fatal complication of alcoholism generally correlates with duration and amount of alcohol consumption, and according to Lieber and associates seems not to be related to the nutritional status of the individual (90). Excess deposition of iron in the liver occurs in some cases of alcoholic cirrhosis (84), which in turn may increase the rate of fiber deposition in the liver. If they continue heavy drinking, individuals with alcoholic cirrhosis often die of hemorrhage from portal hypertension or of hepatic failure. However, despite the fact that the basic distortion of the hepatic architecture is irreversible, the outlook is strikingly improved with complete cessation of alcohol intake. A risk which accompanies cirrhosis, more commonly in its late stage and regardless of its cause, is the development of cancer of the liver. This occurs even in alcoholic persons who have not consumed alcohol for many years.

Another complication of alcoholic liver injury, fraught with the danger of severe vascular disturbance, is central sclerosing hyalin necrosis (66). This involves scarring around small veins in the liver, resulting in their fibrosis, narrowing and occlusion of their channels, and eventual distortion of the liver tissue. This process may lead to hypertension of the veins feeding the liver, even in the absence of cirrhosis.

In summary, alcoholic liver disease is one of the most serious consequences of alcohol abuse. Its progressively serious manifestations take the form of fatty liver, alcoholic hepatitis, and cirrhosis.

Etiology of Alcoholic Liver Injury

Ever since the observation that alcoholism is associated with liver disease (60, 107), it was generally assumed that the cause was a toxic effect of alcohol itself. Thus Heberden in 1802 wrote that "the most common cause [of 'scirrhous livers'] is an intemperate use of spirituous liquors, which specifically hurt the liver . . ." (60). Despite F. B. Mallory's early attempts to incriminate other agents, such as copper, this view of alcohol as the toxic agent was widely held until the 1930's, when nutritional defects began to be suspected. In the 1940's, Best and his associates (12) concluded, on the basis of experiments in rats, that "there is no more evidence of a specific toxic effect of pure ethyl alcohol on liver cells than there is for one due to sugar." In Best's studies, alcohol accounted for only about 18 percent of the calories in the diets of the animals. In more recent experiments, when alcohol was incorporated in totally liquid diets given to rats, the amount consumed was increased to constitute 36 percent of the daily calories (87, 88). These studies demonstrated that heavy alcohol intake even without nutritional deficiency could produce fatty liver and changes in liver cells similar to those seen in alcoholic hepatitis. Liver injury by such amounts of alcohol was demonstrated in both alcoholic and nonalcoholic volunteers, even when a diet adequate or enriched with respect to protein and vitamins was being consumed (87, 91, 142). In fact, an increase in liver fat and damage to liver cells were consistently produced after heavy alcohol ingestion for as little as 2 days. All the changes produced by alcohol in the volunteers were rapidly reversible as soon as alcohol was discontinued. Liver injury was produced also by amounts of alcohol that did not cause intoxication—the equivalent of between 7 and 13 ounces of whiskey within 24 hours—such as are commonly consumed by many so-called social drinkers. This is consistent with the pattern of many individuals who drink considerably in the course of their work and social relationships, but who are rarely drunk, and who are not considered to be alcoholic persons by their associates. Such individuals, if they consume sufficient alcoholic beverages, appear to increase their susceptibility to liver injury.

Although alcoholic fatty liver is not an inflammatory condition, and is distinguishable from alcoholic hepatitis by light-microscopy, the remarkable similarity of the electron-microscope features suggests that the former may be the precursor of the latter. The chain of events from fatty liver to alcoholic hepatitis and cirrhosis is still hypothetical, however, and has not yet been verified in laboratory animals. This may be due to the fact that even with improved feeding techniques, alcohol intake by the rat is still below that commonly associated with cirrhosis in man; alcoholic cirrhosis usually requires 10 to 15 years of heavy drinking, a period that has not been reproduced experimentally. Though the deposition of excess fat in the liver almost invariably follows heavy alcohol intake, relatively few alcoholic persons develop cirrhosis. It is therefore thought that moderate or intermittent fatty liver probably does not lead to cirrhosis.

The determinants for the development of cirrhosis are still unclear. In addition to the amount and duration of alcohol consumption, other factors could modify the ultimate response of the liver to alcohol. These include contaminants and flavorings of alcoholic beverages, the pattern of alcohol intake, genetic and constitutional predisposition, and malnutrition or the imbalance between nutrition and alcohol intake.

ALCOHOL AND THE HEART

The occurrence of heart disease in connection with heavy drinking was described nearly 100 years ago (176). Later reports of the frequent occurrence of beriberi heart disease in alcoholic patients (14, 178) suggested to many that in this condition alcohol itself might not be the injurious factor. Rather, a nutritional defect, especially deficiency of thiamin (vitamin B_1), was postulated (56). In recent years a distinction between nutritional heart disease and alcoholic cardiomyopathy has been reported with persistence of the latter after administration of thiamin (135). Alcoholic cardiomyopathy occurs usually in men with a long history of alcohol abuse. The clinical characteristics include either slow or sudden onset of left- and right-sided congestive heart failure. A large heart, distended neck veins, narrow pulse pressure, elevated diastolic blood pressure, and peripheral edema are characteristic. Severe liver disease or neurological manifestations of vitamin deficiencies are not usually seen in these patients.

The experimental administration of intoxicating amounts of alcohol to men results in increases in the resting cardiac output, heart rate, and myocardial oxygen consumption, without a change in the stroke volume (117, 134). The increase in oxygen consumption after acute intoxication suggests a decrease in the mechanical efficiency of the heart. This action of alcohol has also been produced in experimental animals (115, 168). In men, experimental blood alcohol levels lower than 0.065 percent increased the effective coronary blood flow. However when the alcohol was 0.19 percent, a marked diminution of the velocity of the left ventricular contraction was observed (112). In alcoholic persons, catheterization of the coronary sinus blood showed a consistently altered balance of oxidative overt enzymes, suggesting that enzymes within the mitochondria are affected in these patients, even when they do not have manifest heart disease (179, 180). These effects were obtained in experiments with intoxicating amounts of alcohol.

Although the appearance of the heart in alcoholic cardiomyopathy is characteristic, neither the gross nor the microscopic findings are specific. Usually the coronary arteries are free of significant arteriosclerosis or other occlusive changes, and the valves are entirely normal. In most cases the heart is large and flabby, with focal myocardial fibrosis and endocardial thickening. In some instances, only cardiac enlargement is seen. Under the microscope the heart muscle cells may reveal loss of striations, pyknotic nuclei, vacuolization, and hydropic change. From studies using the higher resolving power of the electron microscope, ultrastructural changes remarkably similar to those seen in the alcohol-damaged liver have been reported (41, 62).

The clinical, biochemical, pathological, and ultra-structural data all provide evidence that alcoholic cardiomyopathy is indeed a distinct entity. This concept is supported by the report that administration of alcohol to a patient receiving a good, vitamin-supplemented diet for 5½ months produced the clinical syndrome of alcoholic cardiomyopathy, which improved after alcohol was discontinued (132). The administration of alcohol with an adequate diet to rats led to the consistent accumulation of fat in the heart (95), and similar treatment over a period of months produced a decrease in cardiac function. Under electron-microscope examination, the same sort of studies in mice demonstrated changes in the heart similar to those observed in human alcoholic cardiomyopathy (17).

The mechanism and pathogenesis of alcoholic heart disease are unknown at this time. Whether a direct effect of ethanol on heart cells plays a role, or whether a metabolic product such as acetaldehyde does, remains to be seen. Patients with alcoholic cardiomyopathy are treated conservatively with the usual measures for congestive heart failure. As in the case of liver cirrhosis, absolute abstinence from alcohol is a prerequisite for successful treatment. Mural thrombi on the diseased endocardium represent an occasional complication, which may lead to strokes. Prolonged bed rest which "unloads" the heart appears to be highly beneficial (110). Most patients who are treated with bed rest and adjunct therapy will recover if they abstain from alcohol. A small number of patients, however, have irreversible heart disease by the time they are seen by a physician.

ALCOHOL AND THE GASTROINTESTINAL TRACT

The effects of alcohol on other parts of the gastrointestinal tract have not been as intensively studied as those on the liver, but sufficient knowledge is available to indicate that chronic heavy drinking has a variety of injurious effects on the gastrointestinal system. The association of diarrhea with alcohol intoxication was noted by Hippocrates, who prescribed wine as a purgative (60).

Although most of the harm associated with heavy drinking occurs after its absorption, when strong alcoholic beverages are taken the irritating effect may cause direct local injury. The possible sites of such injury are the mouth, the stomach, and the esophagus. An increased frequency of cancer of these parts of the digestive tract has indeed been reported among alcoholic persons (182, 183, 184). The possible relationship to the irritative effect of alcohol is complicated, however, by the fact that alcoholic persons are usually also heavy smokers.

Stomach

Ingestion of alcoholic beverages stimulates acid production in the stomach, presumably by enhancing the secretion of the hormone gastrin (3, 34). In addition, emptying of the stomach is delayed (8), and from animal experiments it appears that strong alcohol solutions may damage the gastric mucosal barrier. In that event, back diffusion of acid would occur, damaging the lining of the stomach. The combination of salicylate and alcohol (24, 25, 26) or alcohol alone (22), has been shown to cause a movement of hydrogen ions out of the stomach, and the passage of sodium and potassium ions into it. Since alcohol leads to alteration in the electrical properties of the stomach wall, a direct injury by the alcohol has been suggested (48).

Gastritis and achlorhydria are common chronic conditions in alcoholic persons, and gastric ulcers have been reported frequently (30, 48, 119, 123). One of the life-threatening emergencies in medical practice is massive upper gastrointestinal hemorrhage (98). More than half of the patients with hemorrhagic erosive gastritis had ingested alcohol or aspirin or both shortly before the onset of bleeding. Both superficial and atrophic gastritis were more frequent in the alcoholic patients than in a control population examined by Dinoso and associates (29, 30). However, whether either the superficial or the atrophic gastritis are direct sequels of alcoholic beverages has not been settled.

Small Intestine

Maladies of the small intestine are not often a medical complication in alcoholism, but occasionally they are troublesome. Malabsorption of various substances (72, 73) such as thiamin (162), folic acid (59), xylose (136), fat (136), and vitamin B_{12} (97, 136), have been reported in alcoholic patients. The administration of large doses of alcohol experimentally has been reported to interfere with intestinal transport of amino acids both in test-tube experiments and in studies in animals (67) and man (97). Prolonged heavy intake of alcohol by human volunteers, together with excellent protein and vitamin intake, resulted in depression

91

of vitamin B_{12} absorption from the ileum, the distal part of the small intestine. This suggests that alcohol can impair the function of the ileum even when nutrition is adequate (97). Since alcohol is generally absorbed before reaching the ileum, its interference with vitamin B_{12} absorption seems to be dependent upon an indirect effect. Specimens of intestinal tissue from alcoholic patients have not usually appeared abnormal when examined by light-microscopy (67). However, administration of alcohol to volunteers for 3 to 4 weeks resulted in changes of the small intestine, revealed by electron-microscopic examination (140). All the intestinal injuries associated with chronic alcohol abuse appear to be rapidly reversible. The mechanism by which alcohol affects small-intestine ultrastructure, absorption, and transport is at present unknown.

Pancreas

Alcoholism is occasionally associated with pancreatitis and pancreatic insufficiency (146). Individuals with a long history of alcohol abuse show a diminished response to pancreatic stimulation in volume, bicarbonate concentration, and amylase secretion (114). Moreover, a provocation test in alcoholic patients leads to increased amylase and lipase activity in the serum, indicating subclinical pancreatic damage (52). These abnormalities appear to be reversible when alcohol is discontinued. It is not feasible to perform pancreatic biopsy in volunteers, but studies in rats given heavy alcohol doses over long periods have disclosed ultra-structural changes reminiscent of those seen in the liver (23). A decrease in pancreatic lipase may secondarily lead to malabsorption of fat in the small intestine.

The occurrence of pancreatitis may be related to a direct effect of alcohol or to spasm of the sphincter of Oddi, which would increase pressure in the pancreatic duct (130). Since alcohol increases gastric acidity, a greater elaboration of secretin may follow, which would result in increased secretion against an obstructed duct. This situation is known to favor the development of pancreatitis (32). In addition, the metabolism of pancreatic cells may be disturbed, as evidence by the report of decreased protein synthesis in animals after prolonged treatment with alcohol (145).

ALCOHOL AND MUSCLE

Although muscle weakness in alcoholic persons has been known for almost 150 years (68), a well-defined syndrome of muscle disease associated with chronic alcohol abuse was described in Russia (149) in 1928 and reconfirmed there (99) in 1962. In the United States this syndrome was first recognized in 1957 (40) and since then has been increasingly accepted as a complication of alcoholism (126). The disorder has been classified into three general forms: (a) subclinical myopathy; (b) acute alcoholic myopathy; and (c) chronic alcoholic myopathy (126).

The subclinical variety combines a lack of symptoms with alterations in the levels of certain enzymes in the blood serum, of which creatine phosphokinase (CPK) is the most important. A majority of patients admitted to the hospital following prolonged consumption of large amounts of alcohol show increased serum CPK, but in the largest reported series (127) about 40 percent had a normal serum CPK. In addition, a majority of the alcoholic patients exhibit a diminished rise of lactic acid in the blood as a response to ischemic exercise (127, 170).

Acute alcoholic myopathy may present itself in several different forms. In some patients, the only symptom is sudden muscle cramps which occur from a few minutes to a few hours apart, but usually last for only about a day. Although the cramps are most common in muscles of the extremities, isolated contraction of various muscles, particularly of the abdominal wall, have been reported. Perhaps the most dramatic form of acute alcoholic myopathy—certainly one of the most striking complications of alcoholism—is associated with a severe myoglobinuria, that is, the occurrence of muscle pigment in the urine. An alcoholic debauch is followed by severe pain and swelling of involved muscles, together with a pronounced weakness. Arms and legs may both be involved, the latter more frequently. This form of alcoholic myopathy is generally seen in patients with long histories of alcoholism, and consequently may be associated with severe liver disease. Recovery is the rule if alcohol is discontinued, although acute renal failure may be precipitated by myoglobinuria. In recovered individuals, pain and swelling of muscles generally disappear after several days or weeks but the basic process may progress inexorably to chronic myopathy, without further symptoms of the acute phase. Laboratory examination of patients with acute alcoholic myopathy generally discloses increased serum CPK and a diminished rise in blood lactic acid after ischemic exercise.

Persons with a history of prolonged severe alcoholism may develop chronic alcoholic myopathy insidiously or after one or more episodes of clinically recognizable acute myopathy. The principal findings then are weakness and atrophy, which may affect almost any muscle in the body but are most common in the legs. Proximal muscles are generally involved to a greater extent than distal ones. Episodes of acute myopathy may also occur in patients who are suffering from the chronic form. Since chronic alcoholic myopathy is usually found after a long history of alcoholism, it is important, on medical examination, to distinguish the muscle disease from peripheral neuropathy or encephalopathy associated with nutritional disturbances or acute effects of alcohol on the central nervous system.

Acute and chronic alcoholic myopathy are associated with pathological changes observable by both light-microscopic and electron-microscopic examination of muscle tissue. Focal atrophy of individual muscle cells has been seen in the subclinical form of the disease. Severe acute myopathy, usually with myoglobinuria, results in necrosis, edema, and fragmentation of muscle fibers.

The pathogenesis of alcoholic myopathy has not yet been elucidated. Both ischemia (31) and nutritional deficiency (170) have been suggested as possible causes. An etiology other than a direct effect of alcohol was supported by a lack of increase in CPK after infusion of alcohol into dogs, and a similar response when normal human subjects were tested after social drinking (126). However, administration of alcohol to rats for 9 months showed decreased substrates of the citric acid cycle in muscle, when compared with pair-fed controls (126). A recent experiment in human volunteers suggests a direct toxicity of alcohol. In three volunteers, intake of alcohol sufficient to provide 42 percent of the total calories for 4 weeks led to increased serum CPK and striking ultrastructural changes in muscle, similar to those observed in patients with acute alcoholic myopathy (156). In these studies, the volunteers received adequate amounts of all dietary constituents, including vitamins, folic acid, and minerals.

In summary, chronic heavy alcohol ingestion is associated with an acute and chronic disease of muscle which may be independent of nutritional factors, but in some clinical cases the condition has been connected with water and electrolyte imbalance (109).

ALCOHOL AND THE ENDOCRINES

The endocrine system is an exquisitely sensitive apparatus, essential to maintain the constancy of the internal environment of the organism. Thus, when a compound such as alcohol, which has characteristics of both a drug and a food and which markedly affects bodily functions, is taken by man, the endocrine system can be expected to react. When such a compound is ingested repeatedly, adaptive changes in the system will occur to maintain the body's internal balance.

The greatest attention to date has been focused on the effects of alcohol on the hypothalamic-pituitary-adrenal (HPA) axis. It was postulated in the late 1940's and early 1950s (13, 152, 165) that preexisting deficiencies in this axis predispose some people to consume alcohol to eventual adrenal exhaustion. Because of certain similarities between Addison's disease and delirium tremens, adrenocortical insufficiency was seen as the end stage of alcoholism. Indeed, with little supporting data, a flurry of essentially uncritical reports appeared, proclaiming the efficacy of adrenocortical extracts in treating the acute stages of alcoholism, including delirium tremens, and in maintaining sobriety (13, 70, 154). With more careful observation and critical examination of the data (69, 181), serious questions were raised about the value of indiscriminate use of hormones in the treatment of alcoholic patients.

The effect of alcohol on the HPA axis has been the subject of a recent review (121). Current studies in both animals and man indicate that alcohol stimulates the adrenal cortex, resulting in the release of its hormones. This stimulation is probably mediated via the pituitary gland, which releases adrenocorticotropic hormone—the hormone that activates the adrenal cortex. Various defects in the HPA axis and metabolism of adrenal hormones in alcoholic persons have been described (70, 79, 108, 113). There are few consistent findings, however, and any comparison between the HPA status of control subjects and alcoholic patients is complicated by many uncontrolled variables; these include organ pathology and disease states, nutrition, drugs (both illicit and prescription), stress, and emotional factors. There is no convincing evidence that abnormalities in the HPA system are causally related to alcoholism, rather than being associated with or consequences of prolonged alcohol abuse.

Data are accumulating which suggest that alcohol affects the metabolism of another adrenal hormone, aldosterone, which induces retention of sodium, potassium, and chloride (120, 148). Other hormones that are known to be influenced by alcohol are the catecholamines, such as epinephrine (adrenalin) (1, 128),

95

norepinephrine, and dopamine (4). Animal and clinical studies indicate that acute administration of alcohol increases the excretion of catecholamines. The metabolism of catecholamines and serotonin has also been shown to be affected by alcohol (27, 28, 151).

The powerful effect of alcohol on urinary excretion is an old observation, confirmed by experiments (35). The effects of alcohol on water balance occur partly through the inhibition of the antidiuretic hormone by the posterior pituitary (35, 157, 169), thus facilitating water excretion by the kidney (144).

The release of oxytocin, a hormone which stimulates contraction of the uterus, from the posterior pituitary is also inhibited by the administration of alcohol (46, 47, 174).

In men, the clinical triad of alcoholic liver cirrhosis, testicular atrophy, and enlargement of the breast is called the Silvestrini-Corda syndrome (150). Unfortunately, the notion that high estrogen levels affect the endocrine organs of alcoholic persons with cirrhosis has not been convincingly demonstrated. Since the liver inactivates estrogen, the female hormone, it was supposed that the imbalance of gonadal function observed in these alcoholic patients was secondary to cirrhosis of the liver (58). In an extensive study of cirrhotics suffering from gynecomastia, testicular atrophy, and loss of potency, Lloyd and Williams (100) found low levels of certain sex hormones. In a recent study, Brown (16) reported that the recovery of injected estrogens in alcoholic persons with cirrhosis was within the normal range. Furthermore, quantities and ratios of estrogens in these patients were normal during the preterminal state. The endocrine mechanism underlying the sexual dysfunction in some alcoholic patients still remains an open question.

Information on the effects of alcohol on the other endocrine systems is either scanty and impressionistic, or totally lacking. Thus, while alcoholic hypoglycemia (low blood sugar) is a well-recognized clinical entity (45), little or no information is available on the role of insulin and glucagon in this phenomenon.

While there have been some clinical assessments to support the observation of hypothyroidism in alcoholic persons (54, 55), this theory (133) is currently under investigation.

ALCOHOL AND NUTRITION

Malnutrition is commonly observed among alcoholic persons. In recent years this has been more true of those found on skid row, but it is by no means rare among those in better circumstances. One of the main reasons for this is the fact that alcohol itself represents an important source of calories. Each gram of alcohol provides 7.1 calories, which means that a pint of 100-U.S.-proof distilled spirits represents more than 1,300 calories, possibly half to two-thirds of the normal daily caloric requirement of many people. Therefore, heavy drinkers need less food to fulfill their caloric needs. Since alcoholic beverages do not contain significant amounts of protein, vitamins, minerals, and amino acids, they provide only "empty calories," and the intake of the vital elements of nutrition by a heavy drinker may readily become borderline or insufficient. Economic factors may also reduce the consumption of nutrient-rich food by the alcoholic person.

In addition, even in a person consuming a good diet, heavy alcohol intake can result in malnutrition by interfering with the normal processes of food digestion and absorption (114). As a consequence, there is inadequate digestion of the food actually consumed. Some of the side effects of gastritis also reduce appetite, thereby lessening food intake. Moreover, alcohol appears to affect the capacity of the intestine to absorb various nutrients, including vitamins—especially vitamins B_1 (163, 164) and B_{12} (97) and amino acids (67). In addition, malnutrition itself further reduces the capacity of the intestine to absorb nutrients.

Some of the important diseases associated with defective nutrition in alcoholic persons have already been noted in the sections of this chapter dealing with the alcoholic encephalopathies, liver, and heart. Others long known to afflict these individuals are polyneuropathy (associated chiefly with deficiency of vitamin B_1); pellegra, due to deficiency of niacin and other fractions of the vitamin B complex, with symptoms of dermatosis, digestive disorder, and mental dysfunction; anemia, due to deficiency of iron and cobalamin (vitamin B_{12}); and, less often, scurvy, due to deficiency of Vitamin C; and other hypovitaminoses which result in defective bodily functioning of the organism (14, 56, 71, 72, 73).

In addition, an adequate supply of nutrients, especially protein and vitamins, is needed for the normal maintenance of liver function. The role that protein deficiency may play in the development of liver disease in adult humans has not been clarified. In experimental animals, however, severe protein deficiency has been shown to aggravate the pathological effects on tissues of an alcoholized diet (96).

One of the significant recent findings concerning the development of injury from alcohol has been the observation that, although nutritional deficiency states can aggravate the effect of alcohol upon the liver, sufficient alcohol—even in the absence of malnutrition—can have a deleterious effect upon that organ (87, 92, 93, 142).

A particularly dramatic complication of alcohol intoxication is low blood sugar (hypoglycemia) which, if unrecognized, may be responsible for some of the "unexplained" sudden deaths observed in acutely intoxicated alcoholic patients. This complication occurs in individuals whose liver glycogen stores are depleted by fasting or starvation, or in those who have preexisting abnormalities of carbohydrate metabolism.

INTERACTION OF ALCOHOL AND OTHER DRUGS

In light of the current interest in drug abuse generally, and the particular emphasis being accorded the problems of alcohol as the most commonly abused drug, it is pertinent to consider the status of the interrelationships of the use of alcohol in combination with other drugs. An interaction between alcohol and other drugs may contribute to fatal automobile accidents and accidental or suicidal deaths in individuals who have consumed barbiturates or tranquilizers while they were intoxicated. Indeed, more alcoholic persons die from intoxication by drugs other than alcohol, than from alcohol intoxication (158). Moreover, both alcohol intoxication and alcoholism may affect the dosage requirements and safety limits of medically indicated drugs—for example, anesthetics in surgery, oral medications for diabetes, anticonvulsants in epilepsy, and anticoagulants after heart attacks (44).

The interaction of alcohol and drugs appears paradoxical. While intoxicated, individuals are more sensitive to many drugs—for example, sedatives and tranquilizers (44). When sober, alcoholic persons are unusually tolerant to many drugs (155). In the past, these interactions have been explained as due to the additive actions of drugs and alcohol and by adaptation of the brain to increasing amounts of the drugs (44).

Drug Metabolism in the Liver

Alcohol bears many similarities to other drugs that are metabolized by the liver (143). The prolonged use of such drugs, exemplified by phenobarbital, leads to acceleration of the metabolism not only of the administered drug but also of many others. A single dose of one drug decreases the metabolism of others by competing for the same detoxification mechanism.

In rats fed an adequate diet, prolonged administration of alcohol results in an increased rate of elimination of other drugs in the liver (116, 137, 139). Studies in human volunteers maintained with adequate nutrients and vitamins showed essentially the same response to the administration of alcohol—namely, an increase in the capacity of liver tissue to metabolize drugs (116, 139). These findings suggest that the increased rate of drug metabolism in patients who are hospitalized for the treatment of alcoholism (77) is a consequence of their prolonged heavy alcohol intake rather than of nutritional factors or the intake of other drugs.

The similarity of alcohol to other drugs has also been found to be true in studies of inhibition of drug metabolism. Alcohol intoxication in both rats and men conspicuously delayed the elimination of pentobarbital and meprobamate from the blood; that is, it inhibited drug metabolism (138). An explanation for the similarity of alcohol to other drugs metabolized by the liver was the finding that alcohol is partially metabolized in the liver by a system similar to that which metabolizes other drugs (85).

In summary, alcohol is one of the drugs metabolized by the liver. A single large dose of alcohol leads to the inhibition of the metabolism of other drugs, while prolonged heavy intake leads to accelerated drug metabolism. These findings on the combined effects of alcohol and drugs explain, in part, the accentuated tolerance of alcoholic persons, when sober, to other drugs, as well as the enhanced effect of other drugs in persons intoxicated by alcohol.

Drugs and the Central Nervous System

On the behavioral level, many other drugs when used simultaneously with alcohol are capable of grossly distorting the usual responses expected from alcohol consumption alone. This is due to the combined effects exerted by alcohol and other drugs on the central nervous system.

The interactive result of taking alcohol and other drugs that also depress the central nervous system may be either additive or potentiative (sometimes called synergistic) (43). An additive effect is experienced when a half-dose of one drug taken with a half-dose of another similarly acting drug produce the same effect as a full dose of either drug alone. A potentiative effect results when half-doses of two drugs taken together produce an exaggerated action that is grossly disproportionate to the effect of a full dose of either drug taken separately. An example of a potentiative effect is the combination of barbiturates and alcohol which produces a depressant effect on the central nervous system that is much greater than would occur from either of these drugs taken alone (74).

During the past several decades, hundreds of new drugs have been produced and introduced to the public. Their judicious use by physicians has revolutionized the practice of medicine, affording great relief from suffering and saving countless lives. Many of these drugs are legally obtained only through medical prescription. Others are freely available on drug store, supermarket, and specialty-shop counters.

Some of these drugs are central nervous system depressants, acting on the same brain structures as alcohol (75). They include drugs for inducing sleep, tranquilization, sedation, and for relief of pain, motion sickness, or head cold and allergy symptoms. The drugs used for these purposes in the United States—both by prescription and for self-medication—are too numerous to name. But they can be classified according to the principal purpose of their use: narcotics; hypnotic-sedative drugs (including barbiturates); tranquilizers; antihistamines; and volatile solvents.

Narcotics are mainly opium, morphine, heroin, codeine, and synthetic drugs such as Demerol (meperidine hydrochloride) and methadone. Next to alcohol, narcotics have been the most widely abused drugs. The general action of all narcotics on the central nervous system, and their major medical use, is to depress the sensory area of the cerebral cortex, resulting in relief of pain. The general depressant action of these drugs also includes sedation, apathy, drowsiness, sleep, and—with high enough dosage—respiratory failure and death.

Hypnotic-sedative drugs (including barbiturates) are primarily general central nervous system depressants that exercise a broad range of suppression of brain function. These drugs differ from each other in the degree of depression they produce. Increasing dosages of all hypnotic-sedative drugs, however, produce a continuum of effects, from tranquilization and sedation . . . to motor and intellectual impairment . . . to stupor, coma, and death. This is similar to the progression seen with alcohol.

In the past, hypnotic-sedative drugs such as chloral hydrate, paraldehyde, and bromides were widely used in medicine and by the general public for sedation and inducing sleep. They are often replaced in medicine by the more efficient and easily controlled barbiturates, which can produce the entire range of depressant effects, from mild tranquilization to deep anesthesia. A person under the influence of barbiturates acts exactly like one under the influence of alcohol. Depending on the dose, his speech is thick and slurred; he sways; he staggers; he falls; he loses consciousness. As explained previously, alcohol and barbiturates when combined enhance each other's effects. The consumption of even small amounts of both drugs in close order can be particularly dangerous and may result in death (74).

Tranquilizers are drugs used mainly to relieve or prevent uncomfortable emotional feeling, reduce tension and apprehension, and promote a state of calm and relaxation. The effects overlap with those of depressant drugs such as alcohol. Some sedative and hypnotic effects from tranquilizers are similar to those of barbiturates which, in turn, have tranquilizing actions.

Tranquilizing drugs vary widely in potency. If used without medical direction, the stronger tranquilizer drugs such as Compazine (prochlorperazine) and Thorazine (chlorpromazine), can be dangerous even in low dosages, with effects ranging from marked depression to deep sleep. The weaker tranquilizers such as Miltown (meprobamate), Valium (diazepam), and Librium (chlordiazepoxide) are considerably less severe in their effects. Because the effect of tranquilizers combined with alcohol may be potentiative, patients for whom they are prescribed should be instructed about the heightened danger of their drinking and particularly about the increased risks in operating motor vehicles or machinery.

Antihistamines block the action of histamine in the body. Histamine is a substance produced in the body under certain pathological conditions such as head colds and allergies, and is responsible for the congestion, bronchial spasm, and unpleasant tissue inflammations characteristic of these conditions. Antihistamines prevent or relieve these symptoms. The drugs in this group are numerous, and include Dramamine (dimenhydrinate), Benadryl (diphenhydramine hydrochloride), Phenergan (promethazine hydrochloride), and Pyribenzamine (tripelennamine). Some of the antihistamine drugs also have the ability to diminish or abolish the symptoms of motion sickness, and many drugs marketed for this purpose contain moderate to large doses of antihistamines. The antihistamines are included among the hypnotic-sedative drugs because they act as central nervous system depressants (53). In ordinary dosages they cause drowsiness. Larger amounts produce sleep. Because of their depressant action, these drugs are the major ingredients in most of the nostrums advertised as "tension" relievers and sleep-inducers, and are freely dispensed without prescription. Their potential additiveness with alcohol often goes unrecognized.

Volatile solvents include compounds of volatile substances such as isoamyl acetate, ethyl acetate, toluene, methanol, and many others, which are additive or potentiative with alcohol. As such, these compounds have a depressant effect on the central nervous system similar to barbiturates and narcotics. Apart from a small population of "glue-sniffers," there are large numbers of persons who are exposed for many hours to inhalation of these vapors in industrial situations. Intoxication due to the interaction of such exposure to drugs and a relatively small amount of alcohol has frequently been reported (124), especially in the courts, when an intoxicated driver was a victim of this interaction phenomenon.

The use of any drug that has a depressant effect on the central nervous system in combination with alcohol represents an extra hazard to health and safety and, in some cases, to life itself.

SUMMARY AND CONCLUSION

Alcohol abuse and alcoholism are implicated as primary or related causal factors in many pathological conditions. These include:

- Brain disorders such as Wernicke's syndrome, Korsakoff's psychosis, niacin-deficiency encephalopathy, and Marchiafava's disease.
- Disorders of the digestive system, such as malabsorption of vital nutrients, gastritis, pancreatitis, fatty liver, hepatitis, and cirrhosis.
- Generalized myopathy and cardiomyopathy, numerous nutritional diseases in addition to some of the encephalopathies, including polyneuropathy, beriberi heart, pellagra, scurvy, and anemia.
- Atrophy of some endocrine glands, disturbances of metabolism that may aggravate or precipitate such conditions as

gout and hypoglycemia, and disturbance of metabolism of other drugs.

• Increased risk of accident, injury, and death from intake of other drugs that interact additively or potentiatively with alcohol.

These disorders undoubtedly exacerbate other illnesses when they occur in alcoholic persons, and contribute to the substantial reduction of their lifespan.

REFERENCES

(1)   Abelin, I., Herren, C., and Berli, W. Uber die erregende Wirkung des Alkohols auf den Adrenalin-und Noradrenalinhaushalt des menschlichen Organismus. Helv. Med. Acta 25:591–600, 1958.

(2)   Adams, R.D. Nutritional diseases of the nervous system in the alcoholic patient. Trans. Amer. Climat. (Clin.) Ass. 71:59–94, 1959.

(3)   Anderson, S. Gastric and duodenal mechanisms inhibiting gastric secretion of acid. In: Handbook of Physiology. Vol. II, Secretion, Chapter 48, Section 6. Washington, D.C.: American Physiological Society, 1967, pp. 869–877.

(4)   Anton, A.H. Ethanol and urinary catecholamines in man. Clin. Pharmacol. Ther. 6:462–469, 1965.

(5)   Bacon, S.D., ed. Studies of Driving and Drinking. Quarterly Journal of Studies on Alcohol. Supplement No. 4, 1968.

(6)   Baisset, A., Montastruc, P., and Garrigues, M. Recherches sur les interactions de l'alcool et de la secretion antidiuretique neuro-hypophysaire. Influence des preparations post-hypophysaires sur la soif provoquee par l'ingestion d'alcool. (Research on the interaction of alcohol and neurohypophyseal antidiuretic secretion. Influence of posthypophyseal preparations on thirst induced by the ingestion of alcohol.) Pathol. Biol. (Paris) 13:241–251, 1965.

(7)   Baraona, E. and Lieber, C.S. Effects of chronic ethanol feeding on serum lipoprotein metabolism in the rat. J. Clin. Invest. 49:769–778, 1970.

(8)   Barboriak, J.J. and Meade, R.C. Effect of alcohol on gastric emptying in man. Amer. J. Clin. Nutr. 23:1151–1153, 1970.

(9)   Barchha, R., Stewart, M.A., and Guze, S.B. The prevalence of alcoholism among general hospital ward patients. Amer. J. Psychiat. 125:681–684, 1968.

(10)   Barry, H., III and Miller, N.E. Effects of drugs on approach-avoidance conflict tested repeatedly by means of a "telescope alley." J. Comp. Physiol. Psychol. 55:201–210, 1962.

(11)   Beard, J.D., Barlow, G., and Overman, R.R. Body fluids and blood electrolytes in dogs subjected to chronic ethanol administration. J. Pharmacol. Exp. Ther. 148: 348–355, 1965.

(12) Best, C.H., Hartroft, W.S., Lucas, C.C., and Ridout, J.H. Liver damage produced by feeding alcohol or sugar and its prevention by choline. Brit. Med. J. 2:1001–1006, 1949.

(13) Bettencourt-Gomes, S.C. A.C.T.H. in delirium tremens. Brit. Med. J. 2:339, 1953.

(14) Blankenhorn, M.A. Diagnosis of beriberi heart disease. Ann. Intern. Med. 23:398–404, 1945.

(15) Bowman, K.M. and Jellinek, E.M. Alcoholic mental disorders. Quart. J. Stud. Alc. 2:312–390, 1941.

(16) Brown, J.B., In: Paulsen, C.A., ed. Estrogen Assays in Clinical Basis and Methodology; A Workshop Conference; Medicine. Seattle: University of Washington Press, 1965, pp. 295–297.

(17) Burch, G.E. and DePasquale, N.P. Alcoholic cardiomyopathy. Amer. J. Cardiol. 23:723–731, 1969.

(18) Burch, G.E. and Giles, T.D. Editorial: Alcoholic cardiomyopathy. Concepts of the disease and its treatment. Amer. J. Med. 50:141–145, 1971.

(19) Cameron, C.B. Brit. Med. Bull. 13:119, 1957.

(20) Carlsson, C. and Haggendal, J. Arterial noradrenaline levels after ethanol withdrawal. Lancet 2:889, 1967.

(21) Cathell, J.L. The occurrence of certain psychosomatic conditions during different phases of the alcoholic's life. N.C. Med. J. 15:503–505, 1954.

(22) Dagradi, A.E., Stempien, S.J., Lee, E.R. et al. Hemorrhagic-erosive gastritis. Gastroint. Endosc. 14:147–150, 1968.

(23) Darle, N., Ekholm, R., and Edlund, Y. Ultrastructure of the rat exocrine pancreas after long term intake of ethanol. Gastroenterology 58:62–72, 1970.

(24) Davenport, H.W. Gastric mucosal injury by fatty and acetylsalicylic acids. Gastroenterology 46:245–253, 1964.

(25) Davenport, H.W. Potassium fluxes across the resting and stimulated gastric mucosa: Injury by salicylic and acetic acids. Gastroenterology 49:238–245, 1965.

(26) Davenport, H.W., Cohen, B.J., Bree, M. and Davenport, V.D. Damage to the gastric mucosa: Effects of salicylates and stimulation. Gastroenterology 49:189–196, 1965.

(27) Davis, V.E., Brown, H., Huff, J.A. and Cashaw, J.L. The alteration of serotonin metabolism to 5-hydroxytryptophol by ethanol ingestion in man. J. Lab. Clin. Med. 69:132–140, 1967.

(28) Davis, V.E., Brown, H., Huff, J.A. and Cashaw, J.L. Ethanol-induced alterations of norepinephrine metabolism in man. J. Lab. Clin. Med. 69:787–799, 1967.

(29) Dinoso, V.P., Chey, W.Y., Siplet, H. et al. Effects of ethanol on the gastric mucosa of the Heidenhain pouch of dogs. Amer. J. Dig. Dis. 15:809–817, 1970.

(30) Dinoso, V.P., Chey, W.Y., Braverman, S. et al. Gastric Secretion and Gastric Mucosal Morphology in Chronic Alcoholics. Arch. Intern. Med. (in press).

(31) Douglas, R.M., Fewings, J.D., Casley-Smith, J.R. and West, R.F. Recurrent rhabdomyolysis precipitated by alcohol: A case report with physiological and electron microscopic studies of skeletal muscle. Aust. Ann. Med. 15:251–261, 1966.

(32) Dreiling, D.A., Richman, A. and Fradkin, N.F. The role of alcohol in the etiology of pancreatitis: A study of the effect of intravenous ethyl alcohol on the external excretion of the pancreas. Gastroenterology 20:636–646, 1952.

(33) Edmondson, H.A., Peters, R.L., Reynolds, T.B. and Kuzma, O.T. Sclerosing hyaline necrosis of the liver in the chronic alcoholic. Ann. Intern. Med. 59:646–673, 1963.

(34) Elwin, C.E. Stimulation of gastric acid secretion by irrigation of the antrum with some aliphatic alcohols. Acta Physiol. Scand. 75:1–11, 1969.

(35) Eggleton, M.G., The diuretic action of alcohol in man. J. Physiol. 101:172–191, 1942.

(36) Evans, W. Alcoholic Cardiomyopathy. Amer. Heart J. 61:556–567, 1961.

(37) Fabre, L.F., Jr., Farmer, R.W., and Davis, H.W. In: Roach, M.K., McIssac, W.M. and Creaven, P.J. eds., Biological Aspects of Alcohol. Austin: University of Texas Press, 1971.

(38) Fabre, L.F., Jr., Farmer, R.W., Pellizzari, E.D. and Farrell, G. The effect of ethanol on human urinary aldosterone excretion. Clin. Res. 18:359, 1970.

(39) Fabre, L.F., Jr., Farmer, R.W., Pellizzari, E.D., and Mendelson, J.H. Adrenal response to alcohol mineral corticoid metabolism. In: Mello, N.K. and Mendelson, J.H., eds., Recent Advances in Studies of Alcoholism. Washington, D.C.: U.S. Government Printing Office, in press.

(40) Fahlgren, H., and Hed, R. and Lundmark, C. Myonecrosis and myoglobinuria in alcohol and barbiturate intoxication. Acta Med. Scand. 158:405–412, 1957.

(41) Ferrans, V.J., Burch, G.E., Walsh, J.J., Hibbs, R.G. Alcoholic cardiomyopathy. Bull. Tulane, Med. Fac. 24:119–124, 1965.

(42) Fischbach, K., Simmons, E.M. and Pollard, R.E., Delirium tremens treated with intravenously administered corticotropin (ACTH). J.A.M.A. 149:927–928, 1952.

(43) Forney, R.B. and Hayer, R.N. Toxicology of ethanol. Amer. Rev. Pharmacol. 9:379, 1969.

(44) Forney, R.B., and Hughes, F.W. Combined Effects of Alcohol and Other Drugs. Springfield, Ill.: Charles C. Thomas, 1968.

(45) Freinkel, N., Arky, R.A., Singer, D.L., Cohen, A.K., Bleicher, S.J., Anderson, J.B., Silbert, C.K. and Foster, A.E. Alcohol hypoglycemia, IV: Current concepts of its pathogenesis. Diabetes 14:350–361, 1965.

(46) Fuchs, A.R., Coutinho, E.M., Xavier, R., Bates, P.E., and Fuchs, F. Effect of ethanol on the activity of the nonpregnant human uterus and its reactivity to neurohypophyseal hormones. Amer. J. Obstet. Gynec. 101:997–1000, 1968.

105

(47) Fuchs, A.R. and Fuchs, F. Alcohol effect on oxytocin release and uterine mobility. In: Sardesai, V.M., ed., Biochemical and Clinical Aspects of Alcohol Metabolism. Chapter 13. Springfield, Ill.: Charles C. Thomas, 1969, pp. 105–114.

(48) Geall, M.G., Phillips, S.F. and Summerskill, W.H.J. Profile of gastric potential differences in man. Effects of aspirin, alcohol, bile, and endogenous acid. Gastroenterology 58:437–443, 1970.

(49) Giacobini, E., Izikowitz, S. and Wegmann, A. The urinary excretion of noradrenaline and adrenalin during alcohol intoxication in alcoholic addicts. Experientia 16:467, 1960.

(50) Giacobini, E., Izikowitz, S. and Wegmann, A. Urinary norepinephrine and epinephrine excretion in delirium tremens. Arch. Gen. Psychiat. 3:289–296, 1960.

(51) Gitlow, S.E., Bertani, L.M., Dziedzic, S.W. and Wong, B.L. Metabolism of norepinephrine (NE) in the alcoholic during ethanol ingestion, the withdrawal syndrome and sobriety. Clin. Res. 19:349, 1971.

(52) Goebell, H., Bode, C.H., Bastian, R. and Strohmeyer, G. Klinische asymptomatische Funktionsstorungen des exokrinen Pankreas bei chronischen Alkoholikern. (Asymptomatic abnormalities of exocrine pancreatic functions in chronic alcoholics.) Dtsch. Med. Wochenschr. 95:808–814, 1970.

(53) Goldberg, L. Alcohol, tranquilizers and hangover. Quart. J. Stud. Alc. Suppl. No. 1, pp. 37–56, 1961.

(54) Goldberg, M. The occurrence and treatment of hypothyroidism among alcoholics. J. Clin. Endocrin. 20:609–621, 1960.

(55) Goldberg, M. Thyroid impairment in chronic alcoholics. Amer. J. Psychiat. 119:255–256, 1962.

(56) Goodhart, R. and Jolliffe, N. The role of nutritional deficiencies in the production of cardiovascular disturbances in the alcohol addict. Amer. Heart J. 15:569–581, 1938.

(57) Gray, S. Epigastric symptoms in alcoholics with and without gastritis. Gastroenterology 1:221–226, 1943.

(58) Hall, P.F. Gynaecomastia. Monographs of the Federal Council of the British Medical Association in Australia, No. 2. Glebe, Australia: Australasian Medical Pub. Co., 1959.

(59) Halsted, C.H., Griggs, R.C., Harris, J.W. The effects of alcoholism on the absorption of folic acid (H^3–PGA) evaluated by plasma levels and urine excretion. J. Lab. Clin. Med. 69:116–131, 1967.

(60) Heberden, W. Commentaries on the History and Cure of Diseases. London: Payne, 1802.

(61) Hetherington, E.M. and Wray, N.P. Aggression, need for social approval, and humor preferences. J. Abn. Soc. Psychol. 68:685–689, 1964.

(62) Hibbs, R.G., Ferrans, V.J., Black, W.C., Weilbaecher, D.C., Walsh, J.J. and Burch, G.E. Alcoholic cardiomyopathy: An electron microscopic study. Am. Heart J. 69:766–779, 1965.

(63) Huang, K.C., Knoefel, P.K., Shimoura, L. and Buren King, N. Some effects of alcohol on water and electrolytes in the dog. Arch. Int. Pharmacodyn. 109:90–98, 1957.

(64) Irgens-Jensen, O. Problem Drinking and Personality; A Study Based on the Draw-a-Person Test. Publication No. 9, National Institute for Alcohol Research. Oslo: Universitetsforlaget, 1971.

(65) Iseri, O.A., Lieber, C.S. and Gottlieb, L.S. The ultrastructure of fatty liver induced by prolonged ethanol ingestion. Amer. J. Path. 48:535–555, 1966.

(66) Iseri, O.A. and Gottlieb, L.S. Alcoholic hyalin and megamitochondria as separate and distinct entities in liver disease associated with alcoholism. Gastroenterology 60:1027–1035, 1971.

(67) Israel, Y., Salazar, I., Rosenmann, E. Inhibitory effects of alcohol on intestinal amino acid transport in vivo and in vitro. J. Nutr. 96:499–504, 1968.

(68) Jackson, J. On a peculiar disease resulting from the use of ardent spirits. New Engl. J. Med. Surg. 2:351–353, 1822.

(69) Jellinek, E.M. The Disease Concept of Alcoholism. New Haven: Hillhouse Press, 1960, pp. 99–110.

(70) Jenkins, J.S. and Connolly, J. Adrenocortical response to ethanol in man. Brit. Med. J. 2:804–805, 1968.

(71) Jolliffe, N., Goodhart, R., Germis, J. and Cline, J.K. The experimental production of vitamin B_1 deficiency in normal subjects; the dependence of the urinary excretion of thiamin on the dietary intake of vitamin B_1. Amer. J. Med. Sci. 198:198–211, 1939.

(72) Jolliffe, N., Wortis, H. and Stein, M.H. Vitamin deficiencies and liver cirrhosis in alcoholism. Pt. IV. The Wernicke syndrome. Pt. V. Nicotinic acid deficiency encephalopathy. Quart. J. Stud. Alc. 2:73–92, 1941.

(73) Jolliffe, N., Wortis, H. and Stein, M.H. Vitamin deficiencies and liver cirrhosis in alcoholism. Pt. VI. Encephalopathies with possible nutritional involvement. Quart. J. Stud. Alc. 2:92–97, 1941.

(74) Jones, K.L., Shainberg, L.W. and Byer, C.O. Drugs and Alcohol. New York: Harper and Row, 1969, p. 45.

(75) Kalant, H. The pharmacology of alcohol intoxication. Quart. J. Stud. Alc. Suppl. No. 1, pp. 1–17, 1961.

(76) Kalin, R., McClelland, D.C. and Kahn, M. Effects of male social drinking on fantasy. J. Pers. Soc. Psychol. 1:441–452, 1965.

(77) Kater, R.M.H., Roggin, G., Tobon, F., Zieve, P. and Iber, F.L. Increased rate of clearance of drugs from the circulation of alcoholics. Amer. J. Med. Sci. 258: 35–39, 1969.

107

(78) Kissin, B., and Begleiter, H., eds. The Biology of Alcoholism. Vol. 2: Neurophysiology and Behavior. New York: Plenum Press, 1972.

(79) Kissin, B., Schenker, V. and Schenker, A.C. The acute effect of ethanol ingestion on plasma and urinary 17–hydroxycorticoids in alcoholic subjects. Amer. J. Med. Sci. 239:690–705, 1960.

(80) Kissin, B., Schenker, V. and Schenker, A.C. Hyperdiuresis after ethanol in chronic alcoholics. Amer. J. Med. Sci. 248:660–669, 1964.

(81) Kramer, K., Kuller, L. and Fisher, R. The increasing mortality attributed to cirrhosis and fatty liver, in Baltimore (1957–1966). Ann. Int. Med. 69:273–282, 1968.

(82) Leevy, C.M. Fatty liver: A study of 270 patients with biopsy proven fatty liver and a review of the literature. Medicine 41:249–276, 1962.

(83) Lelbach, W.K. Leberschaden bei chronischem Alkoholismus; Ergebnisse einer klinischen, klinisch-chemischen und bioptisch-histologischen Untersuchung an 526 Alkoholkranken wahrend der Entziehungskur in einer offenen Trinkerheilstatte. (Liver damage in chronic alcoholism; result of a clinical, clinical-chemical and bioptic-histologic study of 526 alcoholic patients during withdrawal treatment in a public hospital for alcoholics. III. Bioptic-histologic findings.) Acta Hepatosplenol (Stuttg.) 14:9–39, 1967.

(84) Lieber, C.S. Metabolic effects produced by alcohol in the liver and other tissues. Advances Intern. Med. 14:151–199, 1968.

(85) Lieber, C.S. and DeCarli, L.M. Ethanol oxidation by hepatic microsomes: Adaptive increases after ethanol feeding. Science 162:917–918, 1968.

(86) Lieber C.S. and DeCarli, L.M. Hepatic microsomal ethanol-oxidizing system. In vitro characteristics and adaptive properties in vivo. J. Biol. Chem. 245:2505–2512, 1970.

(87) Lieber, C.S., Jones, D.P. and DeCarli, L.M. Effects of prolonged ethanol intake: Production of fatty liver despite adequate diets. J. Clin. Invest. 44:1009–1021, 1965.

(88) Lieber, C.S., Jones, D.P., Mendelson, J.H. and DeCarli, L.M. Fatty liver, hyperlipemia and hyperuricemia produced by prolonged alcohol consumption, despite adequate dietary intake. Trans. Ass. Amer. Physicians 76:289–300, 1963.

(89) Lieber, C.S., Jones, D.P., Losowsky, M.S. and Davidson, C.S. Interrelation of uric acid and ethanol metabolism in man. J. Clin. Invest. 41:1863–1870, 1962.

(90) Lieber, C.S., Lefevre, A., Spritz, N., Feinman, L. and DeCarli, L.M. Difference in hepatic metabolism of long- and medium-chain fatty acids; the role of fatty acid chain length in the production of the alcoholic fatty liver. J. Clin. Invest. 46:1451–1460, 1967.

(91) Lieber, C.S. and Rubin, E. Alcoholic fatty liver in man on a high protein and low fat diet. Amer. J. Med. 44:200–206, 1968.

108

(92) Lieber, C.S. and Rubin, E. Alcoholic fatty liver. N. Engl. J. Med. 280:705–708, 1969.

(93) Lieber, C.S., Rubin, E. and DeCarli, L.M. Respective role of dietary and metabolic factors in the pathogenesis of the alcoholic fatty liver: The biochemical basis for the ethanol-induced liver injury. In:Sardesai, V.M., Biochemical and Clinical Aspects of Alcohol Metabolism. Chapter 19. Springfield, Ill,: Charles C. Thomas, 1969, pp. 176–188.

(94) Lieber, C.S. and Spritz, N. Effects of prolonged ethanol intake in man: Role of dietary, adipose, and endogenously synthesized fatty acids in the pathogenesis of the alcoholic fatty liver. J. Clin. Invest. 45:1400–1411, 1966.

(95) Lieber, C.S., Spritz, N. and DeCarli, L.M. Accumulation of triglycerides in heart and kidney after alcohol ingestion. J. Clin. Invest. 45:1041, 1966.

(96) Lieber, C.S., Spritz, N. and DeCarli, L.M. Fatty liver produced by dietary deficiencies: Its pathogenesis and potentiation by ethanol. J. Lipid Res. 10:283, 1969.

(97) Lindenbaum, J. and Lieber, C.S. Alcohol-induced malabsorption of vitamin B_{12} in man. Nature 224:806, 1969.

(98) Lipp, W.F. and Lipsitz, M.H. The clinical significance of the coexistence of peptic ulcer and portal cirrhosis; with special reference to the problem of massive hemorrhage. Gastroenterology 22:181–191, 1952.

(99) Litvak, L.M. Alkogol' irritatsionnyi neiro-vegetativni sindrom. (The alcoholic irritative neurovegetative syndrome.) Zh. Nevropat. 59:649–656, 1959; 62:440–443, 1962.

(100) Lloyd, C.W. and Williams, R.H. Endocrine changes associated with Laennec's cirrhosis of the liver. Amer. J. Med. 4:315–330, 1948.

(101) Lolli, G. Marchiafava's disease. Quart. J. Stud. Alc. 2:486–495, 1941.

(102) Lucia, S.P. A History of Wine as Therapy. Philadelphia: Lippincott, 1963, p. 37.

(103) MacAndrew, C. and Edgerton, R.B. Drunken Comportment. Chicago: Aldine, 1969.

(104) MacDonald, R.A. and Baumslag, N. Iron in alcoholic beverages; possible significance for hemochromatosis. Amer. J. Med. Sci. 247:649–654, 1964.

(105) MacDonald, R.A. and Mallory, G.K. Hemochromatosis and hemosiderosis. Arch. Intern. Med. 105:686–700, 1960.

(106) Maines, J.E., III, and Aldinger, E.E. Myocardial depression accompanying chronic consumption of alcohol. Amer. Heart J. 73:55–63, 1967.

(107) Mallory, F.B. Cirrhosis of the liver; five different types of lesions from which it may arise. Bull. Hopkins Hosp. 22:69–75, 1911.

(108) Margraf, H.W., Moyer, C.A., Ashford, L.E. and Lavalle, L.W. Adrenocortical function in alcoholics. J. Surg. Res. 7:55–62, 1967.

(109) Mayer, R.F., Garcia-Mullin, R. and Eckholdt, J.W. Acute "alcoholic" myopathy. Neurology 18:275, 1968.

109

(110) McDonald, C.D., Burch, G.E. and Walsh, J.J. Alcoholic cardiomyopathy managed with prolonged bed rest. Ann. Int. Med. 74:681–691, 1971.

(111) Mendelson, J.H., Stein, S. and Mello, N.K. Effects of experimentally induced intoxication on metabolism of ethanol-I-C^{14} in alcoholic subjects. Metabolism 14:1255–1266, 1965.

(112) Mendoza, L.C., Hellberg, K., Rickart, A., Tillich, G. and Bing, R.J. The effect of intravenous ethyl alcohol on the coronary circulation and myocardial contractility of the human and canine heart. J. Clin. Pharmacol. 11:165–176, 1971.

(113) Merry, J. and Marks, V. Plasma-hydrocortisone response to ethanol in chronic alcoholics. Lancet 1:921–923, 1969.

(114) Mezey, E., Jow, E., Slavin, R.E. and Tobon, F. Pancreatic function and intestinal absorption in chronic alcoholism. Gastroenterology 59:657–664, 1970.

(115) Mierzwiak, D.S., Wildenthal, K. and Mitchell, J.H. Effect of ethanol on the canine left ventricle. Clin. Res. 15:215, 1967. (Abst.)

(116) Misra, R.S., Lefevre, A., Ishii, H., Rubin, E. and Lieber, C.S. Increase of ethanol, meprobamate and pentobarbital metabolism after chronic ethanol administration in man and in rats. Amer. J. Med. 51:346–351, 1971.

(117) Mitchell, H.G. and Cohen, L.S. Alcohol and the heart; Hemodynamic effects of alcohol-animal studies. Mod. Conc. Cardiovasc. Dis. 39:109–113, 1970.

(118) Moskow, H.S., Pennington, R.C. and Knisely, M.H. Alcohol, sludge and hypoxic areas of nervous system, liver and heart. Micro-vascular Research 1:174–185, 1968.

(119) Navratil, L. On the etiology of alcoholism. Quart. J. Stud. Alc. 20:236–244, 1959.

(120) Nicholson, W.M. and Taylor, H.M. The effect of alcohol on the water and electrolyte balance in man. J. Clin. Invest. 17:279–285, 1938.

(121) Noble, E.P. In: Fox, R. and Bourne, P., eds., Alcoholism: Progress in Research and Treatment. New York: Academic Press, in press.

(122) Ogata, M., Mendelson, J.H., Mello, N.K. and Majchrowicz, E. Adrenal function and alcoholism. II. Catecholamines. Psychosom. Med. 33:159–180, 1971.

(123) Palmer, E.D. Gastritis: A revaluation. Medicine (Balt.) 33:199–290, 1954.

(124) Patty, F.A., ed. Industrial Hygiene and Toxicology. Vol. 2. New York: Interscience, 1965.

(125) Pearson, W.S. The "hidden" alcoholic in the general hospital; a study of hidden alcoholism in white male patients admitted for unrelated complaints. N. C. Med. J. 23:6–10, 1962.

(126) Perkoff, G.T. Alcoholic myopathy. Ann. Rev. Med. 22:125–132, 1971.

(127) Perkoff, G.T., Dioso, M.M., Bleisch, V. and Klinkerfuss, G. A spectrum of myopathy associated with alcoholism. Ann. Intern. Med. 67:481–492, 1967.

(128) Perman, E.S. The effect of ethyl alcohol on the secretion from the adrenal medulla in man. Acta Physiol. Scand. 44:241–247, 1958.

(129) Phillips, G.B. and Davidson, C.S. Acute hepatic insufficiency of the chronic alcoholic. Clinical and pathological study. Arch. Intern. Med. 94:585–603, 1954.

(130) Pirola, R.C. and Davis, A.E. Effects of ethyl alcohol on sphincteric resistance at the choledocho-duodenal junction in man. Gut 9:557–560, 1968.

(131) Popper, H. and Szanto, P.B. Fatty liver with hepatic failure in alcoholics. J. Mt. Sinai Hosp. 24:1121–1131, 1957.

(132) Regan, T.J., Levinson, G.E., Oldewurtel, H.S., Frank, M.J., Weisse, A.B., and Moschos, C.B. Ventricular function in noncardiacs with alcoholic fatty liver: Role of ethanol in the production of cardiomyopathy. J. Clin. Invest. 48:397–407, 1969.

(133) Richter, C.P. Loss of appetite for alcohol and alcoholic beverages produced in rats by treatment with thyroid preparations. Endocrinology 59:472–478, 1956.

(134) Riff, D.P., Jain, A.C., Doyle, J.T. Acute hemodynamic effects of ethanol on normal human volunteers. Amer. Heart J 78:592–597, 1969.

(135) Robin, E. and Goldschlager, N. Persistence of low cardiac output after relief of high output by thiamine in a case of alcoholic beriberi and cardiac myopathy. Amer. Heart J. 80:103–108, 1970.

(136) Roggin, G.M., Iber, F.L., Kater, R.M.H. and Tabon, F. Malabsorption in the chronic alcoholic. Johns Hopkins Med. J. 125:321–330, 1969.

(137) Rubin, E., Bacchin, P., Gang, H. and Lieber, C.S. Induction and inhibition of hepatic microsomal and mitochondrial enzymes by ethanol. Lab. Invest. 22:569–580, 1970.

(138) Rubin, E., Gang, H., Misra, P.S. and Lieber, C.S. Inhibition of drug metabolism by acute ethanol intoxication. Amer. J. Med. 49:801–806, 1970.

(139) Rubin, E., Hutterer, F. and Lieber, C.S. Ethanol increases hepatic smooth endoplasmic reticulum and drug-metabolizing enzymes. Science 159:1469–1470, 1968.

(140) Rubin, E. and Lieber, C.S. Personal communication.

(141) Rubin, E. and Lieber, C.S. Early fine structural changes in the human liver induced by alcohol. Gastroenterology 52:1–13, 1967.

(142) Rubin, E. and Lieber, C.S. Alcohol-induced hepatic injury in nonalcoholic volunteers. New Engl. J. Med. 278:869–876, 1968.

(143) Rubin, E. and Lieber, C.S. Alcoholism, alcohol and drugs. Science 172:1097–1102, 1971.

(144) Rubini, M.E., Kleeman, C.R. and Lamdin, E. Studies on alcohol diuresis. 1. The effect of ethyl alcohol ingestion on water, electrolyte and acid-base metabolism. J. Clin. Invest. 34:439–447, 1955.

(145) Sardesai, V.M. and Orten, J.M. Effect of prolonged alcohol consumption in rats on pancreatic protein synthesis. J. Nutr. 96:241–246, 1968.

(146) Schapiro, H., Wruble, L.D. and Britt, L.G. The possible mechanism of alcohol in the production of acute pancreatitis. Surgery 60:1108–1111, 1966.

111

(147) Schenkman, J.B. Studies on the nature of the type I and type II spectral changes in liver microsomes. Biochemistry 9:2081–2091, 1970.

(148) Sereny, G., Rapoport, A. and Husdan, H. The effect of alcohol withdrawal on electrolyte and acid-base balance. Metabolism 15:896–904, 1966.

(149) Shumkov, G. [Alcohol zones determined by palpato-reflexological method.] Russian text. Vrach. Gaz. 32:563–665, 1928.

(150) Silvestrini, R. La reviviscenza mammaria nell'uomo affetto da cirrosi del Laennec. Riforma Med. (Napoli) 13:701–704, 1926.

(151) Smith, A.A. and Gitlow, S. Effect of disulfiram and ethanol on the catabolism of norepinephrine in man. In: Maickel, R.P., ed., Biochemical Factors in Alcoholism. New York: Pergamon, 1967, pp. 53–59.

(152) Smith, J.J. The endocrine basis and hormonal therapy of alcoholism. N.Y. St. J. Med. 50:1704–1706, 1711–1715, 1950.

(153) Smith, J.J. A medical approach to problem drinking; Preliminary report. Quart. J. Stud. Alc. 10:251–257, 1949.

(154) Smith, J.J. The treatment of acute alcoholic states with ACTH and adrenocortical hormones. Quart. J. Stud. Alc. 11:190–198, 1950.

(155) Soehring, L. and Schuppel, R. Wechselwirkungen zwischen Alkohol und Arzneimitteln. (Interaction between alcohol and drugs.) Dtsch. Med. Wschr. 91: 1892–1896, 1966.

(156) Song, S.K. and Rubin, E. Ethanol produces muscle damage in human volunteers. Science, in press.

(157) Strauss, M.B., Rosenbaum, J.D. and Nelson, W.P., III. Alcohol and homeostasis, the uncompensated water diuresis induced by whiskey. J. Clin. Invest. 28:813–814, 1949.

(158) Sundby, P.R. Alcoholism and Mortality. Publication No. 6, National Institute for Alcohol Research. Oslo: Universitetsforlaget, 1967.

(159) Svoboda, D.J. and Manning, R.T. Chronic alcoholism with fatty metamorphosis of the liver; mitochondrial alterations in hepatic cells. Amer. J. Path. 44:645–662, 1964.

(160) Takala, M., Pihkanen, T.A. and Markkannen, T. The Effects of Distilled and Brewed Beverages. Physiological, Neurological, and Psychological Study. Helsinki: Finnish Foundation for Alcohol Studies. Publ. No. 4, 1957.

(161) Terris, M. Epidemiology of cirrhosis of the liver: National mortality data. Amer. J. Public Health 57:2076–2088, 1967.

(162) Thomson, A.D., Baker, H., Leevy, C.M. Thiamine absorption in alcoholism. Amer. J. Clin. Nutr. 21:537–538, 1968.

(163) Thomson, A.D., Baker, H. and Leevy, C.M. Patterns of 35S-thiamine hydrochloride absorption in the malnourished alcoholic patient. J. Lab. Clin. Med. 76:34–45, 1970.

(164) Tomasulo, P.A., Kater, R.M.H. and Iber, F.L. Impairment of thiamine absorption in alcoholism. Am. J. Clin. Nutr. 21:1340–1344, 1968.

112

(165) Tintera, J.W. and Lovell, H.W. Endocrine treatment of alcoholism. Geriatrics 4:274–280, 1949.

(166) Tisdale, W.A. Parenchymal sclerosis in patients with cirrhosis after portasystemic-shunt surgery. New Engl. J. Med. 265:928–932, 1961.

(167) U.S. Department of Transportation. Alcohol and Highway Safety. Washington, D.C., 1968.

(168) Valicenti, J.F., Jr. and Newman, W.H. Cardiac size, contractile force and wall tension following ethanol, pentobarbital, and ouabain. Fed. Proc. 27:658, 1968.

(169) Van Dyke, H.B. and Ames, R.G. Alcohol diuresis. Acta Endocr. (Kbh.) 7:110–121, 1951.

(170) Velez-Garcia, E., Hardy, P., Dioso, M. and Perkoff, G.T. Cysteine-stimulated serum creatine phosphokinase: Unexpected results. J. Lab. Clin. Med. 68:636–645, 1966.

(171) Victor, M. Observations on the amnestic syndrome in man and its anatomical basis. In: Brazier, M.A.B., ed., Brain Function. Vol. 2. Berkeley University of California Press, 1965, pp. 311–340.

(172) Victor, M. and Adams, R.D. On the etiology of the alcoholic neurologic diseases, with special reference to the role of nutrition. Amer. J. Clin. Nutr. 9:379–397, 1961.

(173) Von Rokitansky, C. A Manual of Pathological Anatomy. Vol. 2: London: Sydenham Society, 1849, p. 145.

(174) Wagner, G. and Fuchs, A.R. Effect of ethanol on uterine activity during suckling in post-partum women. Acta Endocr. (Kbh.) 58:133–141, 1968.

(175) Wallgren, H. and Barry, H., III. Actions of Alcohol. Vol. 1: Biochemical, Physiological and Psychological Aspects. Vol. 2: Chronic and Clinical Aspects. New York: Elsevier, 1970.

(176) Walshe, W.H. A Practical Treatise on the Diseases of the Heart and Great Vessels, including the Principles of Their Diagnosis. 4th Ed. London: Smith, Elder & Co., 1873.

(177) Wechsler, H., Kasey, E.H., Thum, D. and Demone, H.W. Alcohol level and home accidents. Public Health Reports 84:1043–1050, 1969.

(178) Weiss, S. and Wilkins, R.W. Nature of cardiovascular disturbances in vitamin deficiency states. Trans. Ass. Amer. Physicians 51:341–373, 1936.

(179) Wendt, V.E., Ajiluni, R., Bruce, T.A., Prasad, A.S. and Bing, R.J. Acute effects of alcohol on the human myocardium. Amer. J. Cardiol. 17:804–812, 1966.

(180) Wendt, V.E., Wu, C., Balcon, R., Doty, G. and Bing, R.J. Hemodynamic and metabolic effects of chronic alcoholism in man. Amer. J. Cardiol. 15:175–184, 1965.

(181) Wexberg, L.E. A critique of physiopathological theories of the etiology of alcoholism. Quart. J. Stud. Alc. 11:113–118, 1950.

(182) Wynder, E.L. and Bross, I.J. Aetiological factors in mouth cancer; an approach to its prevention. Brit. Med. J. 1:1139–1143, 1957.

113

(183) Wynder, E.L., Bross, I.J. and Day, E. Epidemiological approach to the etiology of cancer of the larynx. J.A.M.A. 160:1384–1391, 1956.

(184) Wynder, E.L., Bross, I.J. and Feldman, R.M. A study in the etiological factors in cancer of the mouth. Cancer 10:1300–1323, 1957.

(185) Zieve, L. Jaundice, hyperlipemia, and hemolytic anemia; a heretofore unrecognized syndrome associated with alcoholic fatty liver and cirrhosis. Ann. Intern. Med. 48: 471–496, 1958.

114

Chapter V

THEORIES ABOUT THE CAUSES OF ALCOHOLISM

THE CAUSES OF ALCOHOLISM are unknown, although the number of theories that have been advanced are as numerous as the professions and scientific disciplines concerned with the problem. No single theory has yet proved adequate to explain the complex of symptoms which are collectively termed alcoholism, alcohol addiction, or alcohol dependence. Most probably, the condition reflects a form or response to an interactive combination of physiological, psychological, and sociological factors in an individual and his environment (8).

Experimental Animal Models of Addiction

The importance of central nervous system alterations in the development of alcoholism can be inferred from the demonstration of behavioral tolerance or adaptation to alcohol in persons dependent on or addicted to the drug, which cannot be explained by metabolic factors (46, 48, 52, 53, 54, 55, 56). Yet progress in understanding the central nervous system mechanisms involved in the phenomenon of alcohol dependence has been limited because many types of experiments cannot be performed with human subjects. Only the development of an alcohol-dependent animal might permit study of the development of the dependency (the addictive process) at behavioral, biochemical, and neurophysiological levels.

In man, the development of alcohol dependence usually extends over many years and, consequently, its developmental antecedents are obscured by time. The more rapid induction of alcohol dependence in experimental animals could clarify the neural, endocrine, or metabolic changes which may be critical for expression of the dependent state. Testing the efficacy of new therapeutic interventions in animal models of disease processes is an established practice in medical science. The testing of new pharmacotherapeutic agents on alcohol-dependent animals would have many advantages, including the possible alleviation of alcohol-related illnesses.

Historically, efforts to develop an animal model of alcohol dependence have failed, partly because most animals dislike the taste of alcohol and partly because even a demonstrated preference for alcohol by experimental animals cannot be equated with alcohol-dependent behavior in humans. Many researchers have tried to devise techniques for inducing a preference for alcohol in animals, sometimes in the hope that from the preference, dependence could be developed. Several groups of investigators have now succeeded in devising techniques to induce an alcohol withdrawal syndrome—regarded as indicative of physical dependence—in a variety of species. Yanagita, Deneau, and Seevers (83) were the first to show that rhesus monkeys could be made alcohol-dependent in this sense. They used an apparatus which was activated by a monkey pressing a lever. Each press delivered a tiny amount of alcohol directly into the animal's bloodstream through a cardiac catheter. Monkeys thus injected enough alcohol into themselves daily so that in about 22 days they became physically dependent; that is, they showed a withdrawal syndrome (14, 83). These original observations have been confirmed and extended by other investigators (79, 81, 82). Using the same technique, they have shown that monkeys can produce sustained self-intoxication, with blood alcohol levels ranging between 0.20 percent to 0.40 percent, that are comparable to those seen in alcohol-dependent people (81).

The comparability was particularly illustrated by the concordance in patterns of alcohol intake between monkeys and alcoholic persons given 24-hour access to alcohol over a period of days. In both instances there was an interesting alternation between 2- to 3-day periods of heavy alcohol intake and 1- to 2-day periods of relative abstinence (81).

116

Another successful method of producing physical dependence on alcohol in rhesus monkeys (16, 17) and in dogs (18) is by forced administration of alcohol through a nasogastric tube. Daily administration of large amounts of alcohol in 2 or 3 divided doses induced alcohol dependence within 2 to 3 weeks. Essig and Lam (18) also obtained similar results by administering the alcohol directly into the stomach through a Pavlov gastric cannlua. Whether an animal thus treated will voluntarily consume large quantities of alcohol once it recovers from the withdrawal sickness, is not yet known.

Orangutans and chimpanzees, given a choice between plain and alcoholized fruit juices, drank considerable amounts of alcohol, the latter enough to become obviously intoxicated (21). But this work has not yet been followed up by experiments to determine whether dependence might be developed. It has been very difficult to produce self-selection of alcohol in rhesus monkeys in the absence of an experimental stressor (such as an electric shock or overcrowding) (47). It is difficult to mask the taste of alcohol effectively and to produce addictive drinking with behavioral techniques (9).

In operant conditioning (learning behavior) situations, where monkeys were required to drink alcohol if they wanted to avoid an unpleasant shock or to obtain food, they consistently learned a variety of techniques which permitted them to get the food or avoid shock without consuming alcohol (50, 51). In addition to the adversive taste of alcohol, the inevitable delay between alcohol ingestion and intoxication probably reduces the potential reinforcing efficacy of alcohol taken by drinking, in contrast to an intravenous infusion paradigm. However, efforts to devise a behavioral technique to produce addictive drinking in monkeys are continuing in many laboratories, since only a behavioral method would permit the identification and the subsequent manipulation of environmental determinants which could affect the acquisition and maintenance of alcohol dependence.

Attempts to examine the effects of early experience with alcohol on the subsequent development of preference, tolerance, and physical dependence in primates have only just begun. Infant rhesus monkeys, separated from their mothers immediately after birth and maintained under conditions of maternal and peer deprivation, were given increasing concentrations of alcohol in their diets as the only fluid for 1½ years. None of these monkeys showed evidence of physical dependence when withdrawn from alcohol, despite living with stable blood alcohol levels as high as

117

0.20 percent (49). Using the same techniques as in dogs, however, Ellis and Pick (17) demonstrated the withdrawl syndrome in primates, observing tremors and convulsions in rhesus monkeys after only 10 to 18 days of administering alcohol. Pieper and associates (62) achieved withdrawal reactions in infant chimpanzees after six to 10 days with large amounts of alcohol (blood alcohol levels up to 0.3%). When alcohol was stopped, all the animals showed at least increased reflexes and irritability; some exhibited severe convulsions. Although the discrepancies between these data may be attributed to a species difference, the extent to which prolonged drinking of alcohol in a developing monkey is sufficient to produce physical dependence is still open to question.

Although a primate model of alcohol addiction would be the most useful, its development in rodents is potentially valuable for neurochemical and neurophysiological research. Using a forced ingestion technique, LeBlanc and associates (31) have demonstrated the induction of behavioral tolerance in rats following 20 days of alcohol administration. Freund (22) reported severe withdrawal symptoms in mice when, following a 30 percent weight reduction, they were maintained for a period of 4 days with a liquid diet in which 35 percent of the calories came from alcohol. A replication and extension of Freund's study found that forced ingestion of a liquid diet was effective in producing the withdrawal signs of physical dependence only in severely starved mice. But mice maintained with an adequate diet, even though they were induced to consume more alcohol over a longer period of time—using the behavioral technique of polydipsia—did not show similiar signs of physical dependence (60). The critical factors contributing to the potency of a combination of alcohol plus dietary deficiency in producing alcohol withdrawal signs and symptoms remain to be determined. These findings serve to reemphasize that the crucial determinants in the development of the signs of physical dependence upon alcohol are unknown and that the nature of the addictive process remains a matter of conjecture.

There is a vast literature on attempts to induce preference for alcohol through a variety of behavioral, physiological, dietary, genetic, pharmacological, and surgical manipulations. Many of these are dealt with in the following sections on the physiological and psychological theories of the etiology of alcoholism. Only the intravenous infusion or nasogastric administration procedures have been successful in producing signs attributed to physical dependence or addiction. Our understanding of the biological bases of addiction to all drugs, including alcohol, awaits further research.

PHYSIOLOGICAL THEORIES

Some researchers explain chronic heavy alcohol intake in terms of physiological or biochemical mechanisms. They try to come to grips with such phenomena as addiction, habituation, tolerance, physical dependence, loss of control, and craving and "appetite" for alcohol by examining physiological functions and processes, either by experimental studies or by observations of naturally occurring cases.

Genetotrophic Theory

The genetotrophic theory of alcoholism, advanced by R. J. Williams (75, 76, 77, 78) combines the concept of a genetic trait and nutritional deficiency. It is postulated that, owing to an inherited defect or "error" of metabolism, some people require unusual amounts of some of the essential vitamins. Since they do not get these unusual amounts in their normal diet, they have a genetically caused nutritional deficiency. In those who have become acquainted with alcohol, this results in the development of an abnormal craving for the substance, and the consequence is alcoholism.

Two lines of research are related to the genetotrophic theory. One is concerned with manipulating nutritional (vitamin) status as a means of influencing alcohol intake. The other is concerned with developing a strain of rodents with a strong tendency to drink alcohol.

In one early line of research preceding the genetotrophic theory (41) animals (usually rats or mice) were provided with a choice of two fluids: water and an alcohol solution. Those animals which were fed a deficient diet tended to drink larger proportions of the alcohol solution than their counterparts fed a normal diet. In similar experiments in Williams' laboratory, Beerstecher and associates (5) reported that alcohol consumption increased when rats were deprived of the following vitamins: thiamin, riboflavin, pyridoxine, and pantothenate.

Lester and Greenberg (35), however, provided their rats with a triple choice: water, an alcohol solution, and a sugar solution. Their nutritionally deprived animals demonstrated no preference

119

for the alcohol solution; they chose the sugar solution. These findings were confirmed in the laboratories of Mardones (40). Thus it seemed that the increased alcohol consumption under vitamin-deprived conditions could not adequately explain the cause of alcoholism.

The second line of research focused on genetic factors and the preference for alcohol, with or without nutritional control. Mardones and his associates (39, 40, 68) selectively bred two strains of rats, one consisting of alcohol "nondrinkers" and the other of alcohol "drinkers." After 25 or 30 generations, neither a high alcohol-preferring strain nor a low alcohol-preferring strain was developed. The investigators concluded that alcohol preference was not inherited in a simple genetic manner.

Nevertheless, related studies suggested that animals showing an increased appetite for alcohol may have inherited an enzymatic system different from nondrinking animals. In this connection, the work of von Wartburg (74) indicates that the primary enzyme involved in the metabolism of ethanol, alcohol dehydrogenase, shows considerable individual variability as well as species differences. He believes that his data comport well with Williams' view that individuals may have individualized nutritional requirements, and that his data provide a biological basis for the disease concept of alcoholism.

Genetic Theory

Some workers in the field theorize that alcoholism may be inherited. Alcoholism appears to run in families; it is, therefore, suggested that an alcoholism-prone individual may have inherited a susceptibility to be influenced adversely by ingested alcohol. Possible genetic links to alcoholism have been studied in animals. The team of McClearn and Rodgers (42, 43, 66) found several strains of inbred mice that show a relatively high preference for alcohol solutions, while other strains avoid alcohol. The work on preference for alcohol, however, has not been linked with quantities consumed, a correlation that would relate to alcoholism.

Other attempts to link alcoholism to heredity involve observations of physical characteristics such as blood group or color blindness, in alcoholic patients. Cruze-Coke and his associates (11) have presented evidence suggesting an association between color blindness and cirrhosis of the liver, and between alcoholism and color blindness (12, 13). Fialkow and his associates (20) and

Smith and Brinton (70) however, found that the defective color vision in their patients improved after nutritional treatment, so that there appeared to be no causal connection between alcoholism and color-vision defect.

Attempts to correlate alcoholism and blood groups (7, 59) have proved uninformative. Studies that gave positive findings were inadequately controlled for such variables as nationality or racial origin.

Another approach to finding a genetic basis in alcoholism is the study of twins and families. On the basis of his review of studies of heredity, Jellinek (26) suggested that persons might inherit a constitution which serves as a breeding ground for alcoholism. He thought, however, that certain sociocultural factors must also be concurrently present. Roe (67) showed that children of alcoholic parents placed in foster homes before the age of 10 were no more likely to become alcoholic individuals than children of nonalcoholic parents. An elaborate study of 902 male twin pairs by Partanen, Bruun, and Markkanen (61) identified three factors: (a) amount consumed on a single occasion; (b) frequency of alcohol use; and (c) lack of control. They concluded that heredity may influence the use of alcohol but not its social consequences, and that the factors of frequency of drinking and lack of control over drinking may themselves be influenced by environmental factors.

In summary, the evidence thus far for a genetic inheritance of alcoholism is unsatisfactory. The possibility that humans may inherit a predisposition for alcoholism or an immunity to it, however, has not been ruled out. This suggests that the onset and development of alcoholism is not solely under biological control. A critique of studies on the genetics of alcoholism has been published recently by Edwards (15).

Endocrine Theory

Another major physiological theory of the cause of alcoholism indicates a dysfunction of the endocrine system (24, 38, 69, 73). Through glandular symptoms of its hormones, this system is important in helping maintain a balance in the body's functions. Similarities between the symptoms seen in alcoholic patients and in patients with endocrine disorders suggest that some failure of the endocrines might be causally related to the onset of alcoholism. If alcohol ingestion stresses the organism, chronic heavy drinking could cause a hyperactivity of the pituitary gland, eventual exhaustion of the adrenal cortex, and, consequently, a breakdown in the functions regulated by the adrenal hormones.

Zarrow and his associates (84) studied the effects of alcohol intake in rats by manipulating the endocrine system. Using the three-choice self-selection technique (water, alcohol solution, and sugar solution), no preference for alcohol resulted from castration, drug-induced diabetes, surgical removal of the adrenal gland, or drug-induced stresses that might exhaust the adrenals.

Richter (65) showed that animals fed thyroid preparations did reduce their alcohol intake. He also noted that alcoholism is rare in hyperthyroid individuals, while hypothyroidism is found in alcoholism. However, Augustine (2) reported that in 109 acutely intoxicated male and female alcoholics, none was hypothyroid.

A case for an association of alcoholism and endocrine function can thus be made out. The experimental clinical evidence, however, does not provide unequivocal support for a theory of causality. The available information suggests that the endocrine characteristics associated with alcoholism may be a result of chronic heavy drinking rather than its cause.

PSYCHOLOGICAL THEORIES

Theorists in this area assume that alcoholism is a symptom of an underlying personality or emotional disorder. The three main psychological approaches are based on psychoanalysis, learning theory, and personality trait.

Psychoanalytic Theory

Psychodynamic explanations of the causes of alcoholism rest on three major theoretical positions, as expressed by McCord and McCord (45): (a) the Freudian view that alcoholism results from one or more of three unconscious tendencies, including self-destruction, oral fixation, and latent homosexuality; (b) the Adlerian view that alcoholism represents a struggle for power; and (c) the view that alcoholism develops as a response to an inner conflict between dependency drives and aggressive impulses.

Early psychoanalytic writers—Freud, Abraham, Ferenczi, and Knight—emphasized the release from inhibition afforded by alcohol, allowing expression of repressed urges. The repressed tendencies of prime importance to this school of thought are oral dependency and latent homosexuality. These traits are presumed to develop because of defects in the parent-child relationship, which preclude the child's learning self-control, fix his development at the oral stage, and lead to overidentification with the father.

Another analyst espousing the oral-dependent view is Fenichel (19), who maintained that underlying alcoholism are passive, dependent, narcissistic urges and a wish to use the mouth as the primary means to achieve gratification. Lolli (37) views alcoholism similarly: The alcoholic person experiences overwhelming unconscious longings for warmth and nurture, equivalent to longings for security and self-respect, which cannot be satisfied in ordinary relationships.

Menninger (57) places prime importance on a self-destructive tendency. In his view, a person resorts to alcoholism to avert a greater self-destruction. His drinking arises from guilt associated with his anger toward his parents, whose behavior toward him during childhood frustrated his need for oral gratification. In adulthood, his theory holds, the person may abuse alcohol to accomplish three purposes: (a) oral gratification; (b) self-punishment for his anger toward his parents; and (c) symbolic revenge against his parents.

The Adlerian view is that alcoholism represents a striving for power, which compensates for a pervasive feeling of inferiority. It is assumed that the alcoholic person derives his feelings of inferiority from a childhood in which overindulgent parents did not permit him to learn how to cope with the problems of adult life. The alcoholic person turns to alcohol to enhance his feelings of self-esteem and prowess.

Recent studies by McClelland and associates (44) suggest that frustrated ambitions may play a role in the development of an alcohol problem. It is suggested that the alcoholic person may have an enhanced need for power, but finds himself inadequate to achieve his goals. He resorts to alcohol because it provides a sense of release, of power, and feelings of achievement. Since overindulgence in alcohol precludes an effective coping with the problems needing solution and leads to additional problems, this vicious cycle results in confirmed alcoholism.

Evidence to support the psychoanalytic views is necessarily inconclusive, since it is difficult to devise experimental tests of these theories. In a retrospective study, McCord and McCord (45) found that boys with oral tendencies were more likely to develop alcoholism than others; and Witkin and his associates (80) found

123

alcoholic patients to be more field dependent by the Rod-and-Frame test. But evidence of latent homosexuality was not found in the studies of McCord and McCord (45) and Landis (30). Nevertheless, the application of psychoanalytic ideas in the treatment of alcoholism has been reported to give successful results. Thus Knight (29) reported considerable improvement through psychoanalytic therapy.

Learning Theory

Learning and reinforcement theory explains alcoholism by considering alcohol ingestion as a reflex response to some stimulus and as a way to reduce an inner drive state such as fear or anxiety. Characterizing life situations in terms of approach and avoidance, this theory holds that persons tend to be drawn to pleasant situations or repelled by unpleasant or tension-producing ones. In the latter case, alcohol ingestion is said to reduce the tension or feelings of unpleasantness and to replace them with the feeling of well-being or euphoria generally observed in most persons after consuming one or two drinks.

Some experimental evidence tends to show that alcohol reduces fear in an approach-avoidance situation. Conger (10) trained one group of rats to approach a food goal and, using aversive conditioning, trained another group to avoid electric shock. After an injection of alcohol, the pull away from the shock was measurably weaker, while the pull toward the food was not stronger. Thus, alcohol seemed to decrease an avoidance response based on fear rather than to enhance the approach to a pleasant situation.

The obvious troubles experienced by alcoholic persons appear to contradict the learning theory in the explanation of alcoholism. The discomfort, pain, and punishment they experience should presumably serve as a deterrent to drinking. The fact that alcoholic persons continue to drink in the face of family discord, loss of employment, illness, and other sequels of repeated bouts is explained by the proximity of the drive reduction to the consumption of alcohol; that is, alcohol has the immediate effect of reducing tension while the unpleasant consequences of drunken behavior come only later. The learning paradigm, therefore, favors the establishment and repetition of the resort to alcohol.

In fact, the anxieties and feelings of guilt induced by the consequences of excessive alcohol ingestion may themselves be-

124

come the signal for another bout of alcohol abuse. The way in which the cue for another bout could be the anxiety itself is explained by the process of stimulus generalization: Conditions or events occurring at the time of reinforcement tend to acquire the characteristics of stimuli. When alcohol is consumed in association with a state of anxiety or fear, the emotional state itself takes on the properties of a stimulus, thus triggering another drinking bout.

The role of punishment is becoming increasingly important in formulating a cause of alcoholism based on the principles-of-learning theory. While punishment may serve to suppress a response, experiments have shown that under some circumstances it can serve as a reward and reinforce the behavior (71). Thus if the alcoholic person has learned to drink under conditions of both reward and punishment, either type of condition may precipitate renewed drinking.

Ample experimental evidence supports the hypothesis that excessive alcohol consumption can be learned. By gradually increasing the concentration of alcohol in drinking water, psychologists have been able to induce the ingestion of larger amounts of alcohol by an animal than would normally be consumed. Other researchers have been able to achieve similar results by varying the schedule of reinforcement; that is, by requiring the animal to consume larger and larger amounts of the alcohol solution before rewarding it. In this manner, animals learn to drink large amounts of alcohol to obtain the reward. Nevertheless, the animals in these studies do not drink enough to become dependent on alcohol in terms of demonstrating withdrawal symptoms. The learning-theory explanation, therefore, is not universally acceptable as the answer to alcohol addiction.

The application of learning-theory in treatment has been discussed by Kepner (28) and demonstrated with varying degrees of success and failure by many different techniques of aversive conditioning (1, 32).

Personality Trait Theory

Psychological research has also attempted to define the causes of alcoholism in terms of an "alcoholic personality." Though it is conceded that all alcoholic persons need not all have the same characteristics, it is postulated that in the prealcoholic stage a personality pattern or constellation of characteristics should be discernible and should correlate with a predisposition toward

125

alcoholism. One of the main difficulties in this approach is that the population ordinarily available for study is already in trouble with alcohol. The question, not easy to answer, is whether the personality traits observed in these people predate the onset of the alcoholism, or are a consequence of alcoholism.

Blane (6) has set forth some of the personality characteristics commonly seen in alcoholism, suggesting they are relevant to treatment and rehabilitation of alcoholic persons. The characteristics include low frustration tolerance, sociability, feelings of inferiority combined with attitudes of superiority, fearfulness, and dependency.

Lisansky (36), summarizing her review, suggested that the predisposed personality type has: (a) an intensely strong need for dependency; and (b) a weak and inadequate defense mechanism against this excessive need, leading, under certain conditions, to (c) an intense dependence-independence conflict. There is also (d) a low degree of tolerance for frustration or tension; and (e) unresolved love-hate ambivalences. This is the predisposed personality constellation awaiting the stresses and strains of the environment and the possible resort to alcohol.

Using objective and projective tests, researchers have attempted to identify an underlying personality disorder. As yet, these approaches have failed to identify a common personality structure of the alcoholic patient which would be predictive of alcoholism. There is evidence that alcoholic patients exhibit some personality traits in common. Once the addiction has been established, these patients show some common behavioral and trait manifestations which appear to be more relevant to alcoholism than to other psychological disorders. Alcoholic persons have most frequently—though not universally—been characterized as dependent personality types, perhaps forming an analogy to their apparent physical dependence upon alcohol.

The Minnesota Multiphasic Personality Inventory (MMPI) is a widely used test to assess the similarities of individuals to psychiatric diagnostic groups. Alcoholic persons characteristically show an elevated Pd (psychopathic deviate) trait score on the MMPI, which is related to the category sometimes labeled "psychopathic personality." Although such individuals have not lost touch with reality, they seem unable to profit from experience and come into conflict with societal norms in a variety of ways, including the abuse of alcohol.

126

As a group, alcoholic individuals so diagnosed in a psychiatric facility show higher Pd scores than do other types of psychiatric patients. This does not mean, however, that a high Pd score is predictive of later alcoholism. Pd is suggestive of classifying an individual as an alcoholic person only when he has arrived at a psychiatric facility. Furthermore, elevated Pd scores are also characteristic of heroin addicts within a psychiatric setting, and criminals in an enforcement setting. Thus, at most, Pd scores are suggestive but neither predictive of alcoholism, nor specific to it.

The MMPI has also been used in an effort to develop alcoholism scales; that is, each of the 566 items of the MMPI have been analyzed in terms of the proportion of alcoholic respondents who respond True or False to the items. Response patterns which differentiate alcoholic persons from others have been selected on a statistical basis for inclusion in an alcoholism scale. Several such scales have been developed—by MacAndrew, Hoyt and Sedlacek, Holmes, Hampton, and Linden and Goldstein. The MacAndrew and the Hoyt-Sedlacek alcoholism scales in particular have shown a capacity to discriminate alcoholic psychiatric patients from nonalcoholic psychiatric patients. This statistical discrimination by these alcoholism scales does not prove that there is, in fact, an underlying personality trait common to alcoholic patients. One of the anomalies of the success of the MacAndrew and Hoyt-Sedlacek alcoholism scales is that despite their separate validities, they do not correlate with each other and appear, therefore, to be measuring different sets of traits.

SOCIOLOGICAL THEORIES

Cultural and national groups have different rates of alcoholism. Some of the groups with apparently high rates of alcoholism are Americans, northern French, Poles, northern Russians, Swedes, and Swiss. Groups with an apparently low incidence include Chinese, southern French, Greeks, Italians, Jews, Portuguese, and Spaniards. Sociologists and therapists have sought to explain these differences by examining the attitudes and values of the different populations.

Cultural Theory

From the viewpoint of drinking as a symptom, Horton (25) noted that its nearly universal occurrence and its survival as a

127

custom suggest its high acceptability and utilitarian function in society. He proposes that alcohol use in primitive societies provides for relief of anxiety. Primitive man constantly lives at the margin of existence; under threat and danger from many sources; and constantly experiencing anxieties, fears, and tensions. The key to the universal use of alcohol, therefore, is its anxiety-reducing capacity.

Bales (3) proposed three ways in which culture and social organization can influence the rates of alcoholism:

- The degree to which the culture operates to bring about inner tensions or acute needs for adjustment in its members;
- The sort of attitudes toward drinking the culture produces in its members;
- The degree to which the culture provides suitable substitute means of satisfaction.

In support of the first point, he cites the previously mentioned Horton study (25) of the function of alcohol in primitive societies. With respect to the second point, Bales (3) distinguishes four different kinds of attitudes which seem to affect rates of alcoholism: (a) complete abstinence, as, for example, among religious groups to which the use of alcohol is forbidden, although sometimes this taboo is unevenly observed and difficult to enforce; (b) ritual drinking, as the use of alcohol in many religious ceremonies by orthodox Jews, among whom researchers have noted a low incidence of alcoholism; (c) convivial drinking, tending toward the ritual in its seeming symbolism of solidarity expressed on such occasions as births, marriages, and wakes, with utilitarian implications in the expected feeling of camaraderie—a type of drinking common among the Irish who may drink on all occasions, be it the launching of a ship or the chance meeting of a friend; and (d) utilitarian drinking, such as may be seen at the consummation of a business deal, or as a hangover remedy, or in other medicinal use to alleviate or prevent some illness.

With respect to the third cultural factor that can influence rates of alcoholism, Bales suggests that societies may provide alternatives to or substitutes for alcohol use. Some societies have less stringent sanctions against narcotic drugs and therefore have a lower alcoholism rate. Others permit emotional outlets through ceremonies and rituals and thereby provide culturally accepted means of anxiety reduction.

Deviant Behavior Theory

Depending on the context, the use of alcohol can be illegal or only illegitimate . . . acceptable or even sanctified . . . forbidden or abominated. Thus, the concept of alcohol abuse as deviant behavior is receiving increasing attention by researchers. Jessor and his co-workers (27) suggest three main reasons for social concern about alcohol: (a) the intrinsic properties of alcohol as a drug which may eventuate in loss of control; (b) the symbolic or cultural definitions attached to drinking which permit relaxation of social and personal controls; and (c) the widely held view that alcohol use is associated with socially undesirable behavior. These concerns provide a base for norms and regulations of alcohol use; each society, however, defines for itself its attitude toward alcohol use, intoxication, and drunken behavior.

From the perspective of viewing alcoholism as deviant behavior, the societal reaction or labeling theory represents the alcoholic person as someone who, through a set of circumstances, becomes publicly labeled a deviant and is forced by society's reaction into playing a deviant role (4, 33, 34). Lemert (33), however, makes a distinction between primary deviance, which may cause someone to be labeled as a deviant, and secondary deviance, which is the behavior produced by being placed in a deviant role. Little significance is attached to the primary deviance except that reactions are elicited from society as a consequence of the deviant behavior. In reviewing the societal reaction view, Gove (23) states that primary deviance is attributed to hedonistic variables or to ignorance; when psychological characteristics such as personality have been identified and labeled as such, however, society responds to that person as a deviant. This typically forces him into a deviant group and makes it increasingly difficult for him to return to society.

The anomie theory of deviant behavior is another sociocultural explanation (58). Merton postulates that anomie is brought about by a disjunction between goals shared by persons in the same society and the means for achieving them. As a basic postulate of anomie theory, deviant behavior (such as alcoholism) results from the strain between perceived goals and means. Merton suggests that modes of adaptation to this conflict include conformity, ritualism, retreatism, and rebellion. In particular, alcoholism may represent one of the latter two modes.

129

Another sociological view applicable to alcoholism as deviant behavior has been referred to as social and cultural support theory (63, 72). In this view, a subculture may condition its members to perform behaviors classified by another subculture as deviant. The significant other or other reference group in a person's life encourages such deviant behavior because of its own need to be permissive or to otherwise reward the behavior.

Sociological theories of the etiology of alcoholism are steadily coming under more rigorous testing, resulting in revisions and modifications. The development of a more generalized sociocultural explanation of alcoholism would have considerable relevance to programs of prevention. A detailed evaluation of sociological theories relevant to alcoholism is included in the works of Gove (23) and Reiss (64).

SUMMARY AND CONCLUSION

The search for a single cause of alcoholism may be an unrealistic goal. Nevertheless, researchers with specialized interests, and with needs to define alcoholism from their own perspectives, will probably continue to look for a unitary answer to solve the problem of how alcohol addiction occurs and to identify the crucial factors associated with its onset and progression.

Many theorists, however, suggest a multifaceted approach which incorporates elements from two or more hypotheses. Generally, such an approach selects from each of the broad areas discussed: physiology, psychology, and sociology. A tentative model may be developed as suggested by Plaut (63):

An individual who (1) responds to beverage alcohol in a certain way, perhaps physiologically determined, by experiencing intense relief and relaxation; and who (2) has certain personality characteristics, such as difficulty in dealing with and overcoming depression, frustration, and anxiety; and who (3) is a member of a culture that induces guilt and confusion regarding what kinds of drinking behavior are appropriate, is more likely to develop trouble than will most other persons.

More research will have to be done to gain deeper insight into the causes of alcoholism. Work is needed to identify better the association between alcohol use and all aspects of physiological responses, predispositions and attitudes, and the social context and consequences of drinking.

130

Nevertheless, enough is known at present about the treatment and rehabilitation of alcoholic persons to make a difference in their lives and that of their families. Even without knowing the underlying causes of alcoholism, a wide variety of treatment methods are available to help the alcoholic individual to overcome his alcoholism and the other problems associated with it. The need is, therefore, urgent to bring persons suffering from alcoholism into the treatment system without waiting for the full understanding of the basic causes (8). As further research is conducted and the causes of alcoholism are better understood, more specific and effective treatments may be devised.

REFERENCES

(1) Abrams, S. An evaluation of hypnosis in the treatment of alcoholics. Amer. J. Psychiat. 120:1160–1165, 1964.

(2) Augustine, J.R. Laboratory studies in acute alcoholics. Canad. Med. Ass. J. 96:1367, 1967.

(3) Bales, R.F. Cultural difference in rate of alcoholism. In: McCarthy, R.G., ed., Drinking and Intoxication. New York: Free Press, 1959, pp. 263–277.

(4) Becker, H.S. Outsiders: Studies in the Sociology of Deviance. New York: Free Press, 1963.

(5) Beerstecher, E., Jr., Reed, J.G., Brown, W.D. and Berry, L.J. The effect of single vitamin deficiencies on the consumption of alcohol by white rats. In: Individual Metabolic Patterns and Human Disease. University of Texas Publication No. 5109. Austin: University of Texas, 1951, pp. 115–138.

(6) Blane, H.T. The personality of the alcoholic. In: Chafetz, M.E., Blane, H.T. and Hill, M.J., eds., Frontiers of Alcoholism. New York: Science House, 1970, pp. 16–28.

(7) Camps, F.E. and Dodd, B.E. Increase in incidence of non-secretors of ABO blood group substances among alcoholic patients. Brit. Med. J. 1:30, 1967.

(8) Chafetz, M.E. and Demone, Jr., H.W. Alcoholism and Society. New York: Oxford University Press, 1962.

(9) Clark, R. and Polish, E. Avoidance conditioning and alcohol consumption in rhesus monkeys. Science 132:223–224, 1960.

(10) Conger, J.J. The effects of alcohol on conflict behavior in the albino rat. Quart. J. Stud. Alc. 12:1–29, 1951.

(11) Cruz-Coke, R. Colour-blindness and cirrhosis of the liver. Lancet 2:1064, 1964. 1:1131, 1965.

(12) Cruz-Coke, R. and Varela, A. Colour-blindness and alcohol addiction. Lancet 2:1348, 1965.

(13) Cruz-Coke, R. and Varela, A. Inheritance of alcoholism; its association with colour-blindness. Lancet 2:1282–1284, 1966.

(14) Deneau, G., Yanagita, T. and Seevers,, M.H. Self-administration of psychoactive substances by the monkey. Psychopharmacologia 16:30–48, 1969.

(15) Edwards, G. The status of alcoholism as a disease. In: Phillipson, R.V., ed., Modern Trends in Drug Dependence and Alcoholism. New York: Appleton-Century Croft, 1970, pp. 140–163.

(16) Ellis, F.W. and Pick, J.R. Ethanol-induced withdrawal reactions in rhesus monkeys. Pharmacologist 11(2):256, 1969.

(17) Ellis, F.W. and Pick, J.R. Ethanol intoxication and dependence in rhesus monkeys. In: Mello, N.K. and Mendelson, J.H., eds., Recent Advances in Studies of Alcoholism. Washington, D.C.: U.S. Government Printing Office, 1971, in press.

(18) Essig, C.F. and Lam, R.C. Convulsions and hallucinatory behavior following alcohol withdrawal in the dog. Arch. Neurol. Psychiat. 18:626–632, 1968.

(19) Fenichel, O. The Psychoanalytic Theory of Neurosis. New York: W.W. Norton Co., 1945.

(20) Fialkow, P.J., Thuline, H.C. and Fenster, F. Lack of association between cirrhosis and common types of colour-blindness. New Engl. J. Med. 275:584, 1966.

(21) Fitz-Gerald, F.L., Barfield, M.A. and Warrington, R.J. Voluntary alcohol consumption in chimpanzees and orangutans. Quart. J. Stud. Alc. 29:330–336, 1968.

(22) Freund, G. Alcohol withdrawal syndrome in mice. Arch. Neurol. 21:315–320, 1969.

(23) Gove, W.R. Societal reaction as an explanation of mental illness: An evaluation. Amer. Sociol. Rev. 35:873–874, 1970.

(24) Gross, M. The relation of the pituitary gland to some symptoms of alcoholic intoxication and chronic alcoholism. Quart. J. Stud. Alc. 6:25–35, 1945.

(25) Horton, D. Primitive societies. In: McCarthy, R.G., ed., Drinking and Intoxication. New York: Free Press, 1959, pp. 251–262.

(26) Jellinek, E.M. Heredity of the alcoholic. In: Alcohol, Science and Society. New Haven: Quarterly Journal of Studies on Alcohol, 1945, pp. 105–114.

(27) Jessor, R., Graves, T.D., Hanson, R.C. and Jessor, S.L. Society, Personality and Deviant Behavior. New York: Holt, Rinehart and Winston, 1968.

(28) Kepner, E. Application of learning theory to the etiology and treatment of alcoholism. Quart. J. Stud. Alc. 25:279–291, 1964.

(29) Knight, R. The psychoanalytic treatment in a sanitarium of chronic addiction to alcohol. J.A.M.A. 111:1443–1446, 1938.

(30) Landis, C. Theories of the alcoholic personality. In: Alcohol, Science and Society. New Haven: Quarterly Journal Studies on Alcohol, 1945.

(31) LeBlanc, A.E., Kalant, H., Gibbins, R.J. and Berman, N.D. Acquisition and loss of tolerance to ethanol by the rat. J. Pharmacol. Exp. Ther. 2:168–244, 1969.

(32) Lemere, F. and Voegtlin, W.L. An evaluation of the aversion treatment of alcoholism. In: Podolsky, E., ed., Management of Addictions, New York: Philosophical Library, 1955, pp. 238–243.

(33) Lemert, E. Human Deviance, Social Problems and Social Control. Englewood Cliffs, N.J.: Prentice Hall, 1967.

(34) Lemert, E.M. Sociocultural research on drinking. In: Keller, M. and Coffey, T.G., eds., 28th International Congress on Alcohol and Alcoholism, Vol. 2. Highland Park, N.J.: Hillhouse Press, 1969, pp. 56-64.

(35) Lester, D. and Greenberg, L. Nutrition and the etiology of alcoholism. The effect of sucrose, saccharin and fat on the self-selection of ethyl alcohol by rats. Quart. J. Stud. Alc. 13:553, 1952.

(36) Lisansky, E.S. The etiology of alcoholism: The role of psychological predisposition. Quart. J. Stud. Alc. 21:314–343, 1960.

(37) Lolli, G. Alcoholism as a disorder of the love disposition. Quart. J. Stud. Alc. 17:96–107, 1956.

(38) Lovell, L.H. and Tintera, J.W. Hypoadrenalism in alcoholism and drug addiction. Geriatrics 6:1–11, 1951.

(39) Mardones, J. Experimentally induced changes in the free selection of ethanol. In: Pfeiffer, C.C. and Smythies, J.R., eds., International Review of Neurobiology, Vol. II, 1960, pp. 41–76.

(40) Mardones, J., Segovia-Riquelme, N., Hederra, A. and Alcaino, F. Effect of some self-selection conditions on the voluntary alcohol intake of rats. Quart. J. Stud. Alc. 16:425–437, 1955.

(41) Mardones, R.J. and Onfray-B., E. Influencia de una substancia de la levadura (¿elemento del complejo vitaminico B?) sobre el consumo de alcohol en ratas en experimentos de auto-seleccion. Rev. Chilena Hig. Med. Prev. 4:293–297, 1942.

(42) McClearn, G.E. and Rodgers, D.A. Differences in alcohol preference among inbred strains of mice. Quart. J. Stud. Alc. 20:691–695, 1959.

(43) McClearn, G.E. and Rodgers, D.A. Genetic factors in alcohol preference of laboratory mice. J. Comp. Physiol. Psychol. 54:116–119, 1961.

(44) McClelland, D.C., Davis, W.N., Kalin, R. and Wanner, H.E. Alcohol and Human Motivation. New York: Free Press, in press.

(45) McCord, W. and McCord, J. Origins of Alcoholism. Stanford University Press, 1960, p. 28.

(46) Mello, N.K. Some aspects of the behavioral pharmacology of alcohol. In: Efron, D.H., ed., Psychopharmacology. A Review of Progress, 1957–1967. PHS Publ. No. 1836. Washington, D.C.: U.S. Govt. Printing Office, 1968, pp. 787–809.

(47) Mello, N.K. and Mendelson, J.H. Factors affecting alcohol consumption in primates. Psychosom. Med. 28:529–550, 1966.

(48) Mello, N.K. and Mendelson, J.H. Alterations in states of consciousness associated

with chronic ingestion of alcohol. In: Zubin, J. and Shagass, C., eds., Neurobiological Aspects of Psychopathology. New York: Grune & Stratton, 1969, pp. 183–218.

(49) Mello, N.K. and Mendelson, J.H. Effects of prolonged exposure to ethanol in infant monkeys. Fed. Proc. 30(2): Abstract No. 2084, p. 568, 1971.

(50) Mello, N.K. and Mendelson, J.H. Polydipsia as a technique to induce alcohol consumption in primates. Physiol. Behav., 1971, in press.

(51) Mello, N.K. and Mendelson, J.H. The effects of drinking to avoid shock on alcohol intake in primates. In: Creaven, P.J. and Roach, M.K., eds., Biological Aspects of Alcohol. Austin: University of Texas Press, 1971, in press.

(52) Mendelson, J.H., ed., Experimentally Induced Intoxication and Withdrawal in Alcoholics. Quart. J. Stud. Alc., Supplement No. 2, 1964.

(53) Mendelson, J.H. Biochemical pharmacology of alcohol. In: Efron, D.H., ed., Psychopharmacology. A Review of Progress, 1957–1967. PHS Publ. No. 1836. Washington, D.C.: U.S. Govt. Printing Office, 1968, pp. 769–785.

(54) Mendelson, J.H. Biological concomitants of alcoholism. New Engl. J. of Med. 283:24–32, 71–81, 1970.

(55) Mendelson, J.H. Biochemical mechanisms of alcohol addiction. In: Begleiter, H. and Kissin, B., eds., The Biology of Alcoholism, Vol. I: Biochemistry. New York: Plenum Press, 1971.

(56) Mendelson, J.H., Stein, S. and Mello, N.K. The effects of experimentally induced intoxication on metabolism of ethanol–1–C^{14} in alcoholic subjects. Metabolism 14:1255, 1965.

(57) Menninger, K. Man Against Himself. New York: Harcourt, Brace and Company, 1938, p. 149.

(58) Merton, R.K. Social Theory and Social Structure. New York: Free Press, 1957.

(59) Nordmo, S.M. Blood groups in schizophrenia, alcoholism and mental deficiency. Amer. J. Psychiat. 116:460, 1959.

(60) Ogata, H., Ogata, F., Mendelson, J.H. and Mello, N.K. A comparison of techniques to induce alcohol dependence in mouse. J. Pharmacol. Exp. Ther., 1972, in press.

(61) Partanen, J., Bruun, K. and Markkanen, T. Inheritance of Drinking Behavior; A Study on Intelligence, Personality and Use of Alcohol of Adult Twins. Helsinki: Finnish Foundation for Alcohol Studies, 1966.

(62) Pieper, W.A., Skeen, M.J., McClure, H.M., and Bourne, P.G. The chimpanzee as an animal model for investigating alcoholism. Science. In press, 1972.

(63) Plaut, T.F.A. Alcohol Problems: A Report to the Nation by the Cooperative Commission on the Study of Alcoholism. New York: Oxford University Press, 1967.

(64) Reiss, I.L. Premarital sex as deviant behavior: An application of current approaches to deviance. Amer. Soc. Rev. 35:78–87, 1970.

134

(65) Richter, C.P. Loss of appetite for alcohol and alcoholic beverages produced in rats by treatment with thyroid preparations. Endocrinology 59:472–478, 1956.

(66) Rodgers, D.A. and McClearn, G.E. Mouse strain differences in preference for various concentrations of alcohol. Quart. J. Stud. Alc. 23:26–33, 1962.

(67) Roe, A. The adult adjustment of children of alcoholic parents raised in foster homes. Quart. J. Stud. Alc. 5:378–393, 1944.

(68) Segovia-Riquelme, N., Hederra, A., Anex, M., Barnier, O., Figuerola-Camps, I., Campos-Hoppe, I., Jara, N. and Mardones, J. Nutritional and genetic factors in the appetite for alcohol. In: Popham, R.E., ed., Alcohol and Alcoholism. Chapter 12. Toronto: University of Toronto Press, 1970.

(69) Smith, J.J. A medical approach to problem drinking: Preliminary report. Quart. J. Stud. Alc. 10:251–257, 1949.

(70) Smith, J.W. and Brinton, G.A. Color-vision defects in alcoholism. Quart. J. Stud. Alc. 32:41–44, 1971.

(71) Solomon, R.L. Punishment. Psychologist 19:239–253, 1964.

(72) Sutherland, E.H. and Cressley, D.R. Principles of Criminology. Chicago: Lippincott, 1960.

(73) Tintera, J.W. and Lovell, L.H. Endocrine treatment of alcoholism. Geriatrics 4:274–278, 1949.

(74) von Wartburg, J.P. Alcohol dehydrogenase distribution in tissues of different species. In: Popham, R.E., ed., Alcohol and Alcoholism. Chapter 3. Toronto: University of Toronto Press, 1970.

(75) Williams, R.J. The etiology of alcoholism: A working hypothesis involving the interplay of hereditary and environmental factors. Quart. J. Stud. Alc. 7:567–585, 1946.

(76) Williams, R.J. Nutrition and Alcoholism. Norman, Oklahoma: University of Oklahoma Press, 1951.

(77) Williams, R.J. Biochemical individuality and cellular nutrition: Prime factors in alcoholism. Quart. J. Stud. Alc. 20:452–463, 1959.

(78) Williams, R.J. Alcoholism: The Nutritional Approach. Austin, Texas: University of Texas Press, 1959.

(79) Winger, G., Ikomi, F. and Woods, J.H. Intravenous ethanol self administration in rhesus monkeys. Proceedings of the 32nd annual conference of the Committee on Problems of Drug Dependence. NAS–NRC, 1970, pp. 6598–6605.

(80) Witkin, H.A., Karp, S.A. and Goodenough, D.R. Dependence in alcoholics. Quart. J. Stud. Alc. 20:493–504, 1959.

(81) Woods, J.H., Ikomi, F. and Winger, G. The reinforcing properties of ethanol. In: Creaven, P.J. and Roach, M.K., eds., Biological Aspects of Alcohol. Austin: University of Texas Press, 1971, in press.

(82) Woods, J.H. and Winger, G. A critique of methods for inducing ethanol self-intoxication in animals. In: Mello, N.K. and Mendelson, J.H., eds., Recent

Advances in Studies of Alcoholism. Washington, D.C.: U.S. Govt. Printing Office, 1971, in press.

(83) Yanagita, T., Deneau, G.A. and Seevers, M.H. Evaluation of pharmacologic agents in the monkey by long-term intravenous self or programmed administration. Abstract No. 66, 23rd International Congress of Physiological Sciences, Tokyo, 1965.

(84) Zarrow, M.X., Addus, H. and Denison, M. Failure of the endocrine system to influence the alcoholic drive in rats. Quart. J. Stud. Alc. 21:400–413, 1960.

Chapter VI

TREATMENT OF ALCOHOLISM

THE CAUSES OF ALCOHOLISM are so many and appear in such differing constellations from person to person that one cannot consider treating alcoholism as if it were a single illness with an identifiable and specific etiology, a known course, and a proven response to a particular chemical agent or medical treatment. Alcoholism is the result of complex and interacting factors. About the only characteristic shared by most of the alcoholic population is some pattern of repeated alcohol abuse that acts as a form of "self-treatment" for the sufferer.

The variety of people afflicted with alcoholism is probably as varied as humanity itself, and a variety of treatment techniques have been developed and, hopefully, are waiting to be developed for this field. Although each technique has its partisans, the critical research has not been done to demonstrate convincingly which approach works best with which specific person.

There is some general misunderstanding about the pain experienced by the alcoholic person. Sometimes we forget this, however, and view the alcoholic person only as a fun-loving, irresponsible, and childish person who is given over to the immediate gratification of every impulse. As a matter of fact, such a being exists within every one of us. Yet on reaching maturity we have to deny this part of ourselves. Thus when it looks as though the alcoholic

137

person is not playing the game of adulthood fairly, we get angry with him and attempt to teach him a lesson or give him the "good-old-kick-in-the-pants" treatment. Sometimes this creates an ambivalence in those who treat the alcoholic patient—an ambivalence based on an overt and conscious wish to help the alcoholic patient, and a covert and unconscious wish to punish him. These conflicting feelings may distort a treatment program.

Pain of Alcoholism

The pain the alcoholic person feels is the pain of self-loathing and humiliation . . . from loss of the respect of his family and friends . . . from growing isolation and loneliness . . . from the awareness that he is throwing away much of his unique and creative self and gradually destroying his body and soul. He doesn't usually mean to get drunk, really drunk—he just wants to take the value from alcohol. Getting drunk, really drunk as only an alcoholic person becomes, is a nightmare of lost memories, retching, vertigo, the shakes, and a profound melancholy of regret. Sometimes it becomes a living nightmare of terrifying visions, screaming accusatory voices, and convulsions.

Who would seek such experiences knowingly? From the intra-psychic viewpoint, heavy drinking is a form of adaptation or adaptive repair that has gotten out of control. Maladaptive symptoms are developed and maintained tenaciously because they are useful. For example, phobia is developed as a way to hide a serious neurotic fear behind some foolish fear, such as fear of heights or of closed spaces or of water. The foolishly feared thing is then avoided so that awareness of the underlying neurotic fear can be avoided. In addition, once stuck with such a problem-solving technique, the unhealthy coping mechanism can be used for secondary advantages such as avoiding responsibilities.

Value of Alcoholism

Alcohol has many such advantages. Indeed, it is the ubiquitous and quick problem-solving potential of this substance which is our major problem. In small doses for social drinkers, it gives a pleasantly softening and mood-elevating effect that facilitates social interaction. A slight "buzz" is experienced as pleasurable. For the alcoholic person, however, a "big bust" has become a necessity for survival. It may provide euphoria to relieve apathy

138

and sadness, a reduction of apprehension when more and more of life seems too stressful, or oblivion to blot out loneliness and disappointment. For some, it may provide a deliciously prolonged state of self-pity and destruction with which to punish someone.

More attention needs to be directed to the "value" of alcohol in helping the alcoholic individual cope—albeit in a sick way—with some of his most deeply hurting problems. Therein lies the dilemma: The devastating effects of alcoholism are so obvious that we are bewildered by patients apparently evading or frustrating the best treatment efforts. But when heavy drinking is seen as an adaptive phenomenon, we are not so perplexed that people can actually treat themselves this way. This view opens up therapeutic opportunities. But it also brings a humble sense of respect for the symptom—alcoholism—and the knowledge that the solution will not be simple or easy. A few lectures on the evil effects of alcohol will not suffice, nor will increasing life's pain by punishment. Having accepted the reality of alcoholism as a chronic and often recurring sickness, one becomes more tolerant of relapses—the so-called "slips"—by the patient and, at the same time, more optimistic about the long-range benefits of treatment.

General Systems Theory

A general systems theory approach can help to clarify the complexities of alcoholism (26). In the field of human actions, the general systems theory holds that behavior is composed of several layers of action and reaction, with each layer related to other layers that are more or less complex . . . or above or below it . . . in a systems hierarchy. Thus we cannot treat disordered behavior by assigning ultimate cause to one system, and then treating that system. Rather, multiple interacting systems must be taken into account.

Unfortunately, the systems approach precludes any easy answer. But the process of searching for answers is the "childhood" of any science and may be the forerunner of successful solutions.

The systems to be reviewed for therapeutic opportunities in the field of alcoholism are:

- Biological
  - Biochemical-cellular
  - Organ-body
- Intrapsychic

139

- Interpersonal
- Social
  - Small group
  - Large group
- Society

BIOLOGICAL

Biochemical-Cellular

The ill effects of alcohol on the body rather than the basic phenomenon of alcoholism itself have been of greatest interest to medical investigators and physicians, possibly because they feel more at home in this field. Some physicians confuse the treatment of alcohol intoxication with the treatment of alcoholism; non-medical people are as much in error by thinking that the treatment of intoxication is not important in the treatment of alcoholism itself. Nevertheless detoxification, which is actually only the treatment of acute medical symptoms, is a vital first step in helping alcoholic individuals.

Treatment. Much is known today about the metabolism of alcohol and its pharmacological, metabolic, physiological, and biochemical effects on the human body. Improved detoxification processes have reduced the mortality and morbidity rate of severe intoxication and postintoxication states. The usual procedure is to use anticonvulsant drugs and sedative compounds to prevent seizures and delirium tremens during the period when alcohol-withdrawal symptoms are manifest (11, 19, 34, 40, 44). High-potency vitamins and general supportive care are also standard components of treatment at this stage.

Patients must be examined carefully to detect possible head injuries, tuberculosis, the development of pneumonia or other infection, or metabolic or electrolyte disorders. Sound sleep is sought with compounds that increase dream sleep, since a deficit in dream sleep during and immediately following intoxication may be a factor in acute agitation, hallucinosis, or delirium tremens (33, 35).

For many years, a medical axiom held that alcoholic patients are dehydrated. The patients were therefore treated with large amounts of intravenous fluids. Recent research (5, 45) has demonstrated that a rising blood alcohol concentration does indeed lead to dehydration. But if there is no diarrhea, vomiting, or unusual degree of perspiration, a drop or flattening curve of blood alcohol actually leads to overhydration. Thus, fluids are now given orally in many small drinks according to the patient's need to slake his thirst.

Ending the after-pains of intoxication more quickly has long been a goal of everyone who ever got drunk. Many home remedies exist; none are effective. Administration of fructose sometimes speeds the metabolism of alcohol (47, 75). But the central nervous system disorders and metabolic symptoms of acute postintoxication states may require a week or more—long after the alcohol has disappeared from the body—for complete physiological recovery.

Hospitals that accept alcoholic patients for detoxification are reducing both illness and death following acute alcoholic episodes. Despite positions taken by the American Medical Association (4) and the American Hospital Association (3) however, some hospitals and physicians still avoid the responsibility for detoxification (78), and health insurance is often inadequate to cover its costs (65).

Organ-Body

Long, excessive use of alcohol has deleterious effects on the various organ systems such as the heart, pancreas, liver, peripheral nerves, brain, and body cells in general. Alcoholic hepatitis is now thought to be the precursor of cirrhosis. Acute heart failure in alcoholism has a very poor prognosis if the individual continues to drink.

The general social and physical deterioration of the alcoholic person finally results in the "skid row" bum caricature. Only a small minority of alcoholic individuals ever reach this level. Because of their utter helplessness and visibility, however, large amounts of money have been spent in their incarceration and arrest, while little treatment effort has been expended in their service (13). While the future of these forlorn people is not bright (9), their further deterioration might be halted by setting up long-term facilities (8, 32) that offer roofs and food and people-who-care, as well as relief from loneliness, to these unfortunate individuals without homes.

Treatment. For the great majority of alcoholic persons whose fate is by no means sealed, prompt and continued medical supervision is essential. Cessation of drinking and nutritional rehabilitation are the first order of treatment. Those who have

141

suffered injuries to the central nervous system may need organ retraining to help compensate for irreversible damage. Failure to provide adequate medical care may result in premature death in many individuals (67, 72), possibly by an average of 10 to 12 years.

INTRAPSYCHIC

Many professionals treating persons with alcoholism base their techniques on the assumption that the disorder is a result of emotional or unconsciously motivated factors. This assumption is controversial. Since intrapsychic factors are studied by inference and other indirect means, hard confirming information on the validity of this theory is difficult to collect. The view that alcoholism is an intrapsychic disorder is involved in the same debates as those surrounding the typology of emotional and mental disorders, and is subject to the same degree of criticism by many persons who object to seeing it thus classified.

Treatment. At this time, well thought-out and conclusive studies on the effects of various psychological treatment techniques are lacking, equivocal, or contradictory (28, 37, 62). The poor design of followup studies is discouraging (14, 53), making it difficult to practice effective matching of patients and techniques (31, 73).

Putting aside parochial arguments among psychotherapeutic schools, however, most therapists agree that a vital part of any treatment program is the opportunity offered the alcoholic person to develop trust in someone. The alcoholic individual generally appears to be lonely and guilt-ridden. Beneath a facade of conviviality, he yearns for a trusting and non-judgmental helping person upon whom to become dependent. This dependency is often accompanied by such distrust from earlier disappointments in life that the alcoholic person must challenge any new-found helper to see if this caregiver will be found wanting—like all others who came before.

Individual therapy is the preferred mode of therapy for some people. But the course of individual treatment is often rocky and fraught with peril to the therapeutic alliance. For example, the alcoholic patient's repeated testing of the relationship is often so intense and continuous, it may result in fulfillment of the patient's fear and in reinforcing his view that no one can be trusted (7), no one can help. Another way of explaining this interaction is gleaned

142

from the transactional analysis viewpoint that sees the alcoholic person engaged in a game or series of manipulations to accomplish his goal of making human contact. For the alcoholic patient to recover, the therapist must be a better game-player and be able to block destructive moves (70).

Psychotherapists do not agree whether total abstinence is an absolutely necessary goal and the only measure of success in the treatment of alcoholism (10, 58). The abstinent alcoholic patient may present so many other disabilities that just giving up drinking may be an inadequate criterion for recovery (29). Abstinence has long been deemed the first essential step in psychological rehabilitation, but opinions keep appearing to suggest that some alcoholic persons can become normal drinkers while, at the same time, increasing their psychological and interpersonal health in other areas (17, 18, 63). This viewpoint disturbs many therapists who fear that each alcoholic patient will see himself as the exception who can become a controlled drinker. The diagram on the following page gives a schematic representation of this dilemma.

Who is qualified to treat the alcoholic patient (46)? Some feel that an alcoholic person who has recovered from the illness is best qualified since he has a deep, personal understanding of the problem. Members of many professional disciplines disagree with this viewpoint. They agree that the recovered alcoholic person may have an initial advantage in establishing rapport, but fear that the depth of his understanding will be limited by the blind spots and prejudices of his own battle with the disorder.

This controversy is less partisan today than formerly. In our guild partisanship, we must not lose sight of one fact: In the foreseeable future, sufficient numbers of trained professionals will not be available to care for the nation's mental health needs, including the control of alcoholism. We must train sufficient paraprofessional personnel to augment professional manpower. Recognition of the value of volunteer and indigenous groups is growing; no better example exists than Alcoholics Anonymous. Fortunately, the therapeutic disciplines and Alcoholics Anonymous have met, heard, and learned from each other.

Most therapists agree that recovered alcoholic persons can be of great value as counselors, but that professional guidance is essential. The risk of having alcoholic individuals (or, for that matter, any person suffering an intrapsychic illness) treated by inadequately trained personnel is that the latter may, often unconsciously, develop strong feelings that can be destructive to

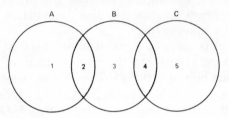
the patient. The inclination of the alcoholic patient to continuously challenge his therapeutic helper, plus his tendency to relapse, can be a severe test for anyone (55). These acts on the part of the patient may provoke destructive hostility (68), or defensive permissiveness to cover the hostility (54), on the part of counselors improperly prepared to recognize and handle these feelings. And permissiveness can be just as destructive as hostility since it does not permit the therapist to set realistic and firm limits on the patient.

Group therapy has a wide acceptance in alcoholism treatment programs (36, 56, 57, 60). This type of treatment is attractive for today's developing community alcoholism programs because it is usually less expensive than individual therapy. But group therapy should be attractive not because it costs less but because it can prove effective in treating alcoholism. It cuts across three systems —intrapsychic, interpersonal, and the social small group— permitting the alcoholic patient to see himself more honestly, to view his relationship to other important figures more clearly, and to feel he is an integral part of a social system.

This type of therapy ranges from groups with intensive psycho-analytic orientation where unconscious motivations (even utilizing dream analyses of both patients and therapists) are probed . . . to community groups where problems of group living are paramount and the group itself has the function of effecting significant changes in the lifestyles of its members.

A form of group therapy now increasingly used with alcoholic patients is one involving a confrontation process. At some level of understanding, the alcoholic person himself is quite aware that he is destroying his life's potential. Alcohol, however, has become such a vital self-treatment he dares not admit the harm inflicted upon himself by use of alcohol. He tries to kid others so they will reflect back to him his own hope that drinking is not really such a serious problem. This denial of his drinking problem is so obvious it may simply look like a lie to an observer.

The inability to face up to the reality, however, is largely an unconscious mechanism and needs to be attacked as the first order of therapeutic business (59). An individual psychotherapist may find his attempts to break through the patient's defenses deflected by the desperate alcoholic patient who reasons, "After all, what does he really know about it?" In the group setting, however, similarly afflicted people confront each other with the fact that each one is, indeed, in the same boat. How obvious the rationalizations of someone else seem! Confrontation with these trans-parencies by one's own peers seems less threatening and is easier to accept, especially when a patient can move back and forth between being the confronter and the confronted. The presence of the professional therapist prevents the session from deteriorating into scape goating or ganging up on a patient who is not yet ready to "take on" the full implications of this type of therapy.

Sometimes role-playing or psychodrama (77) facilitates group therapy. Let's just pretend, the therapist suggests, you are the rebellious son, the cast-out daughter, the long-suffering wife, the overprotective mother, the indifferent father. Roles are inter-changed skillfully. This is make-believe and patients can "ham it up," playing the roles as they appear in their imaginations. They are assuming the parts of other people, and thus they do not bear the threat of self-revelation. But how real and revealing the stage action is to both the group-audience and the players! Poignant and change-effecting therapeutic sessions often involve a sudden coalescence of love and support by the group, sometimes follow-ing a tearful breakthrough of long-hidden emotions revealed by an actor.

Varities of sensitivity training and marathon techniques have also emerged in recent years to be incorporated in some therapy groups. These techniques increase the feeling, tone, and intimacy of groups of alcoholic patients. These modifications seem to fit in with theoretical assumptions about the group therapy process. The only reservations in applying these methods more often are adequate screening of patients who can benefit from these group therapy methods and the need for trained group leaders.

Sensitivity groups have the general purpose of exploring the here and now of how the members feel about each other. The members gain a learning experience by seeing how each comes across to others. This encourages the patients to drop their individual facades and to become more honest in their interpersonal relations, first within and then outside of the group.

As its title implies, the marathon group meets over a prolonged period, lasting perhaps 40 hours. A patient may be able to keep his mask intact over a short interval, but this becomes increasingly difficult to maintain as time lengthens. Pretenses tend to break down and real feelings come out.

Learning theory (41, 43, 51) has been brought into the field of alcoholism treatment with the hypothesis that alcoholism is maintained because it is learned and reinforced as a behavior that engenders important rewards. In trying to account for the persistence of alcohol dependence or addictive drinking, it is always tempting to extrapolate from common experience of alcohol-induced euphoria and to imagine that for the alcoholic person the immediate pleasure of drinking negates the prospect of its many aversive social and health consequences. The profound depression, dysphoria, and anxiety observed in the alcohol-dependent person during the course of chronic heavy alcohol ingestion challenges this type of simplistic explanation. Instead, some learning theorists hold that acceptance by the alcohol-dependent person of the consequences of his gross use of alcohol suggests that the pain he is seeking to assuage is extreme, and that it is this assuagement which constitutes the "immediate reward," thus overriding the foreseeable but delayed punitive consequences.

Treatment based on learning theory (25) involves the use of positive or negative reinforcement techniques, or both kinds, as the behavioral therapist tries to help the patient alter his alcoholic behavior by retraining his form of learning response. Aversive therapy is a form of negative reinforcement; it consists of giving the patient a painful experience and associating it with the use of

146

alcohol. If successful, any consideration of drinking thereafter reflexly evokes a mental association with the painful or aversive stimulus, and the idea of drinking is rejected.

Examples of aversive stimuli are painful electric shocks, drugs that produce violent vomiting, or a drug that paralyzes the musculature and produces a sense of suffocation (15, 16, 26, 49). As is true of other aversive techniques, the enduring effectiveness of these negative reinforcement methods is unsure unless they are backed up with other forms of help. They are not popular with some professionals for fear they might be unknowingly used to vent unconscious hostile feelings toward alcoholic patients.

Modes of positive reinforcement based on learning theory, which would make not-drinking a more rewarding experience than drinking, could be expected to prove more effective in altering behavior. Specific techniques in applying this aim have only begun to be developed experimentally by behavior therapists (42, 61), although in essence this aim underlies most psychotherapeutic programs as they try to develop increased self-esteem, group approval, and renewal of human contacts.

Conflicts that arise between behavioral therapists and other psychological schools are not over the question whether reward reinforces while punishment deters behavior. That is self-evident. The issue concerns what really constitutes reward and punishment. The psychoanalytic theorist would hold that for the obsessively guilty, pain and punishment could be rewarding while success could be painful.

Much accommodation is being made today between learning and other motivational theories. The difference, as well as the growing accommodation between the schools of thought, may be illustrated by the following models: In an attempt to bring about certain responses, the behavioral therapist manipulates the stimuli to be fed into the "black box" (the brain with all its complexities and unknowns) and the responses that are emitted; the black box itself does not interest him. On the other hand, the concerns of the psychoanalytically oriented therapist and his patient are with the black box itself and with the conflicts and motivations contained in it. This therapist avoids applying stimuli, and does not try to establish desirable responses; his quest is for insight, which he believes will allow the needed behavioral changes.

Other techniques that have been tried in the treatment of alcoholism include the use of hypnosis (21, 76) and LSD (16, 48, 74). Hypnosis can be used to explore feelings and memories that

147

are not readily available to conscious experience but play an important role in precipitating drinking episodes. Post-hypnotic suggestions can be given that make abstinence seem pleasurable and drinking painful. This use of hypnosis is an extension of the important impact a therapist can have upon his patient through suggestion and exhortation.

LSD has been utilized to evoke dramatically the patient's awareness of his buried emotions and his human qualities. While some controversy remains, LSD treatment does not appear to offer significant help to alcoholic patients (69), and surveys of hospital-based programs show that LSD, hypnosis, and aversive therapies are not widely used (56, 57).

Psychoactive drugs have made a major impact on the treatment of important psychiatric disorders since the early 1950s. These drugs, along with changes in community attitudes about mental illness, have been significantly responsible for the steady decline in the number of hospitalized psychiatric patients. Most impressive has been the impact of the phenothiazines, a group of major tranquilizers, on schizophrenia and, more recently, lithium salts in the treatment and prevention of manic-depressive psychosis. Less certain is the relative balance of good and harm from the use of the minor tranquilizers in softening the blows of everyday life that are experienced in an exaggerated way by neurotic patients.

Thus, enthusiasm over the antidepressant or mood-elevating drugs has diminished. Much uncertainty exists about the use of chemical compounds to modify the anxiety and depression that reflect the intrapsychic stress experienced by alcoholic persons. The use of sedative and tranquilizing compounds may be essential in treating alcohol-withdrawal syndromes and to prevent delirium tremens; their long term use, however, is fraught with a risk of addiction in the very individuals who are already prone to an addictive response. Therefore, most experienced physicians use such drugs judiciously, usually reserving them for crisis situations. Which drugs are best is controversial, and the placebo effects of drugs are sufficiently high to make it difficult to demonstrate a superiority for any one drug that can be repeated by many investigators and clinicians (19, 44).

Since 1948, one drug—disulfiram (Antabuse)—has had a major impact on the treatment of alcoholism. It remains the favorite of many physicians (23, 39) though others seem reluctant to use it. Disulfiram is, in itself, a relatively inert compound. But it has the effect of interfering with the metabolism of alcohol after its first conversion to acetaldehyde in the liver, by blocking the further breakdown of the acetaldehyde. This results in an increased amount of acetaldehyde in the blood. Since acetaldehyde is very toxic, severe and even dangerous symptoms develop if alcohol is consumed when disulfiram is present in the body. Disulfiram is slowly removed from the body, and a patient who has taken this medication must wait several days after discontinuing it before he can drink safely.

Physicians who prescribe this drug might demonstrate the danger of drinking to the patient by having him undergo a mild disulfiram-alcohol reaction under carefully controlled conditions, but usually a careful explanation is adequate.

The drug itself is not a sufficient therapeutic program. Combined with other psychological rehabilitative techniques, disulfiram can be a most useful tool, but it is not a panacea. In the motivated alcoholic patient, it can "buy time" for him when he has an impulse to drink. During that interval he has time to reconsider his best long-range interests.

Disulfiram is not a drug to be used without careful concern for the medical state of the patient. While it causes relatively few serious side effects in itself, a person in a weakened state might have an attack of acetaldehyde poisoning if he drank an alcoholic beverage while taking disulfiram. This could be dangerous for a person suffering from such conditions as arteriosclerotic heart disease, cirrhosis, severe kidney disease, diabetes mellitus, or any serious debilitating medical disorder. Careful medical examination and psychological considerations should precede the prescription of this compound.

The question of hospitalization for the alcoholic patient is usually generally agreed on when he is acutely intoxicated, or suffering from serious medical complications that would require hospital care even if he did not abuse alcohol or suffer from alcoholism. The reluctance of many general hospitals and physicians to accept this responsibility discriminates, in effect, against the indigent patient. The private patient, who usually has a family doctor, can gain admission to a hospital—though his diagnosis may be masked by vague phrases such as gastrointestinal disorder or fever of undetermined origin. A psychiatric hospital may admit him as having an acute depressive reaction.

Sometimes, the indigent patient may be cared for in a detoxification center operated by city authorities, such as in St. Louis (64) or Washington, D.C. (32). A local city or county hospital may also have a detoxification center. Too often, however, the unofficial detoxification center is the city jail, where medical care for the person in an acute alcoholic episode is likely to be a matter of chance.

Whether or not detoxification is needed, hospitalization for rehabilitative and psychological care is not always available in State mental hospitals and private psychiatric hospitals (56, 57). Most specialists agree that hospitalization is indicated if the patient needs detoxification, is suicidal, homicidal, or unable to terminate a drinking bout unless removed from the source of alcohol by temporary confinement. Not all professionals agree, however, that hospitalizing the alcoholic person for other reasons is indicated; they fear a regressive sheltering or institutionalizing effect of the hospital which may run counter to the need to learn to live in the normal community. Uncertainty also exists as to whether the alcoholic patient should be housed with other psychiatric patients or placed in a special hospital or special unit.

Hospitalization does have the major advantage of getting hold of the alcoholic person long enough to begin instituting various therapeutic techniques that can then be continued after discharge (30). For example, interpersonal and social small-group system intervention such as family therapy and Alcoholics Anonymous can be started during this time, and a foundation laid for necessary aftercare.

INTERPERSONAL

This system falls between the intrapsychic and the social small group systems, blending imperceptibly into each. Interpersonal therapy focuses on marital and family disorders and how they relate to the alcoholic person's marital partner or family member. It consists of give-and-take with important people in the patient's life today, rather than in the past, although those early love and hate experiences show up as a shadow over what the patient is doing now.

In caricature, for example, the wife of the alcoholic man is portrayed as a long-suffering, work-worn, red-eyed, self-sacrificing woman forever bewildered by her once-generous husband's alcoholic debauchery and irresponsibility. Scratching the surface a bit in interpersonal therapy, however, may reveal a rather steely woman, contemptuous of her husband and secretly pleased with her dominant role in the family. Surprisingly, this may not be her first marriage to an alcoholic man.

Further investigation might reveal some dynamics of her past relationships—the intrapsychic system. These would suggest she was acting out old shadows of disappointment in her father's failure to be strong and reliable. She neurotically recreates this scene in her present life by choosing alcoholic mates. If her unconscious choice of a mate does not quite meet the picture of her father—for example, if the spouse turned out to be insufficiently weak—she would subtly undercut and push her husband along the desired path to irresponsibility.

These dynamics can be mirrored when the nonalcoholic partner is the husband. Superior and indifferent treatment of a wife can leave a woman with a growing loneliness and rage, finally culminating in her hidden alcoholism—that is, not hidden from her husband, but ignored by him and hidden by both of them from the world. How mismatched this intact and successful man seems to be with his now slovenly and brain-damaged wife. He must keep her from public view.

Yet, after loud proclamations that this drinking will no longer be tolerated, a nonalcoholic spouse may even be detected sympathetically slipping gin into the hospital for the alcoholic partner now under care for alcoholism. Or, take the example of the physician's wife struggling to avoid her destructive drinking which has become a public humiliation to her husband. Her husband asks her to buy champagne for their wedding anniversary because he forgot her problem with alcohol—a lapse of memory taking place after only a month of abstinence on her part!

In this marital situation, one prediction holds: The nonalcoholic spouse will unconsciously resist attempts of the alcoholic partner to recover. Subtle, or even not so subtle, means may be employed to undercut progress. If, despite these pressures, the alcoholic partner manages to recover, the effects may be devastating for the mental health of the spouse.

Attractive as these theoretical assumptions may be, life—fortunately—isn't that simple. Many wives and husbands of recovered alcoholic persons are delighted by the change; marriages are preserved, and great efforts are expended to encourage prolonged recovery. In other words, the variables are too many to allow accurate prediction.

A broader view holds that the nonalcoholic partner, even with many unresolved needs, is faced with an immediate reality: A chronically inebriated husband or wife. Assuming that the causes lie more with the inebriate individual, to what advantage can this situation be used unconsciously by the nonalcoholic spouse? Faced with a painful reality, this spouse may seek some secondary gain to make up somewhat for the losses. Maybe, when intoxicated, the alcoholic spouse is more, or less, sexually directed . . . more, or less, generous . . . more, or less, communicative . . . or more, or less, intimate. Or, the wife may be faced with a great disappointment in her husband: She can no longer depend on him for support. She is forced to assume a greater and greater share of his responsibilities until finally, she is both mother and father in the house—a position she may find herself unconsciously enjoying.

Meanwhile, the alcoholic spouse may painfully be beginning to move toward recovery. The long-term results might be very much to the advantage of the spouse. For the short run, however, she may not be so willing to relinquish the secondary gains. Her husband demands to take back his man-of-the-house responsibilities. But can she be sure? Will this be just another brief attempt on his part, to be followed by another, even more painful disappointment? She hesitates, holds on to the reins, and gives only half-hearted support to his efforts. He wants back now; she isn't sure. He feels rebuffed and hurt and may go back to drinking. This sequence may be repeated several times.

Treatment. Because so many variables are involved in the differing constellations of marriages, the tendency is growing to treat the couple rather than just the alcoholic partner (12, 13). An immediate resistance that has to be resolved is the belief of the nondrinking spouse that he or she isn't really in need of help but is coming just to help the other. A first attack on this resistance is to point out that it is the marriage which is the patient; the alcoholism of one partner is merely the symptom of a sick marriage. Before long, the complementary pathology of the nonalcoholic spouse is usually in full bloom, ready for therapeutic attention.

This approach may be widened to include other or all members of the immediate family (22, 52). What role do children play in perpetuating a parental drinking pattern? A disdainful, "Is Dad drunk again?" could be a startling confrontation leading toward greater motivation to become well. Unfortunately, the question is more likely to be received with shame and resentment, both good reasons "to really tie one on!" The son's loss of self-respect as he sees his identification model crumbling may require painstaking

152

rebuilding, which may be facilitated if he can participate with his father in the therapeutic reconstruction of the self-esteem of the entire family.

Sometimes the significant other, possibly the addictor, needs to be identified and, if possible, brought into the picture. This could be Mom, Dad, or the mistress who finds her lover more responsive when he is drunk. These significant others are more difficult to bring into a therapeutic situation than a spouse. If the addictor cannot be involved and persists in his or her role, the alcoholic patient may have to be helped to make a clean break for self-survival.

Offshoot organizations of Alcoholics Anonymous have been effective in this area of involving family members and helping them. Al-Anon, an organization for spouses of alcoholic patients, is available whether or not the alcoholic partner is in Alcoholics Anonymous or part of some other rehabilitation procedure. The great value derived from such an organization is to learn that one is not alone in this predicament and to take advantage of other spouses' trial-and-error attempts at better adjustment. Hopefully, greater understanding by the spouse may lead to ways to help the alcoholic partner toward treatment. Al-Ateen is a parallel organization for the teen-age children of an alcoholic parent; Al-Atots is for still younger children.

SOCIAL

Small Group

Not only do all us have intrapsychic and intimate interpersonal experiences, but we also live in small social groups such as friends, acquaintances, clubs, neighbors, and interest groups that extend outside our families. Such contacts play a major role in maintaining identification roles and self-esteem, and in offering opportunities for controlled and healthy release of impulses. Unfortunately, the slow progression to alcoholism usually results in a loss of such contacts. Friends cease to be; old drinking buddies can't and don't wish to keep pace; neighbors are disdainful. The alcoholic person, already struggling with his waning sense of personal worth, progressively becomes alienated and lonely. He may project responsibility upon others for his social rejection. Within himself, however, he is only too aware of where the responsibility lies, thus confirming the worst of his already low self-appraisal.

Treatment. The prime example today of treatment provided within small group settings that take these factors into account is Alcoholics Anonymous, the major influence for the past 30-odd years in gaining acceptance of the disease concept of alcoholism. The aim of Alcoholics Anonymous members is to help each other maintain their sobriety, and to share their recovery experience freely with anyone who may have an alcohol-related problem. The Alcoholics Anonymous program basically consists of "Twelve Suggested Steps" designed for personal recovery from alcoholism. Several hundred thousand alcoholic people have achieved sobriety in this way, but members recognize that their program is not always effective with all alcoholic individuals, and that some persons may require professional counseling or treatment.

Alcoholics Anonymous is concerned solely with the personal recovery and continued sobriety of individuals who turn to this fellowship for help. The organization itself engages in no research, no medical or psychiatric treatment, nor endorsement of any causes, although members often participate in such activities as individuals. Organizationally, Alcoholics Anonymous' policy is one of "cooperation but non-affiliation" with other organizations concerned with the problems of alcoholism. Alcoholics Anonymous is self-supporting through its own groups and members; contributions from all outside sources are declined. Members preserve personal anonymity in the press, films, broadcast, and other public information media.

To some, Alcoholics Anonymous has at times appeared defensive about the roles of professional groups in the field of alcoholism. These fears have largely disappeared as Alcoholics Anonymous members and the professions have come to know one another better. Mutual appreciation, cooperation, and understanding have emerged as a result of better communication between Alcoholics Anonymous and other groups in the field of alcoholism.

Alcoholics Anonymous keeps no membership records and provides no hard statistics. Thus, it is sometimes difficult to verify or explain its success in scientific terms. Nevertheless, it is easy to see why Alcoholics Anonymous should and does work so often. The fellowship seems ideally suited for the guilt-ridden and lonely person lying beneath the facade of good-nature assumed by many alcoholic individuals before coming into Alcoholics Anonymous.

This is not surprising, as Alcoholics Anonymous was developed by people who had experienced similar feelings.

Founded in 1935 by two hopeless alcoholic persons—a stockbroker and a surgeon—Alcoholics Anonymous has proved that hundreds of thousands of people can and do recover from alcoholism, and go on to become productive citizens. While Alcoholics Anonymous has no formal religious dogma, most Alcoholics Anonymous members rely on a spiritual approach—a Higher Power greater than themselves. For some, this reliance may well be the most important factor in their recovery. The "Big Book" of Alcoholics Anonymous (1) is well worth reading. Many alcoholic persons, however, are not able to take the first step of Alcoholics Anonymous: "We admitted we were powerless over alcohol—that our lives had become unmanageable." They need other forms of therapy before they can be motivated to accept the Alcoholics Anonymous program.

The person who does stay with the program also relies on the help of other alcoholic individuals as he sets out on a course of making amends for previous wrongs. He turns to helping others (Twelfth Stepping) not only for the sake of others (the professional viewpoint), but for his own continued personal sobriety. All of this activity occurs in a fellowship with others like himself who are in the process of recovering; in this fellowship he is unconditionally accepted as a peer.

Another form of small group therapy for alcoholic persons is represented by the halfway house, which has been developed to fill the serious gap that has arisen between hospital and outpatient services (20, 50, 66). The middleclass patient, for example, usually returns to or continues with his family. Many alcoholic persons, however, have lost old attachments. After detoxification and with good motivation toward rehabilitation, they unhappily run into the demoralizing situation where no one wants them and they have no place to go.

Originally instituted for various types of emotional disorders, the halfway house has probably performed its greatest service for the alcoholic patient. Generally, this patient can look back to a better experience of integration than, for example, the person with a long history of schizophrenia, and has greater potential to return to at least his former level of functioning. The alcoholic individual on the road to recovery may remain in a halfway house from several weeks to several months. Here he has an opportunity to continue confrontation group therapy, obtain proper nutrition, and take a breathing spell while he job-hunts or undertakes a vocational rehabilitation program. At the halfway house he has a built-in group of acquaintances, and is encouraged to extend his social circle. Very often, the halfway house has a strong Alcoholics Anonymous or spiritual orientation that provides him with vital support. Perhaps one of the greatest values of a halfway house is that it offers a "dry island" to which the recovered alcoholic person may retreat. Here, in association with others to whom he relates, he temporarily insulates himself from community, family stresses, and drinking stimuli during his hours away from work.

Halfway houses may be part of a public network of rehabilitation services, or operated by nonprofit voluntary groups. Unfortunately, halfway houses are in short supply. This is especially true for women, for society often forgets that women also have alcohol-related problems.

A day hospital falls between a halfway house and a hospital (24, 38). The halfway house is for the person with no place to go, but who doesn't need a hospital. The day hospital is for the person who does have a place to go, is not quite ready to go there yet, but doesn't need full-time care.

In the day hospital, the alcoholic patient continues with group therapy, engages in resocialization, participates in vocational rehabilitation programs, and gradually increases his community contacts. He returns home nights and weekends, gradually decreasing the proportion of time he spends in the day hospital.

The night hospital or weekend hospital is a reverse variation on this theme. Perhaps the individual can return to a job which presents few stresses for him, yet needs time before he can return to where his real stresses lie—in his marriage and family.

A major roadblock to greater use of halfway houses and day or other partial hospitalization techniques, is the failure of health insurance to realize that these approaches are less expensive alternatives to full-time hospital care. Hopefully, this penny-wise, pound-foolish attitude will be changed.

Large Group

The estimated 9 million people in our midst with alcohol-related problems undoubtedly have a major impact on such large social groups as industry, the military, and our driving, flying, and boating populations. This is especially relevant when we consider the lack of realism in such traditionally held viewpoints as,

"Alcoholics are bums so they don't hold down jobs in our business or factory"; or, "Alcoholics are too poor to own automobiles, and those who do are too foxy to drive after drinking."

The fact that less than 5 percent of people with alcohol-related problems are on skid row makes it obvious that most alcoholic individuals are in the work force. And most of them, like most of us, do own automobiles and do drive.

Treatment. Within the work world, rehabilitation programs have several essential elements: (a) casefinding; (b) confrontation; (c) motivation; and (d) followup. A relatively easy person to identify is the individual whose job performance shows increasing impairment due to a behaviorial problem which expresses itself through such symptoms as recurrent absenteeism, vague physical complaints, poor on-the-job interpersonal relationships, and decreasing efficiency. The issue is not so much the education of supervisors in early casefinding (they have a pretty good idea of who is in trouble), as it is in their companies establishing policies and procedures that allow them to take corrective action. It should be noted that the criterion for company action is the employee's job performance and not his use of alcohol. Similarly, the only criterion of successful response is improved job performance.

When impaired job performance indicates alcohol abuse or alcoholism may be involved, a company with an alcoholism program refers the individual to medical or personnel counseling services. These services may be an integral part of the company, or they may be community-based services that are used by the company under contract or other agreements. Conceptually, the assistance offered to the employee in this instance does not differ from that offered in cases of job impairment due to other disease-related conditions.

As in many other health and welfare plans, labor and management agreement is essential to the development of industrial alcoholism programs. There are several accepted procedures for implementing such programs. In general, an employee is offered and urged to accept a designated health service for diagnosis of a condition that may possibly be affecting his work. Such a health service identifies the nature of the problem and recommends an appropriate treatment course. In the case of alcoholism, this recommendation may be referral to a specified alcoholism clinic, a psychiatrist, Alcoholics Anonymous, or other appropriate caregiver. During this confrontation, the employee is given a clear choice of either improving his job performance or facing admin-

157

istrative disciplinary procedures. The offer to assist him is expressed firmly, but it must be accepted voluntarily. If treatment is accepted, the worker must show a reasonable effort to pursue treatment, and his work performance must also show improvement. If his performance continues impaired and he manifests little concern in obtaining treatment, the normal administrative procedures based on deteriorating work performance take their course. If sincere treatment effort fails to improve his work, then the issue of disability retirement may have to be resolved. In cases where performance improves although no treatment is undertaken, no company action is warranted beyond monitoring the level of work to ensure that the problem does not repeat itself.

Early identification of the alcoholic employee is essential. A program at one company has already resulted in a 63 percent reduction in absenteeism (71); at another company, substantial rehabilitation has been achieved in 65 percent of the workers diagnosed as needing treatment for alcoholism (27). In both companies, early identification was stressed.

The cost of industry alcoholism programs is negligible compared to the cost of no program. The alcoholic worker, for example, is likely to be an older and more experienced employee. Studies in one large company showed that two-thirds of employees identified as alcoholic persons had from 5 to 15 years of service. In another company, such employees averaged 22 years of service (74). Losing such workers is expensive; so is the cost of continued job impairment. But since these employees have much to lose in terms of seniority, the leverage for constructive on-the-job intervention is great.

When it comes to coping with alcohol-related traffic accidents, one form of positive intervention being tried out in many communities is therapy offered as an alternative to punishment, to the person arrested for driving while intoxicated. A full range of community services are being utilized, just as for the worker who is offered treatment instead of immediate job dismissal. Considering all the previously mentioned complexities of therapy, one standard and rigidly applied program is not likely to be successful. The U.S. Department of Transportation is now funding pilot projects to discover what orientation might be effective. Traditional techniques of jail, fine, and license revocation have not been successful. Neither have the well-intentioned but naive attempts to alter this situation by a few lectures on the evils of "Demon Rum." Though they may act as if they didn't know the facts, the bulk of the "students" are all too knowledgeable about the effects of alcohol, but they are caught up in an addictive illness.

SOCIETY

Ours is a society ambivalent about its drinking habits. Nearly one-third of our adult population does not drink at all, but most people drink at least occasionally. Of the population that drinks, an uncertain proportion wonders whether drinking may be morally evil. For many, even social drinking requires a defiant pullaway from old family attitudes of abstinence. On the other hand, we have groups for which controlled drinking is the norm, but some may be undergoing changes from traditional customs toward uncontrolled drinking.

An overall coordinating agency for services is needed in most communities. Otherwise, gaps in service will exist through which many alcoholic persons will fall, or costly duplications will occur. This coordination can be accomplished under the umbrella of a public health department, a comprehensive health or mental health organization, or some similar group. An important part of the coordinating body is a highly visible community education and referral service, similar to those affiliated with the National Council on Alcoholism. This referral service is a place to which to turn for help in finding the right spot to enter the treatment network. It can be used both for self-referrals and to assist clergymen, physicians, courts, teachers, social agencies, and other health professionals coming in contact with people who have drinking problems or are addicted to alcohol.

An essential first level of treatment is detoxification for the acutely intoxicated person. Some communities might prefer a detoxification center, perhaps operated by a public health department, from which a patient can be referred to rehabilitative resources. Others might prefer to develop detoxification treatment at each community general hospital. A psychiatric hospital will be necessary for those who are a risk to themselves or others, or for those who must be hospitalized so they can obtain a handle on the beginning of long-range rehabilitation. A network consisting of general hospital psychiatric units, private free-standing psychiatric hospitals, and publicly supported mental health units—whatever is locally appropriate—must be developed. Detoxification is merely emergency treatment, representing the first step toward recovery for the acutely intoxicated person. Unfortunately, the only medical service offered by many communities to alcohol abusers and alcoholic persons is a detoxification service, and even when continuing services are provided, facilities are so inadequate that they discourage people from seeking, accepting, or continuing treatment.

Alcoholics Anonymous should be encouraged to participate in the system at an early point, and then reintroduced along the way for those who need special help before they can accept the Alcoholics Anonymous fellowship. Alcoholics Anonymous groups can be established at detoxification units, general and psychiatric hospitals, and clinics. As soon as possible, the patient should be out of a hospital; indeed, the majority will not need a hospital at all. For those still requiring much support, or without personal attachments, halfway houses and a partial hospitalization program should be developed.

Outpatient care may run the gamut from Alcoholics Anonymous, to special alcoholism clinics, to general psychiatric clinics, to private practitioners with special interest and skills in treating alcoholic persons. Therapy must be directed at both intrapsychic and interpersonal problems, sometimes with involvement of spouses and other family members.

Community consultation is essential for a well-functioning program. Professionals should be available to offer help at major casefinding points: the municipal court, the city jail, welfare departments, hospital emergency rooms, and social agencies. Consultation for education programs should be available to schools, clergymen, service clubs, and interested social groups.

Despite the best efforts of this community network, some alcoholic persons will be in an irreversible state. For these people, social centers and sheltered living will have to be provided.

Many communities will find it necessary to bring in special organizations that work best with certain minority or ethnic groups. Indigenous workers should be trained and available as therapeutic intervenors at each step in the network of services.

In general, persons who need adequate mental coverage, and health and social resources as a result of their alcoholism, do not have the same services available—either from the private or public sectors of the Nation—as persons with other illnesses. This has been due, in part, to this historic reluctance to commit incentive, personnel, or funds to this area of need. It is also due to the lack of clear-cut diagnostic procedures which can be used to determine the existence of the illness, alcoholism. Surprisingly, an inventory

160

of resources will show that many of the needed treatment facilities actually exist in most communities. What is lacking is organization, coordination, cooperation and, most important, a dedication to see the alcoholic individual as a person worthy of care. Given some outside grant funding, the cost of supplying the missing links may be within grasp. Operational costs for the community will not be heightened; in fact, they will prove much less expensive than failure to operate such a system. Private health insurance carriers, through State regulatory bodies, should be forced to remove clauses in their policies that discriminate against alcoholism. The cost of providing care for the medically indigent patient will be minimal compared to ultimate public costs of neglecting him.

No one knows what proportion of alcoholic patients can be helped by a system providing such continuity of care. As with many medical and social disorders, alcoholism tends to be a chronic ailment with a myriad of causative factors. Control is the practical goal. Recovery may be temporary, but is vital to survival while it lasts, and temporary improvement allows optimism that control can be gained. To date, at any given time, a cross-section of alcoholic patients shows one-third much improved (not only in alcohol-related behavior but in general living comfort), one-third experiencing some lesser benefit, and one-third unchanged. A slice across the sample at another time will show considerable shifting back and forth among these sectors. With such a success rate at present, we can expect our efforts to be correspondingly rewarded as we muster knowledge and resources in the future.

SUMMARY AND CONCLUSION

Alcoholism is a chronic and often recurring illness that has multiple causations including genetic, biological, psychological, and sociological factors. These factors are found in different combinations and with different relative importance in each alcoholic person. To be successful, treatment must take these various issues into account. The body and its chemistry must be considered. So also must the love, hate, and fear that reside in the unconscious level of our minds—between spouses, among children and parents, within social groups and, ultimately, in the broad spectrum of society as it encourages or prevents alcoholism.

Alcoholism is a complicated disorder, but it can be treated successfully. Any technique used indiscriminately will be much less successful. When the proper treatment modalities are utilized

161

for the unique needs of the particular patient, however, we indeed have cause for optimism.

REFERENCES

(1) Alcoholics Anonymous. Alcoholics Anonymous. New York: Alcoholics Anonymous World Services, Inc., 1955.

(2) Allen, R.P. and Faillace, L.A. Intoxication recovery. Modern Medicine, May 17, 1971, p. 47.

(3) American Hospital Association Statement on Admission to the General Hospital of Patients with Alcohol and Other Drug Problems. Chicago: American Hospital Association, November 19–20, 1969.

(4) American Medical Association Committee on Alcoholism and Drug Dependence. Guidelines for admission of alcohol-dependent patients to general hospitals. J.A.M.A. 210:121, 1969.

(5) Beard, J.D. and Knott, D.H. Fluid and electrolyte balance during acute withdrawal in chronic alcoholic patients. J.A.M.A. 204:135–139, 1968.

(6) Blane, H.T. The Personality of the Alcoholic; Guises of Dependency. New York: Harper & Row, 1968.

(7) Blum, E.M. and Blum, R.H. Alcoholism: Modern Psychological Approaches to Treatment. San Francisco: Jossey-Bass Inc., 1967.

(8) Blumberg, L., Shipley, T.E., Jr., Shandler, I.W. and Niebuhr, H. The development, major goals and strategies of a Skid Row program: Philadelphia. Quart. J. Stud. Alc. 27:242–258, 1966.

(9) Blumberg, L.U., Shirley, T.E., Jr. and Moor, J.O., Jr. The Skid Row man and the Skid Row status community; with perspectives on their future. Quart. J. Stud. Alc. 32:909–941, 1971.

(10) Bolman, W.M. Abstinence versus permissiveness in the psychotherapy of alcoholism; a pilot study and review of some relevant literature. Arch. Gen. Psychiat. 12:456–463, 1965.

(11) Brune, F. and Busch, H. Anticonvulsive-sedative treatment of delirium alcoholicum. Quart. J. Stud. Alc. 32:334–342, 1971.

(12) Burton, G., Kaplan, H.M. and Mudd, E.H. Marriage counseling with alcoholics and their spouses. I. A critique of the methodology of a follow-up study. Brit. J. Addict. 63:151–160. II. The correlation of excessive drinking behavior with family pathology and social deterioration. 161–170, 1968.

(13) Chafetz, M.E. New perspectives in the management of the alcoholic. In: Black, P., ed. Drugs and the Brain. Baltimore: Johns Hopkins Press, 1969, pp. 341–347.

(14) Chafetz, M.E., Blane, H.T. and Hill, M.J. Frontiers of Alcoholism. New York: Science House, 1970.

(15) Clancy, J., Vanderhoff, E. and Campbell, P. Evaluation of an aversive technique as a treatment for alcoholism; controlled trial with succinylcholine-induced apneic

paralysis; an analysis of early changes in drinking behavior. Quart. J. Stud. Alc. 28: 476–485, 1967.

(16) Costello, C.G. An evaluation of aversion and LSD therapy in the treatment of alcoholism. Canad. Psychiat. Assn. J. 14:31–42, 1969.

(17) Davies, D.L. Normal drinking in recovered alcohol addicts. Quart. J. Stud. Alc. 23:94–104, 1962. Responses: Quart. J. Stud. Alc. 24:109–121;321–332, 1963.

(18) Davies, D.L., Scott, D.F. and Malherbe, M.E.L. Resumed normal drinking in recovered psychotic alcoholics. Int. J. Addict. 4:187–194, 1969.

(19) Ditman, K.S. Review and evaluation of current drug therapies in alcoholism. Int. J. Psychiat. 3:248–258, 1967. Critical evaluations. Int. J. Psychiat. 3:258–266, 1967.

(20) Donahue, J. A halfway house program for alcoholics. Quart. J. Stud. Alc. 32: 468–472, 1971.

(21) Edwards, G. Hypnosis in treatment of alcohol addiction. Quart. J. Stud. Alc. 27:221–241, 1966.

(22) Esser, P.H. Conjoint family therapy with alcoholics–a new approach. Brit. J. Addict. 64:275–286, 1970.

(23) Fox, R., ed. Alcoholism; Behavioral Research, Therapeutic Approaches. New York: Springer, 1967.

(24) Fox, V. and Lowe, G.D., II. Day-hospital treatment of the alcoholic patient. Quart. J. Stud. Alc. 29:634–641, 1968.

(25) Franks, C.M. Behavior therapy, the principles of conditioning and the treatment of the alcoholic. Quart. J. Stud. Alc. 24:511–529, 1963.

(26) Franks, C.M. Conditioning and conditioned aversion therapies in the treatment of the alcoholic. Int. J. Addict. 1:61–98, 1966.

(27) Gehrmann, G.H. DuPont program for alcoholics. Inventory 3:21, 1953.

(28) Gerard, D.L. and Saenger, G. Out-Patient Treatment of Alcoholism; A Study of Outcome and Its Determinants. Toronto: University of Toronto Press, 1966.

(29) Gerard, D.L., Saenger, G. and Wile, R. The abstinent alcoholic. Arch. Gen. Psychiat. 6:83–95, 1962.

(30) Glasscote, R.A., Plaut, T.F.A., Hammersley, D.W., O'Neill, F.J.,Chafetz, M.E. and Cumming, E. The Treatment of Alcoholism. A Study of Programs and Problems. Washington, D.C.: The Joint Information Service of the American Psychiatric Association and the National Association for Mental Health, 1967.

(31) Goldfried, M.R. Prediction of improvement in an alcoholic outpatient clinic. Quart. J. Stud. Alc. 30:129–139, 1969.

(32) Grant, M. and Tatham, R.J. The District of Columbia's experience with the alcoholic. J.A.M.A. 202:931–934, 1967.

(33) Greenberg, R. and Pearlman, C. Delirium tremens and dreaming. Amer. J. Psychiat. 124:133–142, 1967.

163

(34) Gross, M.M. Management of acute alcohol withdrawal states. Quart. J. Stud. Alc. 28:655–666, 1967.

(35) Gross, M.M. and Goodenough, D.R. Sleep disturbances in the acute alcoholic psychoses. In: Cole, J.O., ed., Clinical Research in Alcoholism. Psychiatric Research Report No. 24. Washington, D.C.: American Psychiatric Association, 1968, pp. 132–147.

(36) Hartocollis, P. and Sheafor, D. Group psychotherapy with alcoholics; a critical review. Psychiat. Dig. 29:15–22, 1968.

(37) Hill, M.J. and Blane, H.T. Evaluation of psychotherapy with alcoholics; a critical review. Quart. J. Stud. Alc. 28:76–104, 1967.

(38) Hudolin, V. The day hospitals in the treatment of alcoholics. Brit. J. Addict. 61:29–33, 1965.

(39) Jones, R.W. and Helrich, A.R. Treatment of alcoholism by physicians in private practice: a national survey. Quart. J. Stud. Alc., in press 1972.

(40) Kaim, S.C., Klett, C.J. and Rothfeld, B. Treatment of the acute alcohol withdrawal state: a comparison of four drugs. Amer. J. Psychiat. 125:1640–1646, 1969.

(41) Keehn, J.D. Translating behavioral research into practical terms for alcoholism. Canad. Psychol. 10:438–446, 1969.

(42) Keehn, J.D., Bloomfield, F.F. and Hug, M.A. Use of reinforcement survey schedule with alcoholics. Quart. J. Stud. Alc. 31:602–615, 1970.

(43) Kepner, E. Application of learning theory to the etiology and treatment of alcoholism. Quart. J. Stud. Alc. 25:279–291, 1964.

(44) Kissin, B. and Gross, M.M. Drug therapy in alcoholism. Amer. J. Psychiat. 125:21–41, 1968.

(45) Knott, D.H. and Beard, J.D. A diuertic approach to acute withdrawal from alcohol. Southern Med. J. 62:485–488, 1969.

(46) Krystal, H. and Moore, R.A. Who is qualified to treat the alcoholic? Quart. J. Stud. Alc. 24:705–720, 1963. Responses: Quart. J. Stud. Alc. 25:347–360; 558–572, 1964; and 26:118–128; 310–318; 506–514, 1965.

(47) Lowenstein, L.M., Simone, R., Boulter, P. and Nathan, P. Effect of fructose on alcohol concentrations in the blood in man. J.A.M.A. 213:1899–1901, 1970.

(48) Ludwig, A.M., Levine, J. and Stark, L.H. LSD and Alcoholism, Clinical Study of Treatment Efficacy. Springfield, Ill.: Charles C. Thomas, 1970.

(49) Madill, M.F., Campbell, D., Laverty, S.G., Sanderson, R.E. and Vandewater, S.L. Aversion treatment of alcoholics by succinylcholine-induced apneic paralysis; and analysis of early changes in drinking behavior. Quart. J. Stud. Alc. 27:483–509, 1966.

(50) Martinson, R. The California Recovery House; a sanctuary for alcoholics. Ment. Hyg. 48:432–438, 1964.

(51) McBrearty, J.F., Dichter, M., Garfield, Z. and Heath, G. A behaviorally oriented treatment program for alcoholism. Psychol. Rep. 22:287–298, 1968.

164

(52) Meeks, D.E. and Kelly, C. Family therapy with the families of recovering alcoholics. Quart. J. Stud. Alc. 31:399–413, 1970.

(53) Miller, B.A., Pokorny, A.D., Valles, J. and Cleveland, S.E. Biased sampling in alcoholism treatment research. Quart. J. Stud. Alc. 31:97–107, 1970.

(54) Moore, R.A. Reaction formation as a countertransference phenomenon in the treatment of alcoholism. Quart. J. Stud. Alc. 22:481–486, 1961.

(55) Moore, R.A. Some countertransference reactions in the treatment of alcoholism. Psychiat. Dig. 26:35–43, 1965.

(56) Moore, R.A. Alcoholism treatment in private psychiatric hospitals: A national survey. Quart. J. Stud. Alc. 32:1083–1085, 1971.

(57) Moore, R.A. and Buchanan, T.K. State hospitals and alcoholism; a nation-wide survey of treatment techniques and results. Quart. J. Stud. Alc. 27:459–468, 1966.

(58) Moore, R.A. and Krystal, H. The problem of abstinence by the patient as a requisite for the psychotherapy of alcoholism. Quart. J. Stud. Alc. 23:105–123, 1962.

(59) Moore, R.A. and Murphy, T.C. Denial of alcoholism as an obstacle to recovery. Quart. J. Stud. Alc. 2:597–609, 1961.

(60) Mullan, H. and Sanquiliano, I. Alcoholism: Group Psychotherapy and Rehabilitation. Springfield, Ill.: Charles C. Thomas, 1966.

(61) Narrol, H.G. Experimental application of reinforcement principles to the analysis and treatment of hospitalized alcoholics. Quart. J. Stud. Alc. 28:105–115, 1967.

(62) Pattison, E.M. A critique of alcoholism treatment concepts. Quart. J. Stud. Alc. 27:49–71, 1966.

(63) Pattison, E.M., Headley, E.B., Gleser, G.C. and Gottschalk, L.A. Abstinence and normal drinking: An assessment of changes in drinking patterns in alcoholics after treatment. Quart. J. Stud. Alc. 29:610–633, 1968.

(64) Pittman, D.J. and Tate, R.L. A comparison of two treatment programs for alcoholics. Quart. J. Stud. Alc. 30:888–889, 1969.

(65) Rosenberg, N. Hospital insurance of alcoholic patients. Quart. J. Stud. Alc. 32:176–179, 1971.

(66) Rubington, E. The future of the halfway house. Quart. J. Stud. Alc. 31:167–174, 1970.

(67) Schmidt, W. and DeLint, J. Mortality experiences of male and female alcoholic patients. Quart. J. Stud. Alc. 30:112–118, 1969.

(68) Selzer, M.L. Hostility as a barrier to therapy in alcoholism. Psychiat. Quart. 31:301–305, 1957.

(69) Smart, R.G., Storm, T., Baker, E.F.W. and Solursh, L. A controlled study of lysergide in the treatment of alcoholism. I. The effects of drinking behavior. Quart. J. Stud. Alc. 27:469–482, 1966.

165

(70) Steiner, C.M. The alcoholic game. Quart. J. Stud. Alc. 30:920–938, 1969. Responses: Quart. J. Stud. Alc. 30:939–956, 1969.

(71) Straus, R. and Bacon, S.D. Recognizing the problem drinker in business and industry. Journal of Business, University of Chicago 25(2): 1952.

(72) Tashiro, M. and Lipscomb, W.F. Mortality experiences of alcoholics. Quart. J. Stud. Alc. 24:203–212, 1963.

(73) Trice, H.M., Roman, P.M. and Belasco, J. Selection for treatment; a predictive evaluation of an alcoholism treatment regimen. Int. J. Addict. 4:303–317, 1969.

(74) Trice, H. The Problem Drinker on the Job.New York State School of Industrial and Labor Relations. Bulletin No. 40. Ithaca Cornell University, 1959.

(75) Tygstrup, N., Winkler, K. and Lundquist, F. The mechanism of fructose effect on the ethanol metabolism of the human liver. J. Clin. Invest. 44:817–830, 1965.

(76) Wallerstein, R.S. Hospital Treatment of Alcoholism. New York: Basic Books, Inc., 1957.

(77) Weiner, H.B. An overview on the use of psychodrama and group psychotherapy in the treatment of alcoholism in the United States and abroad. Group Psychother. 19: 159–165, 1966.

(78) Wolf, I., Chafetz, M.E., Blane, H.T. and Hill, M.J. Social factors in the diagnosis of alcoholism in social and nonsocial situations. Part II. Attitudes of physicians. Quart. J. Stud. Alc. 26:72–79, 1965.

Chapter VII

THE LEGAL STATUS OF INTOXICATION AND ALCOHOLISM

THE LEGAL STATUS OF INTOXICATION AND ALCOHO-LISM* in this country has changed dramatically in the short space of only 5 years. For over 350 years, public intoxication had been handled exclusively under the criminal law. About 25 years ago, alcoholism began increasingly to be recognized as a medical problem under treatment statutes enacted in some States. Those laws, however, had remained largely ignored or poorly implemented. In the past 5 years, following the landmark court decisions in 1966, more progress has been made toward the medical and rehabilitative handling of intoxication and alcoholism under State and Federal law than in the previous 350 years.

THE COURT DECISIONS

The campaign to change the legal status of intoxication and alcoholism in this country began on the streets of the District of Columbia on July 4, 1964, with the seventh arrest that year of Walter Bowles, a derelict alcoholic, for public intoxication. Two days later he was selected out of the "drunk tank" in the basement of the Court of General Sessions to be the first test case

---

*This chapter excludes consideration of the alcoholic beverage control laws.

(1). Although the prosecutor dropped the charges in that case, other test cases immediately followed. The essential principle sought to be established—that alcoholism is a disease, and that public intoxication is properly handled as a public health, welfare, and rehabilitation problem—has prevailed.

The Criminal Cases

The District of Columbia prosecutor dropped the charges in the *Bowles* case and the next three test cases (2), before the court forced discontinuation of this procedure. The fifth case involved DeWitt Easter, a homeless derelict alcoholic who was arrested for public intoxication on September 23, 1964. Easter had been arrested approximately 70 times since 1937 for public intoxication or other minor violations directly attributable to his alcoholism.

Following the nationwide publicity given to Easter's trial in *Time* magazine, a second test effort was started by filing a habeas corpus petition in the United States District Court for the Eastern District of North Carolina, on behalf of another homeless derelict alcoholic, Joe Driver. Driver's 2-year jail sentence for public intoxication in Durham had earlier been upheld by the North Carolina Supreme Court (3). Driver's record showed over 200 arrests for public intoxication and other minor offenses related to his alcoholism. As a result, he had spent at least two-thirds of his adult life in jail for nothing more than public intoxication.

The legal challenge to the public intoxication statutes in the *Easter* and *Driver* cases relied on a fundamental principle of criminal responsibility—that criminal sanctions may be applied only to voluntary action. It was argued that as a result of his disease, an alcoholic drinks involuntarily and therefore cannot be criminally punished for his intoxication. Since both men were homeless derelict alcoholics, it was also contended that their appearance in public was equally not of their own volition.

In early 1966, after adverse decisions in the lower courts, unanimous favorable decisions were handed down in both cases

---

(1) *District of Columbia v. Bowles*, D.C. Ct. Gen. Sess. Crim. No. 17814–64 (1964).

(2) *District of Columbia v. Turner*, D.C. Ct. Gen. Sess. Crim. No. 24734–64 (1964);
     District of Columbia v. Glover, D.C. Ct. Gen. Sess. Crim. No. 24735–64 (1964);
     District of Columbia v. Lowe, D.C. Ct. Gen. Sess. Crim. No. 24736–64 (1964).

(3) *State v. Driver*, 262 N.C. 92, 136 S.E.2d 208 (1964).

(4). The District of Columbia Circuit, sitting *en banc*, rested its decision on the common law principle that a homeless alcoholic's public intoxication does not constitute voluntary action and is therefore not punishable. The Fourth Circuit held that the eighth amendment prohibition against cruel and unusual punishment precludes convicting a homeless alcoholic for his public intoxication. The end result in both cases, however, was the same. The tradition of handling public intoxication by criminal procedures had been found invalid.

Following these two landmark cases, a number of lower State courts began to rule concordantly. In July 1967, the Superior Court of Fulton County, Georgia, reversed the conviction of an alcoholic for his public intoxication, relying upon both common law and constitutional grounds (5). In August 1967, the Philadelphia Court of Common Pleas held that "habitual intoxication is an illness, and as such may not constitutionally be made a criminal offense" (6). In October 1967, the Circuit Court for Montgomery County, Md., reversed the conviction of an alcoholic for public intoxication on the common law and constitutional grounds (7). In California, one municipal court ruled that alcoholism was not a defense to a charge of public intoxication (8), but another held that the constitution requires acquittal of a chronic alcoholic charged with public intoxication (9).

---

(4)   *Easter v. District of Columbia,* 361 F.2d 50 (D.C. Cir. 1966) (*en banc*) rev'g 209 A.2d 625 (D.C. Ct. App. 1965); *Driver v. Hinnant,* 356 F.2d 761 (4th Cir. 1966), rev'g 243 F. Supp. 95 (E.D.N.C. 1965).

(5)   *Dunlap v. City of Atlanta,* Fulton Co., Georgia, Super. Ct. No. B–29126 (July 17, 1967), reprinted in 113 Cong. Rec. 23759 (August 23, 1967).

(6)   *Lee v. Hendrick,* Pa. Common Pleas Ct. (Phil.) No. H.C.-0075 (Ausgust 31, 1967), digested in 1 BNA Crim. L. Reptr. 2364 (September 20, 1967), reprinted in 113 Cong. Rec. 32717 (November 15, 1967).

(7)   *State v. Ricketts,* Montgomery Co., Maryland, Cir. Ct. Crim. No. 8787 (October 25, 1967), reprinted in 113 Cong. Rec. 31561 (November 7, 1967).

(8)   There were no written decisions in this case except the dissent from the denial for a writ of certiorari, *Budd v. California,* 385 U.S. 909 (1966). Petitions for habeas corpus have also subsequently been denied, *Budd v. Madigan,* 418 F.2d 1032 (9th Cir. 1969), cert. denied, 397 U.S. 1053 (1970).

(9)   *State v. Dobney,* Los Ang. Mun. Ct. No. D475555 (May 16, 1966), reprinted in 112 Cong. Rec. 23660 (September 22, 1966), rev'd on other grounds, Los Ang. Super. Ct. App. Div. No. CRA 6963 (October 14, 1966).

In a Wisconsin case (10), alcoholism was recognized as a disabling disease in the context of a different criminal charge. The defendant, charged with failure to support his child, claimed in defense that he was a chronic alcoholic and that his condition was an illness or a disease that prevented him from keeping any employment and from supporting his family. The court agreed that this would be a valid defense. The defendant was convicted, however, when he failed to present competent testimony to establish his defense.

The *Easter* and *Driver* decisions have raised the question whether alcoholism might be regarded, like insanity, as a defense to any criminal charge. As far back as 1869, in the long-forgotten case of *State v. Pike* (11), the Supreme Court of New Hampshire had ruled that alcoholism was available as a defense to the charge of murder. Following *Easter* Judge Murphy of the District of Columbia Court of General Sessions ruled that alcoholism could be a defense to a charge of disorderly conduct (12). In another case, the United States Court of Appeals for the Sixth Circuit described *Driver* and *Easter* as the recent leading cases holding that chronic alcoholism may be a defense to a charge of unlawful conduct, because of lack of responsibility on the part of one so afflicted. The court held that a guilty plea to a charge of bank robbery by an alcoholic who had experienced delirium tremens for several days after his arrest should not have been accepted by the trial court until it had first thoroughly investigated the circumstances under which the guilty plea was made and then determined that it was voluntarily made with an understanding of the nature of the charge (13).

It was at this point that the United States Supreme Court noted probable jurisdiction, on October 9, 1967, on a direct appeal from the county court of Travis County, Texas, in the case of *Powell v. Texas* (14). In the months that followed, while the *Powell* case was being briefed, argued, and decided, two State supreme courts, in deeply divided cases, upheld an alcoholic's conviction for public

---

(10) *State v. Freiberg,* 35 Wis. 2d 480, 151 N.W.2d 1 (1967).

(11) *State v. Pike,* 49 N.H. 399 (1869).

(12) *District of Columbia v. Phillips,* 95 Wash. L. Reptr. 917 (D.C. Ct. Gen. Sess. 1967), reprinted in 113 Cong. Rec. 12793 (May 16, 1967).

(13) *Fultz v. United States,* 365 F.2d 404 (6th Cir. 1966).

(14) 392 U.S. 514 (1968), rehearing denied, 393 U.S. 898 (1968).

intoxication under the facts of those cases (15), foretelling the widely differing views held by the Supreme Court Justices in the *Powell* case.

Leroy Powell, an uneducated laborer who earned about $12 per week, also had an extensive arrest record for nothing other than public drunkenness. On December 19, 1966, Powell was arrested for public intoxication in Austin, Tex. On December 20 he was found guilty and fined $20. His conviction was appealed to the Travis County Court, where the judge found that he was an alcoholic but nevertheless affirmed his conviction. Since he had no other right of appeal within the State court system, he appealed directly to the United States Supreme Court.

In June 1968, the Supreme Court handed down its judgment, affirming Powell's conviction. A full appreciation of the implications of that case, however, requires analysis of the opinions written by members of the Court, none of which represented a majority view.

An opinion by Mr. Justice Marshall, in which Justices Warren, Black, and Harlan concurred, commented that: "The picture of the penniless drunk propelled aimlessly and endlessly through the law's 'revolving door' of arrest, incarceration, release, and rearrest is not a pretty one," and noted the urgent need for some clear promise of a better world for those unfortunate people. These four Justices nonetheless concluded that the development of common law principles of criminal responsibility, and their application to new medical knowledge, should be left to the States and should not be hardened into rigid constitutional principles.

An opinion written by Mr. Justice Fortas, in which Justices Brennan, Douglas, and Stewart concurred, concluded that imposing criminal penalties upon an alcoholic for his public intoxication would violate the eighth amendment, because criminal penalties may not be inflicted upon a person for being in a condition he is powerless to change. This opinion accepted the argument that alcoholism is a disease which renders its victims powerless to avoid intoxication.

Thus, the deciding vote was cast by Mr. Justice White. In a separate opinion, he concurred both with the reasoning expressed in the opinion of Mr. Justice Fortas, and with the disposition of the case expressed in the opinion of Mr. Justice Marshall. In

---

(15) *Seattle v. Hill*, 72 Wash.2d 786, 435 P.2d 692 (1967); *People v. Hoy*, 380 Mich. 597, 158 N.W.2d 436 (1968).

Justice White's view, the controlling issue was whether Powell could avoid being intoxicated *in public*. Because there was no evidence that Powell could not avoid being in public on the occasion on which he was arrested, Mr. Justice White voted to affirm the conviction. At the same time, however, he recognized that homeless derelict alcoholics suffer from a disease and could not properly be convicted for their public intoxication:

> The fact remains that some chronic alcoholics must drink and hence must drink *somewhere*. Although many chronics have homes, many others do not. For some of these alcoholics I would think a showing could be made that resisting drunkenness is impossible and that avoiding public places when intoxicated is also impossible. As applied to them this statute is in effect a law which bans a single act for which they may not be convicted under the eighth amendment—the act of getting drunk.
>
> It is also possible that the chronic alcoholic who begins drinking in private at some point becomes so drunk that he loses the power to control his movements and for that reason appears in public. The eighth amendment might also forbid conviction in such circumstances, but only on a record satisfactorily showing that it was not feasible for him to have made arrangements to prevent his being in public when drunk and that his extreme drunkenness sufficiently deprived him of his faculties on the occasion in issue. 392 U.S. at 551—552.

A careful reading of the case therefore demonstrates that the Supreme Court, by a vote of 5 to 4, agreed with the earlier rulings in *Easter* and *Driver* that a homeless derelict alcoholic may not constitutionally be punished for his public intoxication. As was recently stated in the Senate Report on the Comprehensive Alcohol Abuse and Alcoholism Prevention, Treatment, and Rehabilitation Act of 1970 (16):

> . . . five of the nine Justices agreed that alcoholism is a disease, that an alcoholic drinks involuntarily as a result of his illness, and that an alcoholic who was either homeless or who could not confine his drunkenness to a private place for some other reason could not be convicted for his public intoxication. Powell's conviction was upheld by a 5-to-4 vote, how-

---

(16) S. Rep. No. 91—1069, 91st Cong. 2d Sess. 3 (1970).

ever, because the record failed to show that he was homeless or otherwise unable to avoid public places when intoxicated.

As the law now stands, therefore, a homeless alcoholic cannot constitutionally be punished for his public intoxication.

Unfortunately, the case has not been as widely understood and applied as it should have been.

The Supreme Court of Pennsylvania, after a close analysis of the *Powell* opinions, expressed the same understanding as the Senate report (17):

> As a result, *Powell v. State of Texas* unequivocally holds that to the extent certain behavior is a "characteristic part" of a disease, to the extent it is an actual symptom of the disease, such behavior cannot be criminally proscribed.

In the District of Columbia, the United States Court of Appeals ruled after the *Powell* decision not only that *Easter* remained the controlling law in that jurisdiction, but that alcoholism might properly be a defense to any criminal act caused by that condition (18). The Supreme Court of Minnesota ruled, in 1969, that alcoholism is a defense to a charge of public intoxication (19), but the Supreme Court of Alaska and the Georgia Court of Appeals have ruled that an alcoholic is criminally responsible for his public intoxication (20).

The present state of the law governing intoxication and alcoholism was substantially clarified in a major address delivered on December 10, 1971, by Attorney-General Mitchell (21):

> Fortunately, as many of you know, progress has been made in recent years. In 1966 the District of Columbia Circuit of the United States Court of Appeals ruled in the *Easter* case that the public drunkenness of a homeless alcoholic was involuntary. Therefore, he could not be held accountable

---

(17) *In re Jones,* 432 Pa. 44, 246 A.2d 356, 363 (1968).

(18) *Salzman v. United States,* 405 F.2d 358 (D.C. Cir. 1968).

(19) *State v. Fearou,* 283 Minn. 90, 166 N.W.2d 720 (1969).

(20) *Vick v. State,* 453 P.2d 342 (Alaska 1969); *Berger v. State,* 118 Ga. App. 328, 163 S.E.2d 333 (1968).

(21) "Alcoholism––To Heal, and Not To Punish," reprinted in 117 Cong. Rec. 21499 (December 11, 1971) (daily ed.), and as Appendix B to this report.

before the law. In the same year another Appellate Court made a somewhat similar ruling in the *Driver* case.

In 1967 the United States Supreme Court heard a similar case—*Powell v. Texas*. While it ruled that the defendant was accountable for being drunk in public because he did have a home to go to, a majority of the justices also expressed an opinion that coincided with that of the two appellate decisions—that a homeless alcoholic is not accountable for his act.

The important point is that the courts have decided what the experts had been saying for years—that alcoholism in itself is involuntary and therefore is not a legal offense in the ordinary sense.

Unfortunately, these cases have not been heeded as they should be, and the constitutionality of the related laws in most states has not been challenged.

The Attorney-General concluded that, "Through the processes now at work, the public itself may come to realize that our task is not to punish, but to heal."

It seems inevitable that, at some point in the future, the United States Supreme Court will unequivocally hold that an alcoholic may not be held criminally responsible for his intoxication. Medical, correctional, and other public officials should prepare for this eventuality. As the Senate Report stated:

> Regardless of their views on the criminal law aspects of alcoholism, none of the nine Justices in the *Powell* case disagreed with the fundamental conclusions that "the legislative response to this enormous problem has in general been inadequate," that "facilities for the attempted treatment of indigent alcoholics are woefully lacking throughout the country," that there is an "absence of a coherent approach to the problem of treatment" and that there is an "almost complete absence of facilities and manpower for the implementation of a rehabilitation program."

Finally, the critical importance of all the court decisions in focusing nationwide attention on the problem of alcoholism must be appreciated. They stimulated the Reports of the Crime Commissions, the changes in State and local laws, and even the new Federal statutes.

The Civil Cases

While major emphasis was placed on confronting the handling of alcoholism under the criminal law, the test cases also had a significant beneficial effect on civil law. Further development of the principles established in the criminal law cases may bear even more fruitful results in the future as they are used to obtain adequate and appropriate treatment for alcoholism under existing civil statutes.

One of the earliest civil cases recognizing the compulsive and involuntary aspects of alcoholism was a labor arbitration award (22):

> Problem drinkers do not deliberately or willfully become drunk . . . It is compulsion, not a willful act.

The implications of this decision for employees' alcoholic programs have not yet begun to be realized.

Subsequent to *Easter* and *Driver*, alcoholism was also recognized as a disabling disease in two Social Security cases. The United States Court of Appeals for the Fourth Circuit held that (23):

> . . . where chronic alcoholism alone or in combination with other causes, is shown to have resulted in a medically determinable disability, rendering gainful employment impossible, recovery of benefits under the Act ought not be barred on account of the origin of the disability.

This claimant failed to make the required showing. The plaintiff in a second case, however, was able to establish a clear disability resulting from his alcoholism, and thus prevailed in his action for payments under the Social Security Act (24). These cases demonstrate the possibility of utilizing existing health, welfare, and rehabilitation legislation to obtain adequate treatment for persons disabled as a result of their alcoholism.

---

(22) *News Syndicate Co., Inc.*, 44 L.A. 308 (1964).

(23) *Lewis v. Celebrezze*, 359 F.2d 398 (4th Cir. 1966).

(24) *Schompert v. Celebrezze*, W.D.N.Y. Civil No. 10937 (May 24, 1966), reprinted in 112 Cong. Rec. 23660 (September 22, 1966).

THE CRIME COMMISSION REPORTS

In August 1965, while the *Easter* and *Driver* cases were still being litigated, President Johnson appointed two Crime Commissions, one to study crime in the District of Columbia, and the other to conduct a broad national survey of law enforcement and the administration of justice (25).

The President's charge to the District of Columbia Crime Commission included study of "diagnosis and noncriminal treatment of socio-medical problem offenders (e.g., alcoholics. . .)." After the *Easter* and *Driver* decisions were handed down in early 1966, both Commissions undertook a major review of the handling of intoxication and alcoholism under the criminal law.

The District of Columbia Crime Commission issued its Report in early 1967 (26). The U.S. Crime Commission's Report was made public only a few weeks later (27). Both recommended elimination of public intoxication as a criminal offense throughout the country, and substitution of public health, welfare, and rehabilitation measures to handle the problem.

The importance of these two Crime Commission Reports in carrying on the reform begun by *Easter* and *Driver* should be clearly understood. *Easter* and *Driver* merely prohibited punishment of alcoholics for public intoxication under the criminal law. The courts could not establish a modern public health system as an alternative way to handle people with alcohol-related problems, however, and without the impetus given by prestigious Presidential Commissions, State legislatures would be reluctant to undertake substantial reform in a politically sensitive area such as alcoholism.

The two Crime Commission Reports complemented each other perfectly. The D.C. Commission focused, in detail, on the specific inhumanities perpetrated on derelict alcoholics both before and after the *Easter* decision. The U.S. Crime Commission took a broader look at the problem across the country and, in its

---

(25) 1 *Weekly Compilation of Presidential Documents* 5–9 (August 2, 1965).

(26) *Report of the President's Commission on Crime in the District of Columbia,* ch. 7, sec. 1 (1966), reprinted as Appendix F in the President's Commission on Law Enforcement and Administration of Justice, *Task Force Report: Drunkenness* (1967).

(27) *The Challenge of Crime in a Free Society: A Report by the President's Commission on Law Enforcement and Administration of Justice,* ch. 9 (1967).

overview, found a repetition of the District of Columbia experience.

One often overlooked, but important, aspect of the U.S. Crime Commission Report is that the discussion of the drunkenness offense comprised a separate chapter. In the State crime commissions set up throughout the country to implement the U.S. Crime Commission Report, a separate task force has generally been established to cover the subject matter in each chapter. On a State level, therefore, special reports recommending reform of intoxication and alcoholism statutes have also been issued. These reports, in turn, have led to the development of new statutory approaches to the problem, which will be discussed below.

STATE INTOXICATION AND ALCOHOLISM LEGISLATION

It is useful to sketch the type of legislation that typically existed prior to the *Easter* and *Driver* decisions, and then to discuss in greater detail the newer legislation which has been enacted in response to the court decisions and the Crime Commission reports.

Legislation Before 1966

Criminal Law

Public intoxication was first made a criminal offense in England by a statute enacted in 1606 (28). This approach was carried over to the Colonies, and public intoxication was handled as a criminal offense in all jurisdictions in the United States until 1966.

The variety of State laws prohibiting public intoxication is as great as the number of legislatures which have considered the matter. A general description of the different types of provisions which have been enacted include:

Drunkenness. Some States simply prohibit drunkenness, without specifying that it is a crime only if it occurs in public. Some legal experts question the constitutionality of making a crime out of intoxication in the privacy of one's home.

Public intoxication. The typical legislative enactment prohibits public intoxication. The courts have interpreted this to include virtually every place except a private home.

(28) 4 *James I, c. 5 (1606).*

Habitual or common drunkard. The prohibition against being a common or habitual drunkard still exists in some State laws. Its constitutionality has been questioned both because of its vagueness and because it purports to punish a status rather than an act.

Vagrancy. Derelict alcoholics can readily be picked up under the broadly worded State vagrancy statutes. Recent court decisions, however, held such statutes unconstitutional because of their vagueness.

Loitering. Loitering statutes are also frequently used to handle public intoxication. Their constitutional footing would appear to be as infirm as the vagrancy and common drunkard provisions in State laws.

Drinking in public. Some States prohibit drinking in public, and this activity could also be encompassed within broadly worded loitering and disorderly conduct statutes.

Disorderly conduct. All States prohibit disorderly conduct, and in some instances public intoxication is handled under this provision. In New York City and Illinois, for example, where there were no public intoxication statutes, derelict alcoholics were regularly arrested and convicted for disorderly conduct even though they were not in fact disorderly in their behavior.

Drunk and disorderly. Some States specify being drunk and disorderly as an offense. Since disorderly conduct is an offense, the drunkenness element adds nothing.

Posting the names of alcoholics. Some State laws provide that the names of known alcoholics may be posted publicly, after which no alcoholic beverage may be sold or given to them. The Supreme Court recently declared one such statute unconstitutional because it failed to provide that the individual must be given notice and a hearing prior to posting his name (29). The difficulties and inevitable inequities in enforcing such a statute make it virtually a dead letter, and useless as a preventive measure.

Civil Law

In addition to these criminal provisions, a number of States had enacted civil statutes providing for treatment for alcoholism. Like the criminal laws, their variety is infinite. A brief listing of their characteristics includes:

Alcoholism agency. Most States have established a separate alcoholism agency or a special agency within the department of

---

(29) *Wisconsin v. Constantineau,* **400 U.S. 433 (1971).**

health or mental health which is generally responsible for developing policy on alcoholism and to provide treatment, rehabilitative services, and education.

Civil commitment. Under most State laws, civil commitment for alcoholism is permissible. In some instances, a separate alcoholism commitment procedure has been established. In others, the procedure is included within the general mental health commitment provisions. The provisions often require hospitalization and permit long terms of detention, but in some instances they reflect more modern concepts of voluntary community-based treatment.

Voluntary treatment. A number of State laws specifically provide for voluntary treatment for alcoholism, but many do not. Voluntary treatment may be provided in many instances under general health provisions, even where there is no statute.

Alcoholism is an illness. In several State laws, alcoholism is specifically recognized as an illness or disease. Such a provision in the District of Columbia law was strongly relied upon by the court in the *Easter* decision.

Legislation Since 1966

The response of State legislatures to the test cases and Crime Commission Reports, between 1966 and August 1971, when the Uniform Alcoholism and Intoxication Treatment Act was adopted by the National Conference of Commissioners on Uniform State Laws, was extremely varied. The overall thrust of the State legislation clearly reflected a movement toward reform. Yet it also revealed the need for a comprehensive and uniform approach to intoxication and alcoholism legislation throughout the country.

North Carolina

The first State legislature to respond to the test cases was North Carolina, the State in which the *Driver* case arose. In 1967, a law was enacted providing that any person acquitted of public intoxication by reason of chronic alcoholism shall remain within the jurisdiction of the court for up to 2 years so that appropriate voluntary or involuntary treatment may be instituted (30). The State did not repeal its drunkenness statute, however, or provide for a modern system of detoxification and treatment.

---

(30) N. Car. L. 1967, c. 1256, N. Car. Gen. Stat., Art. 7A, Sec. 122–65.6 *et seq.*

Hawaii

In April 1968, Hawaii became the first State legislature to abolish the offense of public intoxication, and to substitute a civil detoxification system, in response to the Crime Commission Reports (31). The new statute relied upon the following legislative finding:

> At present, public drunkenness is a criminal offense. In addition to its ineffectiveness, the existing system operates to discriminate against the poor, invites disregard of due process safeguards, and ignores the underlying medical, social, and public health problems of drunkenness. It is urgent that a law be enacted immediately to take drunkenness, as an offense in itself, out of the criminal system and to provide for a civil treatment program for drunkenness and alcoholism, including the use of medical facilities to replace the police station or jail as an initial detention unit for inebriates, inpatient medical care beyond a mere drying out process, and aftercare facilities for chronic drunkenness cases.

Rather than rely primarily upon voluntary treatment measures, however, as recommended by the Crime Commissions, the new Hawaii statute relied upon the rather harsh commitment procedures already contained in its mental illness laws.

District of Columbia

In February 1967, in response to the *Easter* decision and the District of Columbia Crime Commission Report, Congress undertook a comprehensive revision of the District of Columbia intoxication and alcoholism law. As finally enacted, the law represents the fullest embodiment of the recommendations of the crime commissions yet to be enacted by any legislature (32). Congress intended the law to provide a model for the States to follow.

> The new District of Columbia statute directed that: ... all public officials in the District of Columbia shall take cognizance of the fact that public intoxication shall be handled as a

---

(31) Laws 1968, Act 6 (April 18, 1968).

(32) District of Columbia Alcoholic Rehabilitation Act of 1967, P.L. 90–452, 82 Stat. 618 (1968). See S. Rep. No. 1435, 90th Cong., 2d Sess. (1968).

public health problem rather than as a criminal offense, and that a chronic alcoholic is a sick person who needs, is entitled to, and shall be provided adequate medical, psychiatric, institutional, advisory, and rehabilitative treatment services of the highest caliber for his illness.

The statute first repealed the public intoxication statute, replacing it with a new provision prohibiting disorderly intoxication. It then established a comprehensive new system, under civil law, for detoxification, inpatient, and outpatient treatment for intoxicated persons and alcoholics. The statute specifically provided that a person found intoxicated on the streets *may* be taken to his home, but if that is not done he *must* be taken for detoxification and emergency medical care to the new detoxification center. Congress made clear its intent that an intoxicated person could not be arrested for any of the usual petty criminal offenses, but must be handled under the new treatment provisions (33).

As recommended by the Crime Commissions, the new law relied almost wholly upon voluntary treatment. A person could be held at the detoxification center only until he was sober, and in any event no longer than 72 hours. Civil commitment at the detoxification center for additional medical care was permitted only when the person is in any danger of substantial physical harm, for 30 to 90 days. Civil commitment for treatment of alcoholism for persons charged with a misdemeanor was permitted, where the court found that "adequate and appropriate treatment ... is available for the person," for a period not to exceed the maximum term of imprisonment that was otherwise authorized. Civil commitment for treatment for alcoholism of persons not charged with a criminal offense was not authorized.

In practice, in the three years during which this statute has been in operation, only a handful of intoxicated persons have been brought to the detoxification center involuntarily. There has been no need whatever for commitment for emergency medical care. The courts have made frequent use of the civil commitment provisions in lieu of criminal punishment for persons faced with

---

(33) Chief Judge Greene of the D.C. Court of General Sessions explicitly ruled that, unless the person were charged with disorderly intoxication, he must be handled under the civil detoxification provisions of the law. *District of Columbia v. Greenwell,* 96 Daily Wash. L. Reptr 2133 (D.C. Ct. Gen. Sess. December 31, 1968).

criminal charges, but most of the persons given treatment under the Act have been voluntary patients. Since the law went into effect, there has been a waiting list of voluntary patients. The procedures established under the new District of Columbia law have thus proved to be eminently workable.

Maryland

Based in part on the bills pending in Congress for the District of Columbia and in part on other proposed model legislation that will be discussed later in this chapter, the Maryland legislature enacted similar legislation in 1968 (34). The statute repealed the public intoxication offense, and established the same type of detoxification, inpatient, and outpatient treatment for intoxication and alcoholism as in the District of Columbia.

Unlike the District of Columbia statute, however, Maryland law left unrevised the older civil commitment provisions for treatment and rehabilitation of alcoholics. If these were to be widely used, they could result in civil detention in lieu of criminal incarceration—a procedure that would be just as punitive and ineffective. In practice, however, treatment under the Maryland law has been provided on the same voluntary basis as treatment has been provided in the District of Columbia. While adequate treatment resources are still lacking, the statutory framework for providing intoxication and alcoholism treatment exists in Maryland.

North Dakota

In 1969, North Dakota abolished intoxication as a criminal offense and enacted new treatment provisions (35). An intoxicated person is to be taken to a jail for up to 24 hours or to a hospital for up to 72 hours for detoxification, or to his home. The existing commitment procedures for alcoholism treatment were not revised.

---

(34) Comprehensive Intoxication and Alcoholism Control Act, Acts 1968, ch. 146 (1968), Md. Code Ann. art. 2C.

(35) S.L. 1969, ch. 91.

Connecticut

New statutory provisions were enacted in Connecticut in 1969 (36). The offense of intoxication was limited to situations where the person endangered himself or other persons or property, or annoyed persons in his vicinity. The new law stated that, in lieu of arrest, a police officer could, in his discretion, take an intoxicated person to a civil facility for the care of alcoholics.

Florida

In 1971, the Florida legislature enacted a comprehensive revision of its State laws dealing with intoxication and alcoholism (37). It repealed the State laws making criminal offenses of public intoxication, public drinking, and being a common drunkard. It also provided that no political subdivision of the State could adopt any law or ordinance making these or similar acts or conditions criminal offenses.

The detoxification, inpatient, and outpatient treatment provisions of the statute were taken from a variety of sources. The findings and declarations of purposes, for example, were adopted verbatim from the bill introduced by Senator Hughes (38) in Congress in May 1970, that later became the Comprehensive Alcohol Abuse and Alcoholism Prevention, Treatment, and Rehabilitation Act of 1970 (39). The detailed medical and rehabilitative treatment provisions were adopted from one of the intermediate drafts of the Uniform Intoxication and Alcoholism Treatment Act.

Massachusetts

In November 1971, after considering proposed new legislation for several years, Massachusetts enacted a comprehensive new statute governing intoxication and alcoholism (40). The new law eliminates public intoxication as a criminal offense, and establishes a broad range of treatment and rehabilitation services to be

(36) Public Act 828 (July 8, 1969), Conn. Penal Code, art. 21, sec. 186.
(37) Florida Statutes, ch. 71–132 (1971).
(38) S. 3835, 91st Cong., 2d Sess. (1970).
(39) P.L. 91–616, 84 Stat. 1848 (1970).
(40) Mass. L. 1971, c. 1076.

administered by a Division of Alcoholism within the Department of Public Health.

Other States

A number of legislatures in other jurisdictions have also considered and enacted progressive new legislation dealing with intoxication and alcoholism. The Senate Report on the Comprehensive Alcohol Abuse and Alcoholism Prevention, Treatment, and Rehabilitation Act of 1970 explicitly pointed out that one of the important functions of the new National Institute on Alcohol Abuse and Alcoholism included "encouraging the enactment of a consistent pattern of State and local legislation throughout the country" (41). Noting the efforts that had been made toward drafting model legislation, and the pending work on the Uniform State Act, the Report stated that NIAAA would "actively cooperate in the efforts to provide such progressive legislation in every jurisdiction." With the recent adoption in August 1971 of the Uniform Act, this charge to NIAAA has now become a major nationwide effort.

MODEL AND UNIFORM LEGISLATION

Following the Crime Commission Reports, three separate drafting teams proceeded to prepare model or uniform legislation governing intoxication and alcoholism—the American Bar Association-American Medical Association Joint Committee on Alcoholism, the Legislative Drafting Research Fund of Columbia University, and the National Conference of Commissioners on Uniform State Laws. In light of the August 1971 adoption of the Uniform Act, the first two efforts are now largely of historic interest, and will be summarized only briefly. The Uniform Act will be discussed in some detail.

The Comprehensive Intoxication and Alcoholism Control Act of the ABA-AMA Joint Committee on Alcoholism

The first model law governing intoxication and alcoholism was prepared by a Joint Committee on Alcoholism formed by the

---

(41) S. Rep. No. 91–1069, 91st Cong., 2d Sess. 17 (1970).

Committee on Alcoholism and Drug Abuse of the American Medical Association's Council on Mental Health, the Committee on Alcoholism of the American Bar Association's Section of Criminal Law, and the Committee on Alcohol and Drug Reform of the American Bar Association's Section of Individual Rights and Responsibilities. It closely followed the approach recommended by the Crime Commission Reports and the legislation then pending in Congress which later became the District of Columbia Alcoholic Rehabilitation Act of 1967.

The ABA-AMA model law repealed the public intoxication offense by adopting a disorderly intoxication provision, and provided that all intoxicated persons who were not actually disorderly must be handled under civil detoxification, inpatient, and outpatient procedures. The treatment procedures specified in the model law closely resemble those in the District of Columbia statute.

The Model Alcoholism and Intoxication Treatment Act of the Columbia University Legislative Drafting Research Fund

Building upon the ABA-AMA model law and the new District of Columbia and Maryland statutes that had already been enacted, the Legislative Drafting Fund of Columbia University, under contract with the National Institute of Mental Health, also prepared a model act (42).

This model simply abolished all criminal offenses relating to intoxication and drinking in public, rather than adopting a disorderly intoxication provision, on the ground that disorderly intoxication was adequately covered by the standard disorderly conduct law. Its treatment provisions were substantially similar to those in the earlier ABA-AMA model, and in the later Uniform Act. Somewhat more limited in scope than the ABA-AMA model or the Uniform Act, it did not deal with some of the problem areas often closely related to intoxication and alcoholism, such as discrimination against alcoholics in hospitals, comprehensive plan-

---

(42) See Grad, Goldberg & Shapiro, *Alcoholism and the Law* (1971), which contains a very useful discussion of legal approaches to intoxication and alcoholism, the text of the model act together with the draftmen's notes, and an informative series of charts setting out pertinent provisions in current State civil and criminal statutes.

ning, and employee alcoholism programs in government and private industry.

The Uniform Alcoholism and Intoxication Treatment Act of the National Conference of Commissioners on Uniform State Laws

The most significant development in the area of model legislation occurred in August 1971 when the National Conference of Commissioners on Uniform State Laws adopted a Uniform Alcoholism and Intoxication Treatment Act. The National Conference is comprised of representatives appointed by the Governor of each State. Adoption of a Uniform Act obligates those representatives to obtain the introduction of the Act in their legislatures, and to press for its early enactment. The Uniform Act, therefore, unquestionably represents a major step forward.*

Section 1 of the Uniform Act enunciates the following declaration of policy:

It is the policy of this state that alcoholics and intoxicated persons may not be subjected to criminal prosecution because of their consumption of alcoholic beverages but rather should be afforded a continuum of treatment in order that they may lead normal lives as productive members of society.

Section 2 contains some 12 definitions. Of particular importance, the term "alcoholic" is defined as:

... a person who habitually (i) lacks self-control with respect to the use of alcoholic beverages, or (ii) uses alcoholic beverages to the extent that his health is substantially impaired or endangered or his social or economic functioning is substantially disrupted.

A person who is "incapacitated by alcohol" is defined to mean that:

... a person who, as a result of the use of alcohol, is unconscious or has his judgment otherwise so impaired that he is incapable of realizing and making a rational decision with respect to his need for treatment.

---

* The Uniform Act is attached to this report as Appendix A.

186

An "intoxicated person" is a person whose mental or physical functioning is substantially impaired as a result of the use of alcohol.

Section 3 establishes a Division of Alcoholism, and sections 4 and 5 specify its powers and duties. These include development of alcoholism plans and programs, coordination of resources, preparation of educational materials, development of training programs, sponsorship of research, maintenance of statistics, preparation of all State alcoholism treatment plans for funding pursuant to Federal legislation, fostering employee alcoholism programs, establishing highway safety alcoholism programs, encouraging general hospital and insurance programs to handle alcoholism problems, and submission of an annual report.

Sections 6 through 9 establish a State Interdepartmental Coordinating Committee and a Citizens' Advisory Council on Alcoholism and require the Division to establish a program for the treatment of intoxicated persons and alcoholics. The program must include "adequate and appropriate" emergency, inpatient, intermediate, outpatient, and followup treatment.

Section 10 authorizes the Division to establish rules and regulations for its treatment programs guided by priorities for voluntary rather than involuntary treatment, and outpatient rather than inpatient treatment. It also mandates the preparation and maintenance of individualized patient treatment plans, the provision of a continuum of coordinated treatment services, and establishment of the patient's right to be admitted for treatment even if he has previously withdrawn against medical advice or has relapsed repeatedly.

Section 11 provides for the voluntary treatment of alcoholics. Any person may voluntarily apply for treatment directly to any public treatment facility.

Section 12 provides that intoxicated persons and those incapacitated by alcohol may be assisted to their homes or to treatment facilities by the police or emergency service patrols in protective custody under civil law. It also limits the detention of an incapacitated person for emergency medical care to 72 hours unless committed under sections 13 or 14. Those two sections provide for civil commitment for emergency medical care for up to 5 days, or civil commitment of dangerous or incapacitated persons for up to 7 months. The Division must provide "adequate and appropriate" treatment to any committed patient.

Sections 15 through 18 protect the confidentiality of patients' records; provide for visitation and communications; authorize the establishment of an emergency service patrol to replace the police in giving assistance to persons intoxicated or incapacitated by alcohol; and deal with reimbursal for services to patients.

Section 19 prohibits political subdivisions from adopting any law making public intoxication, or any related behavior or condition that includes one of its elements, an offense or the subject of a sanction of any kind. Laws and regulations relating to drunken driving, however, are not affected. Sections 20 through 36 contain provisions for severability, and administrative procedures and rules. In section 37, all prior Acts relating to intoxication and alcoholism are repealed.

Work is just beginning to obtain enactment of the Uniform Act throughout the country. In November 1971, the Secretary of the Department of Health, Education, and Welfare wrote to the Governor of each State, endorsing the Uniform Act and urging its early enactment. The results of this effort are expected to become apparent soon.

FEDERAL LEGISLATION

In spite of the large number of Federal health, welfare, and rehabilitation statutes enacted by Congress prior to 1966, not one explicitly referred to the problems of intoxication and alcoholism. The changed national attitude about these problems is reflected in the new legislative initatives taken by Congress during the past 5 years.

The first Federal statute to deal with these problems was the Highway Safety Act of 1966 (43), which required a study and report to Congress on the effects of the consumption of alcohol on highway safety, as well as "State and local programs for the treatment of alcoholism" (44).

The Economic Opportunity Amendments of 1967 included, as one of several special programs to be funded, the support of facilities and services for the prevention of alcoholism and the rehabilitation of alcoholics (45). This provision was strengthened

---

(43) P.L. 89–564, 80 Stat. 731, 736 (1966).

(44) See Department of Transportation, *Report on Alcohol and Highway Safety* (August 1968).

(45) P.L. 90–222, 81 Stat. 672, 697 (1967).

by the Economic Opportunity Amendments of 1969, which established "An 'Alcoholic Counseling and Recovery' program designed to discover and treat the disease of alcoholism" as a new special emphasis program (46). The 1969 amendments required this program to be "community based" and to "emphasize the reentry of the alcoholic into society rather than the institutionalization of the alcoholic," as recommended by the Crime Commissions.

In his February 1967 Message to Congress on "Crime in America," President Johnson cited the drunkenness problem as one example of need for legislation which would utilize the Federal grants mechanism to assist States, cities, and regional bodies to develop plans for improving police, court, and correctional systems (47). This was the first time in history that a President mentioned this problem in a major message to Congress.

In his message of February 1968 to Congress on crime and law enforcement the President called for "enactment of an Alcoholism Rehabilitation Act, to help provide more effective treatment—rather than simple detention—of alcoholics" (48). This was the first time a President recommended new Federal legislation in this field.

In response, Congress enacted the Alcoholic Rehabilitation Act of 1968 (49). In this new statute, Congress made the following important declarations of findings and purposes:

Sec. 240. (a) The Congress hereby finds that--

(1) Alcoholism is a major health and social problem afflicting a significant proportion of the public, and much more needs to be done by public and private agencies to develop effective prevention and control.

(2) Alcoholism treatment and control programs should whenever possible: (A) be community based, (B) provide a comprehensive range of services, including emergency treatment, under proper medical auspices on a coordinated basis, and (C) be integrated with and involve the active participation of a wide range of public and nongovernmental agencies.

(3) The handling of chronic alcoholics within the system of criminal justice perpetuates and aggravates the broad

---

(46) P.L. 91–177, 83 Stat. 827, 829 (1969).

(47) 3 *Weekly Compilation of Presidential Documents* 182 (February 10, 1967).

(48) 4 *Weekly Compilation of Presidential Documents* 233 (February 12, 1968).

(49) P.L. 90–574, 82 Stat. 1005, 1006 (1968).

problem of alcoholism whereas treating it as a health problem permits early detection and prevention of alcoholism and effective treatment and rehabilitation, relieves police and other law enforcement agencies of an inappropriate burden that impedes their important work, and better serves the interests of the public.

(b) It is the purpose of this part to help prevent and control alcoholism through authorization of Federal aid in the construction and staffing of facilities for the prevention and treatment of alcoholism.

(c) The Congress further declares that, in addition to the funds provided for under this part, other Federal legislation providing for Federal or federally assisted research, prevention, treatment, or rehabilitation programs in the fields of health should be utilized to help eradicate alcoholism as a major health problem.

To implement these findings and purposes, the Community Mental Health Centers Act was amended to provide for construction grants, staffing grants, and grants for specialized facilities specifically for alcoholism. This act was further amended and strengthened by the Community Mental Health Centers Amendments of 1970, by authorizing direct grants for special projects outside of community mental health centers (50). The subsequent appropriations, however, were insufficient to implement the act.

It became apparent to the Congress that, if a truly massive Federal effort was to be mounted to combat alcoholism, new legislation was necessary. The Comprehensive Alcohol Abuse and Alcoholism Prevention, Treatment, and Rehabilitation Act of 1970 was therefore enacted (51). It created the National Institute on Alcohol Abuse and Alcoholism to administer all alcoholism programs and authority assigned to the Department of Health, Education, and Welfare, and to coordinate all Federal activities in this field. It also created a National Advisory Council on Alcohol Abuse and Alcoholism, to assist in developing a national policy.

To receive its share of formula grants under the 1970 act, each State is required to develop a comprehensive alcoholism plan. The act also provides for project grants and contracts for the prevention and treatment of alcohol abuse and alcoholism. It contains a

---

(50) P.L. 91–211, 84 Stat. 54, 57 (1970).

(51) P.L. 91–616, 84 Stat. 1848 (1970).

number of substantive provisions such as the establishment of treatment and rehabilitation programs for Federal civilian employees, incentive for private hospitals to admit alcohol abusers and alcoholics, the requirement of an annual report to Congress, and provision for confidentiality of patient records. To ensure that alcoholism would also be encompassed within the actions required by the Comprehensive Health Planning and Public Health Service Amendments of 1966 (52), and the Partnership for Health Amendments of 1967 (53), the 1970 act also explicitly required that such planning "provide for services for the prevention and treatment of alcohol abuse and alcoholism, commensurate with the extent of the problem."

President Nixon further emphasized the priority on alcoholism programs in his February 1971 message to the Congress on National Health Strategy, when he requested an additional $7 million for "alcoholism programs" to "permit an expansion of our research efforts into better ways of treating this disease." NIAAA will expend this additional $7 million of health initiative funds on applied research in the following priority areas: Providing help to employed alcoholics, rehabilitating the public inebriate, delivering comprehensive services to all alcoholic persons, treating alcoholic individuals identified through traffic safety programs, reducing the incidence of alcoholism among American Indians, and preventing alcoholism.

FOREIGN LAW

Foreign statutes governing intoxication and alcoholism exhibit the same ambivalence as those existing in the United States before 1966. Intoxication is almost uniformly made a criminal offense, but provision is frequently made for the treatment of alcoholism.

Throughout Canada, public intoxication remains a criminal offense subject to imprisonment (54). France has no drunkenness statute, but vagrants or vagabonds—defined as "persons who have neither a fixed residence, nor a means of subsistence, nor a trade or profession"—are punishable by jailing from 3 to 6 months (55).

---

(52) P.L. 89–749, 80 Stat. 1180 (1966).

(53) P.L. 90–174, 81 Stat. 533 (1967).

(54) See Alexander, *Responsibility and Addiction: The Law in Canada,* 13 Addictions, No. 4, at 11 (Winter 1966).

(55) French Penal Code, art. 269–271.

This provision undoubtedly covers alcoholic derelicts. In Germany, anyone who "succumbs to gaming, drunkenness or idleness to such an extent that he falls into a state in which he requires the intervention of the authorities in order to obtain the assistance of others to support him or those for whom he has a duty to care" is subject to criminal sanctions for the petty misdemeanor of deterioration (56).

In some countries, public intoxication is punishable only by fine, not incarceration. In Sweden, public drunkenness may result in a fine of no more than 500 kroner (57). In England, simple drunkenness is subject only to a fine of up to 5 pounds, but drunkenness with other unlawful behavior, such as disorderliness or indecency, is subject to a fine up to 10 pounds or imprisonment for up to 1 month (58). In the Soviet Union, drunkenness is considered a civil administrative offense rather than a criminal offense, and a person who appears on the street in an intoxicated condition is subject to a fine of 3 to 5 rubles imposed by an administrative commission (59).

Most foreign countries also have laws providing treatment for alcoholism. In 1954, France enacted provisions for the treatment of "all alcoholics who present a danger to other persons" (60). A comprehensive Swedish law on temperance, also enacted in 1954, provides treatment for any person who overindulges in alcohol "to the manifest detriment of himself or others," in order "to bring him back to a sober and orderly life" (61). A comprehensive new statute was enacted in Australia in 1968 to provide for civil commitment for treatment of a person suffering from alcohol dependency, which is defined as consuming alcohol to excess and thereby being dangerous to oneself or others or incapable of managing one's affairs (62). Various treatment statutes have been enacted in Czechoslovakia (63), South Africa (64), New Zealand

---

(56) German Penal Code, sec. 361 (5).

(57) Penal Code of Sweden, ch. 16, sec. 15.

(58) See *Report of the Working Party on Habitual Drunkenness Offenders* 15 (1971).

(59) The Russian Research Center, *Soviet Criminal Law and Procedure* 6 (1966).

(60) Law No. 54–439 (April 15, 1954), Public Health Code, Part V, reprinted in 7, Int. Dig. Hlth. Leg. 39 (1956).

(61) Law No. 579 (July 27, 1954), reprinted in 6 Int. Dig. Hlth. Leg. 715 (1955).

(62) Act No. 61 (1968), reprinted in 21 Int. Dig. Hlth. Leg. 31 (1970).

(63) Law No. 120 (December 19, 1962), reprinted in 15 Int. Dig. Hlth. Leg. 75 (1964).

(64) Act No. 86 (June 28, 1963), digested in 15 Int. Dig. Hlth. Leg. 85 (1964).

(65), Germany (66), Poland (67), Finland (68), Switzerland (69), and many other countries.

In many foreign countries, as in the United States, awareness is growing of the futility of criminal sanctions against intoxication and alcoholism. As a result, new methods of civil intervention and treatment are being instituted.

Noncriminal detoxification centers were established in Prague, Czechoslovakia, in 1951, and in Warsaw, Poland, in 1956 (70). Both provide emergency care treatment as an administrative solution to a problem which had previously placed an enormous strain on the police. By 1959, the success of the Polish experiments led to legislation requiring detoxification facilities in every city with a population over 100,000. More than 20 such centers now exist throughout Poland. In 1962, Hungary required detoxification for any alcoholic who disrupts his family life, interferes with the moral development of his minor children, jeopardizes the safety of others, or regularly commits a breach of the peace (71).

Section 91 of the English Criminal Justice Act of 1967 abolished imprisonment for being drunk and disorderly, but increased the maximum fine for this offense from 10 to 50 pounds (72). The new law also provides, however, that a statutory order implementing these changes shall not be made until the Home Secretary is satisfied that sufficient suitable accommodation is

(65) Act No. 97 (October 20, 1966), reprinted in 19 Int. Dig. Hlth. Leg. 421 (1968).

(66) Law No. 35 (June 5, 1958), reprinted in 11 Int. Dig. Hlth. Leg. 154 (1960).

(67) Law No. 62 (April 27, 1956), reprinted in 9 Int. Dig. Hlth. Leg. 323 (1958); replaced by Law No. 434 (December 10, 1959), digested in 12 Int. Dig. Hlth. Leg. 202 (1961).

(68) Law No. 96 (February 10, 1961), reprinted in 13 Int. Dig. Hlth. Leg. 249 (1962). A recent Finnish study on a reduction in the number of criminal prosecutions for drunkenness indicated no causal relationship between the drunkenness prosecution policy and the state of public order. Tornudd, *The Preventive Effects of Fines for Drunkenness,* Scandinavian Studies in Criminology 109 (1968).

(69) Canton of Neuchatel Law of May, 21, 1952, reprinted in 6 Int. Dig. Hlth. Leg. 563 (1955); Canton of St. Galler Law of June 18, 1968, digested in 21 Int. Dig. Hlth. Leg. 656 (1970).

(70) See *Report of the Working Party on Habitual Drunkenness Offenders* 144–145 (1971).

(71) Decree-Law No. 18 (July 21, 1962), digested in 14 Int. Dig. Hlth. Leg. 452 (1963).

(72) *Report of the Working Party on Habitual Drunkenness Offenders* 17 (1971).

available within the community for the care and treatment of persons convicted of the offense. During the debate in the House of Lords, the justification for this legislation offered by the Minister of State at the home office was similar to the conclusions of the U.S. and District of Columbia Crime Commissions (73).

To prepare for implementation of this new statute, a Working Party on Habitual Drunkenness Offenders was established. Its report, issued in 1971, recommended immediate constructive action to help the habitual drunkenness offender by providing detoxification and treatment services. It concluded that, until a full range of community facilities has been provided and been in operation long enough for evaluation, any decision as to whether some form of compulsory treatment might be justified would be premature. The conclusions and recommendations were, again, very similar to those reached by the U.S. and District of Columbia Crime Commissions.

A similar report was issued in 1969 by a Swedish Government Commission studying the same problem (74). That commission concluded that the arrest and punishment of acutely intoxicated persons is an outmoded procedure, and that detoxification clinics should be established to provide adequate care and treatment. The commission proposed such clinics in some 15 towns and cities, and recommended that drunken persons be detained for at least 8 hours and a maximum of 24 hours or, in exceptional cases, 48 hours.

Thus, the clear trend abroad closely parallels that in the United States. Legal sanctions to control intoxication and alcoholism have been found ineffective, and public health measures are being adopted to replace the criminal law.

SUMMARY AND CONCLUSION

For many years, progress in the field of treating intoxication and alcoholism has been inhibited by the existence of antiquated civil and criminal laws providing for punitive incarceration rather than rehabilitation. As a result of recent legal developments, an appropriate statutory framework is now available through which proper treatment and rehabilitation can be provided.

---

(73) House of Lords Official Report (10 May 1967), 282, No. 150, col. 1439.

(74) Ministry of Justice, *Detoxification Instead of Fines* (1969). See *Report of the Working Party on Habitual Drunkenness Offenders* 146 (1971).

194

Test cases, Crime Commission Reports, and even adoption of progressive new uniform legislation, do not guarantee the provision of adequate and appropriate treatment and rehabilitation services. They merely help provide the statutory framework within which a State is not only permitted, but encouraged, to handle the problems of intoxication and alcoholism according to the best current knowledge. Implementation is dependent upon the will of the State, as demonstrated by the level of funding appropriated and the dedication of health, welfare, and rehabilitation personnel to do the job that must be done.

Chapter VIII

RESEARCH NEEDS AND FUTURE DIRECTIONS

This chapter is an overview of recent research in the field of alcohol abuse and alcoholism with indications of the important areas requiring further study. Much has already been learned about the biochemistry of alcohol and its acute effects on cells, tissues, organs, and on body processes. Less is known, however, about the long-term health implications of alcohol consumption. Those areas most in need of immediate clarification are highlighted in this chapter, charting some of the needs and future directions of research programs of the National Institute on Alcohol Abuse and Alcoholism.

These research directions have been divided into three areas: studies of acute intoxication, physical dependence, and withdrawal from alcohol; studies of treatment methods; and studies in prevention and education.

STUDIES ON INTOXICATION AND PHYSICAL DEPENDENCE

Although remarkable progress has occurred in identifying the metabolic course of alcohol through the body, much important knowledge is still lacking on the complex and interactive role that it plays in producing some of the biochemical changes and physiological damage seen in heavy drinkers.

The progress which has been made, however, has resulted in significantly increased capabilities in treating the medical complications related to alcohol abuse and alcoholism, and has provided many beneficial outcomes. Since one continuing cause of death among alcoholic persons is advanced cirrhosis of the liver, investigation into alcohol-related liver diseases has been and continues to be of high priority. Further studies are also necessary in the treatment of pancreatitis, gastritis, and withdrawal reactions, since these are among the serious complications of alcoholic people that physicians encounter daily.

In their attempt to shorten the period of alcohol's effect on the brain and body, a number of investigators have focused on increasing the rate of clearance of alcohol from the body. Some (11) have attempted to enhance the production of those enzymes which are responsible for the breakdown of alcohol in the body. Others have combined alcohol with substances to speed up the metabolism of alcohol. In one reported study (13), intravenous administration of a mixture of both fructose and alcohol in volunteers, for example, resulted in lower blood alcohol levels than would be expected from administration of alcohol alone. Subjects also felt and acted less drunk. This study requires replication. Furthermore, fructose does not produce the same effect if taken orally with alcohol. Hemodialysis (19) is another experimental procedure which, in effect, quickly filters alcohol out of the blood. This procedure has been used in emergencies to remove alcohol from a person's body rapidly. Its use is limited because of technical difficulties and expense. Interestingly, none of the small number of patients who have been withdrawn from alcohol by hemodialysis have experienced delirium tremens, although delirium tremens is thought to be a direct result of alcohol withdrawal after prolonged ingestion. These research results require replication and expanded efforts because of their important treatment implications. If it were possible, for example, to remove alcohol from the body rapidly, the care of severely intoxicated individuals would be greatly facilitated. Similarly, the capability to inhibit the rate of absorption of alcohol into the body might result in improved means of self-regulation of alcohol intake as well as improved medical care for life-threatening intoxications.

Some individuals seem able to metabolize more alcohol than others, and this phenomenon is an important area of study. The results of a series of studies (15) conducted with alcoholic individuals suggests that some of them develop overactive enzyme systems, making it possible for them to break down alcohol more rapidly than people who have not been heavy drinkers. Since a changed enzyme system for alcohol may alter the response of the body to other drugs, further investigation in these areas may shed light on the mechanism of cross-tolerance to other drugs which has been observed in many alcoholic persons and has puzzled physicians for many years. This type of research has important implications for medical treatment, since physicians must be able to predict accurately the response of a patient to a particular drug.

Many of the studies on the metabolism and pathological effects of alcohol on body organs are necessarily conducted with animals. In the past several years much work (7, 8, 9) has been done with animals to study the processes of physical dependence on alcohol and of withdrawal. In addition, animals are used in screening new drugs which may prove to be useful in the treatment of alcoholism prior to human testing. Although we have learned a great deal in these areas, more animal studies are necessary—particularly for determining the dosage and intake schedules which produce both dependence and withdrawal symptoms, and for further screening of agents which might be useful in treatment.

One interesting outcome of these animal studies using rat liver tissue is a suggestion that the process of physical dependence on alcohol has biochemical similarities to narcotic addiction (6). A number of objections have been raised to this hypothesis, however, and it has yet to be verified.

An area of research which is important and has received little emphasis is the identification of the mechanisms by which alcohol acts as an intoxicant affecting the brain and behavior. Improved techniques are also needed to measure blood alcohol levels and correlate them with impaired behavior. Improved techniques may reveal the different levels at which behavioral impairment develops in different persons and may serve to determine practical guidelines for law enforcement agencies concerned with legal definition of the relation between blood alcohol and behavioral impairment. Further study is also needed to clarify the effects of alcohol on driving ability.

Understanding of these underlying physiological and biochemical bases in the development of physical dependence may allow new means for initiating intervention in cases of incipient or active alcoholism.

STUDIES OF TREATMENT METHODS

Studies of psychological and social treatment methods for alcoholic persons have received considerably less emphasis over the past several years than has research on biomedical treatment methods. This is true for many reasons—partly because of inadequate financial support, but also because behavioral science research requires highly sophisticated methodologies and well-trained professionals, both of which are in short supply.

Despite these limitations, a number of interesting research studies have been conducted on treatment methods, including the treatment of alcoholism in a tuberculosis hospital (10), the treatment of homeless alcoholic persons (16, 17), the evaluation of community alcoholism clinics, and a study of a community referral service (5). These studies consistently reveal that when a serious effort is made to meet the needs of alcoholic persons and when these efforts are available and accessible to them, the majority of patients respond and improve substantially. Even a significant proportion of homeless alcoholic men are successfully treated and reintegrated into society when a program is designed to meet their needs.

A vitally important aspect of such studies is the comparison of the effectiveness of different treatment methods with different groups of alcoholic persons. The aim of these studies is to match the individual's needs with the particular treatment resources. This approach is consonant with the view of most investigators that alcoholism is not a unitary disease condition treatable by a single therapy. One study (10), for example, in a tuberculosis hospital suggests that a didactic approach—consisting of a combination of confrontation, explanation, and teaching about alcoholism and alcohol—is more successful in changing the attitudes of these patients toward alcoholism and tuberculosis than a therapeutic community setting which stresses a nonauthoritarian, supportive, and permissive atmosphere.

As these subgroups of alcoholic individuals are identified and specific treatments devised which are maximally effective for each group, a higher treatment success ratio can be expected. This potential has already been realized in several industries which have developed alcoholism programs for their employees.

To develop standards for the assessment of new programs, well-designed followup studies are necessary on the best existing treatment services. In addition, the beneficial factors and dimensions of change achieved by these treatment services need to be sorted out—for example, how, why, and in what ways are people helped? Prepaid group health plans may offer a good population of alcoholic people with which to study various treatment methods, as well as for information about the prevalence of alcohol problems.

Further study of treatment methods alone will not necessarily result in better care of alcoholism since even proven treatment techniques have not been widely adopted. It is clear that efforts need to be directed toward increasing the utilization of proven therapies. Systematic sociological studies may be useful to define the organizational structures needed to provide these effective techniques, such as continuity of care, coordination of services, and adequate referral services for alcoholic persons.

There are a number of other important aspects of alcoholism treatment which have received little study in recent years. One aspect is factors related to motivation for entering or dropping out of treatment. Another area of interest is in-depth study of "spontaneous cures"—persons who seem to have self-aborted their alcoholism. Finally, not much is known about the important psychological and social factors in the onset, continuation, and termination of a drinking "spree." Intensive study of "blackouts" also seems advisable, with attention to onset, frequency, character, duration, and possible techniques of prevention.

PREVENTION AND EDUCATION STUDIES

Although it is vitally important to support research both in innovative treatment methods and in studies of how to utilize proven therapies effectively, no illness can be eradicated by treating only the casualties. A foremost aspect of any public health endeavor must be aimed at education and prevention.

Many studies have clearly established the importance of environmental influences (particularly those impinging upon persons early in life) on perceptions, attitudes, and values. Like many other attitudes and values, those concerning the use of alcohol are also learned in childhood, primarily through the processes of imitation, identification, and role modeling of significant persons in the child's environment. When one or both parents are alcoholic persons, severe stresses are imposed on members of a family (4).

Since the effects of these stresses on family members may not be readily revealed, long-term studies are necessary of the children of alcoholic parents.

Other studies (12, 13) have concentrated on the genesis of alcohol-related problems among high school students. These studies have indicated that predictors of alcohol abuse in the young include an alcoholic father and/or mother, deviant behavior in other life areas, parental rejection and deprivation, impulsivity (or the inability to delay gratification), and alienation from family, friends, or society.

Studies (18) of alcohol drinking among college and high school students which, two decades ago, indicated that most students at that time were not getting into serious trouble over their drinking, now need to be followed up to learn whether early indicators of impending alcohol problems were accurate. Since campus drinking behaviors—just as many other campus patterns of life—probably have also changed, alcohol drinking studies among students will need to be replicated.

Further research is needed on effective methods of teaching responsible use and nonuse of alcohol beverages in schools. Educational programs matching the student's level of maturity need to be created for grade schools, high schools, and colleges, so that information and opportunities for discussion can be provided. Evaluation of existing educational programs and the development of community pilot programs using preventive techniques are needed. These programs should be designed to test specific hypotheses—for example, that an alcoholism and drug education program integrated with the rest of the cirriculum is more effective in creating responsible attitudes and behavior than a separated, isolated educational program on alcoholism and drug abuse. This type of research would require measurement of information transmitted, attitudes changed, and long-term behavioral outcomes.

The so-called "counter-culture," an additional group which has not been systematically studied, is important because it may serve to delineate characteristics of social change. Studies of drinking practices in such subcultures, as well as the attitudes and recommendations of their members, should be further studied for their significance. How great the roles drugs and alcohol play in the lives of members of these groups has not received systematic study to date.

202

The importance of focusing preventive and remedial activities upon groups with high rates of alcohol-related problems is obvious. Regional, urban, and social class differences found in recent surveys (1, 2), however, suggest that it is unlikely that any uniform standard program of preventive or remedial measures will be found appropriate for all localities and that these programs will have to be individualized.

The reasons why alcohol-related problems develop and diminish over time will need to be the focus of longitudinal studies. Since it has been shown (2) that peaks in heavy drinking occur in men in their late twenties, early thirties, and late forties, and in women in their early twenties and late forties, more studies are needed on the impact of such variables as lifestyle, life events, and hormonal changes on drinking behavior. In general, more research on the variables that determine alcohol abuse and alcoholism in women is vitally needed, since society tends to forget that women too are victims of this disease.

Cross-cultural or cross-national studies are needed to examine the mores and sanctions which determine pressures for and against different kinds of drinking behavior within different subgroups. It is vital to determine which variables are important in the process of beginning to drink heavily. The clarification of factors relating either to the perpetuation or cessation of heavy drinking is important. We know, for example, that persons of Italian parentage in the United States drink more heavily than Italian people themselves, but we do not know the reasons for such a difference. In addition, preliminary evidence indicates that alcohol drinking among black people is different from drinking patterns among white people. Two studies have already shown (1, 2) for example, that black women have the highest rate of abstinence but, if they drink, they have high rates of heavy drinking. This is also a preliminary finding of the Harris study for NIAAA.

The increase or decrease in alcohol consumption in different sections and within various groups of the nation must be examined. Tax-paid trends alone do not reveal the facts. Both illegal and home production require study and the application of ingenious research methodologies.

Finally, the effects of local alcohol beverage control laws need to be examined to determine if the availability of alcohol—or laws which affect its availability—have any effect on the incidence and prevalence of alcohol abuse and alcoholism in a community.

Results of such studies could provide the background for the development of model community laws.

Although most of the current research emphasizes heavy drinking and alcohol-related problems, there are insufficient insights available concerning the constructive strategies used by the majority of people with respect to their alcohol use. The study of these individuals would permit methods of self-regulation of alcohol intake to be recognized, and also would reveal clearly recognizable early warning signs of intoxication. Further, the socially integrating function of alcohol has been little studied, especially in rural communities or small villages. Systematic study of the constructive personal strategies of using alcohol positively, for those who choose to drink, would have important implications for education and prevention programs.

SUMMARY AND CONCLUSION

In summary, biomedical research on alcoholism, which has received highest priority over the past several years in the field, has contributed significantly to understanding in several areas, especially the mechanisms of cross-tolerance (15). In addition, a provocative hypothesis (6) was generated relating alcohol dependence and opiate addiction, and followup research on the physiology of alcohol withdrawal could have implications for treatment of this condition.

In the area of applied research, which has received proportionately less attention and support, making meaningful distinctions between alcoholic persons and their particular forms of treatment, and further work on categorization of patient subtypes seem important and necessary. There have been, however, few research projects relating directly to the control and prevention of alcoholism and alcohol-related problems. This is particularly true of education and prevention programs, studies on the effective utilization of available effective treatment modalities, and psychosocial determinants of responsible drinking behavior. While continued support for well-designed research projects in the biological sciences is necessary, NIAAA is currently attempting to develop a more balanced research program by giving greater emphasis to behavioral science research.

Further, NIAAA is giving serious consideration to the establishment of six multidisciplinary research centers across the nation in which the attention of various professionals in the health sciences would be focused on serious public health issues related to alcoholism. In these centers, studies could be directed to important aspects of prevention and treatment of alcoholism which have fallen between the cracks of professional disciplines in the past.

With a balanced research program, the National Institute on Alcohol Abuse and Alcoholism hopes to move ahead on devising innovative means of meeting the medical, psychological, social and human needs of ill people, as well as developing ways of preventing alcoholism through education.

REFERENCES

(1) Bailey, M.B., Haberman, P.W. and Alksne, H. The epidemiology of alcoholism in an urban residential area. Quart. J. Stud. Alc. 26:19–40, 1965.

(2) Cahalan, D., Cisin, I.H. and Crossley, H.M. American Drinking Practices: A National Survey of Drinking Behavior and Attitudes. New Brunswick: Rutgers Center of Alcohol Studies, 1969.

(3) Chafetz, M.E. Alcoholism prevention and reality. Quart. J. Stud. Alc. 28: 345–348, 1967.

(4) Chafetz, M.E., Blane, H.T. and Hill, M.J. Children of alcoholics. Observations in a child guidance clinic. Quart. J. Stud. Alc. 32:687–698, 1971.

(5) Corrigan, E.M. Linking the problem drinker with treatment. Social Work, in press 1972.

(6) Davis, V.E. and Walsh, M.J. Alcohol, amines and alkaloids: A possible biochemical basis for alcohol addiction. Science 167:1005–1007, 1970.

(7) Ellis, F.W. and Pick, J.R. Experimentally induced ethanol dependence in rhesus monkeys. J. Pharmacol. Exp. Ther. 175:88–93, 1970.

(8) Essig, C.F. and Lam, R.C. Convulsions and hallucinatory behavior following alcohol withdrawal in the dog. Arch. Neurol. Psychiat. 18:626–632, 1968.

(9) Freund, G. Alcohol withdrawal syndrome in mice. Arch. Neurol. 21:315–320, 1969.

(10) Gluck, S.B. The Olive View Project: A Study of Alcoholism Treatment Methods as Applied to Tuberculosis Patients. Olive View, Calif.: Olive View Hospital, February, 1969.

(11) Hawkins, R.D., Kalant, H., Khanna, J.M. Effects of chronic intake of ethanol on rate of ethanol metabolism. Canad. J. Physiol. Pharmac. 44:241, 1966.

(12) Jessor, R., Graves, T.D., Hanson, R.C. and Jessor, S.L. Society, Personality and Deviant Behavior. New York: Holt, Rinehart and Winston, 1968.

(13) Jessor, R., Young, H.B., Young, E.B. and Tesi, G. Perceived opportunity, alienation, and drinking behavior among Italian and American youth. J. Personality Soc. Psychol. 15:215, 1970.

(14) Lowenstein, L.M., Simone, R., Boulter, P. and Nathan, P. The effect of fructose on alcohol concentrations in man. J.A.M.A. 213:1899, 1970.

(15) Rubin, E. and Lieber, C.S. Alcoholism, alcohol, and drugs. Science 172: 1097–1102, 1971.

(16) Rubington,E. The future of the halfway house. Quart. J. Stud. Alc. 31:167–174, 1970.

(17) Rubington,E. Referral, Post-treatment contacts, and length of stay in a halfway house. Quart. J. Stud. Alc. 31:659–668, 1970.

(18) Straus, R. and Bacon, S.D. Drinking in College. New Haven: Yale University Press, 1953.

(19) Walder, A.I., Redding, J.S., Faillace, L. and Steenburg, R.W. Rapid detoxification of the acute alcoholic with hemodialysis. Surgery 66 (1):201–207, 1969.

(20) Zucker, R.A. Motivational factors and problem drinking among adolescents. Paper presented at 28th International Congress on Alcohol and Alcoholism. Washington, D.C.: September, 1968.

APPENDIX A

UNIFORM ALCOHOLISM AND INTOXICATION TREATMENT ACT

(WITH COMMENTS)

Drafted by the

NATIONAL CONFERENCE OF COMMISSIONERS ON UNIFORM STATE LAWS

and by it

APPROVED AND RECOMMENDED FOR ENACTMENT IN ALL THE STATES

at its

ANNUAL CONFERENCE
MEETING IN ITS EIGHTIETH YEAR
AT VAIL, COLORADO
AUGUST 21 – 28, 1971

SECTION 1. [*Declaration of Policy.*] It is the policy of this State that alcoholics and intoxicated persons may not be subjected to criminal prosecution because of their consumption of alcoholic beverages but rather should be afforded a continuum of treatment in order that they may lead normal lives as productive members of society.

Comment

This section is intended to preclude the handling of drunkenness under any of a wide variety of petty criminal offense statutes, such as loitering, vagrancy, disturbing the peace, and so forth. As the crime commissions pointed out, drunkenness by itself does not constitute disorderly conduct. The normal manifestations of intoxication—staggering, lying down, sleeping on a park bench, lying unconscious in the gutter, begging, singing, etc.—will therefore be handled under the civil provisions of this Act and not under the criminal law. See *District of Columbia v. Greenwell,* **96 Daily Wash. L. Reptr. 2133 (D.C. Ct. Gen. Sess. December 31, 1968).**

SECTION 2. [*Definitions.*] For purposes of this Act:

(1) "alcoholic" means a person who habitually lacks self-control as to the use of alcoholic beverages, or uses alcoholic beverages to the extent that his health is substantially impaired or endangered or his social or economic function is substantially disrupted;

(2) "approved private treatment facility" means a private agency meeting the standards prescribed in section 9(a) and approved under section 9(c);

(3) "approved public treatment facility" means a treatment agency operating under the direction and control of the division or providing treatment under this Act through a contract with the division under section 8(g) and meeting the standards prescribed in section 9(a) and approved under section 9(c);

(4) "commissioner" means the commissioner [or] of the department;

(5) "department" means [the State department of health or mental health];

(6) "director" means the director of the division of alcoholism;

(7) "division" means the division of alcoholism within the department established under section 3;

(8) "emergency service patrol" means a patrol established under section 17;

(9) "incapacitated by alcohol" means that a person, as a result of the use of alcohol, is unconscious or has his judgment otherwise so impaired that he is incapable of realizing and making a rational decision with respect to his need for treatment;

(10) "incompetent person" means a person who has been adjudged incompetent by [the appropriate State court];

(11) "intoxicated person" means a person whose mental or physical functioning is substantially impaired as a result of the use of alcohol;

(12) "treatment" means the broad range of emergency, outpatient, intermediate, and inpatient services and care, including diagnostic evaluation, medical, psychiatric, psychological, and social service care, vocational rehabilitation and career counseling, which may be extended to alcoholics and intoxicated persons.

Comment

The term "alcoholic" is defined in two alternative ways for two different purposes. The first alternative is a relatively narrow definition based on lack of self-control regarding the use of alcoholic beverages. Lack of self-control may be manifested either by the inability to abstain from drinking for any significant time period, or by the ability to remain sober between drinking episodes but an inability to refrain from drinking to intoxication whenever drinking an alcoholic beverage. This relatively narrow definition has been the basis for the court decisions holding an alcoholic not criminally responsible for his intoxication.

The second alternative definition adopts the World Health Organization's broad approach that alcoholism can be defined as the use of alcoholic beverages to the extent that health or economic or social functioning are substantially impaired. The purpose of this broad definition is to make as large a group as possible eligible for treatment for alcoholism and related problems. Encouraging early treatment for drinking problems will ultimately lead to prevention. This broad definition of alcoholism is useful in making voluntary treatment available to as large a group as possible, but would be wholly inappropriate to define those alcoholics who justify civil commitment for involuntary treatment.

The Act defines "treatment" broadly to include a wide range of types and kinds of services to reflect the fact that there is no single or uniform method of treatment that will be effective for all alcoholics. The Act provides a flexible approach with a variety of kinds of medical, social, rehabilitative, and psychological services according to the individual's particular needs.

SECTION 3 [*Division of Alcoholism.*] A division of alcoholism is established within the department. The division shall be headed by a director appointed by the commissioner. The director shall be a qualified professional who has training and experience in handling medical-social problems or the organization or administration of treatment services for persons suffering from medical-social problems.

SECTION 4. [*Powers of Division.*] The division may:

(1) plan, establish, and maintain treatment programs as necessary or desirable;

(2) make contracts necessary or incidental to the performance of its duties and the execution of its powers, including contracts with public and private agencies, organizations, and individuals to pay them for services rendered or furnished to alcoholics or intoxicated persons;

(3) solicit and accept for use any gift of money or property made by will or otherwise, and any grant of money, services, or property from the Federal government, the State, or any political subdivision thereof or any private source, and do all things necessary to cooperate with the Federal government or any of its agencies in making an application for any grant;

(4) administer or supervise the administration of the provisions relating to alcoholics and intoxicated persons of any State plan submitted for Federal funding pursuant to Federal health, welfare, or treatment legislation;

(5) coordinate its activities and cooperate with alcoholism programs in this and other States, and make contracts and other joint or cooperative arrangement with State, local, or private agencies in this and other States for the treatment of alcoholics and intoxicated persons and for the common advancement of alcoholism programs;

(6) keep records and engage in research and the gathering of relevant statistics; and

(7) do other acts and things necessary or convenient to execute the authority expressly granted to it;

(8) acquire, hold, or dispose of real property or any interest therein, and construct, lease, or otherwise provide treatment facilities for alcoholics and intoxicated persons.

SECTION 5. [*Duties of Division.*] The division shall:

(1) develop, encourage, and foster statewide, regional, and local plans and programs for the prevention of alcoholism and treatment of alcoholics and intoxicated persons in cooperation with public and private agencies, organizations, and individuals, and provide technical assistance and consultation services for these purposes;

(2) coordinate the efforts and enlist the assistance of all public and private agencies, organizations, and individuals interested in prevention of alcoholism and treatment of alcoholics and intoxicated persons;

(3) cooperate with the [department of correction and board of parole] in establishing and conducting programs to provide treatment for alcoholics and intoxicated persons in or on parole from penal institutions;

(4) cooperate with the [department of education], [boards of education], schools, police departments, courts, and other public and private agencies, organizations and individuals in establishing programs for the prevention of alcoholism and treatment of alcoholics and intoxicated persons, and preparing cirriculum materials thereon for use at all levels of school education;

(5) prepare, publish, evaluate, and disseminate educational material dealing with the nature and effects of alcohol;

(6) develop and implement, as an integral part of treatment programs, an educational program for use in the treatment of alcoholics and intoxicated persons, which program shall include the dissemination of information concerning the nature and effects of alcohol;

(7) organize and foster training programs for all persons engaged in treatment of alcoholics and intoxicated persons;

(8) sponsor and encourage research into the causes and nature of alcoholism and treatment of alcoholics and intoxicated persons, and serve as a clearing house for information relating to alcoholism;

(9) specify uniform methods for keeping statistical information by public and private agencies, organizations, and individuals, and collect and make available relevant statistical information, including number of persons treated, frequency of admission and readmission, and frequency and duration of treatment;

(10) advise the Governor in the preparation of a comprehensive plan for treatment of alcoholics and intoxicated persons for inclusion in the State's comprehensive health plan;

(11) review all State health, welfare, and treatment plans to be submitted for Federal funding under Federal legislation, and advise the governor on provisions to be included relating to alcoholism and intoxicated persons;

(12) assist in the development of, and cooperate with, alcohol education and treatment programs for employees of State and local governments and businesses and industries in the State;

(13) utilize the support and assistance of interested persons in the community, particularly recovered alcoholics, to encourage alcoholics voluntarily to undergo treatment;

(14) cooperate with [the commissioner of public safety] [highway commission] in establishing and conducting programs designed to deal with the problem of persons operating motor vehicles while [intoxicated] ;

(15) encourage general hospitals and other appropriate health facilities to admit without discrimination alcoholics and intoxicated persons and to provide them with adequate and appropriate treatment;

(16) encourage all health and disability insurance programs to include alcoholism as a covered illness; and

(17) submit to the Governor an annual report covering the activities of the division.

Comment

Section 5(9) gives the division the responsibility of specifying uniform methods for keeping statistical information, and collecting and disseminating such information. Confidentiality of individual patient records will be protected in accordance with Section 15.

Sections 5 (10) and (11) authorize the division to advise the Governor with respect to the inclusion of alcoholism and intoxication under the State comprehensive health plan, and under all other State health, welfare, and treatment plans submitted for Federal funding. Under the Comprehensive Alcohol Abuse and Alcoholism Prevention, Treatment, and Rehabilitation Act of 1970 (Public Law 91—616), each State must prepare a comprehensive alcoholism plan for Federal funding. The Comprehensive Health Planning and Public

Health Services Amendments of 1966 (Public Law 89—749) and the Partnership for Health Amendments of 1967 (Public Law 90—174) have also been amended by the 1970 Act to require that comprehensive State health plans must "provide for services for the prevention and treatment of alcohol abuse and alcoholism, commensurate with the extent of the problem" in order to receive Federal funds. Finally, numerous other relevant State plans, such as for vocational rehabilitation, are submitted for Federal funding. It will be the responsibility of the division to be certain that alcoholism and intoxication are included in all such pertinent State plans.

Section 5(15) gives the division the responsibility of encouraging general hospitals and other appropriate health facilities to admit and provide adequate treatment to alcoholics and intoxicated persons. This provision is particularly important because the 1970 Federal Act includes a provision under which a general hospital can be denied Federal funds under this law for discriminating against alcoholics.

Section 5(16) gives the division the responsibility of encouraging all health and disability insurance programs to include alcoholism as a covered illness. This provision applies to both private and governmental programs.

SECTION 6. [*Interdepartmental Coordinating Committee.*]

(a) An interdepartmental coordinating committee is established, composed of the [commissioners of public health, mental health, education, public welfare, correction, highway, public safety, vocational rehabilitation, and other appropriate agencies] and the director. The committee shall meet at least twice annually at the call of the commissioner, who shall be its chairman. The committee shall provide for the coordination of, and exchange of information on, all programs relating to alcoholism, and shall act as a permanent liaison among the departments engaged in activities affecting alcoholics and intoxicated persons. The committee shall assist the commissioner and director in formulating a comprehensive plan for prevention of alcoholism and for treatment of alcoholics and intoxicated persons.

(b) In exercising its coordinating functions, the committee shall assure that:

(1) the appropriate State agencies provide all necessary medical, social, treatment, and educational services for alcoholics and intoxicated persons and for the prevention of alcoholism, without unnecessary duplication of services;

213

(2) the several State agencies cooperate in the use of facilities and in the treatment of alcoholics and intoxicated persons; and

(3) all State agencies adopt approaches to the prevention of alcoholism and the treatment of alcoholics and intoxicated persons consistent with the policy of this act.

SECTION 7. [*Citizens Advisory Council on Alcoholism.*]

(a) The Governor shall appoint a citizens advisory council on alcoholism, composed of [15] members. The members shall serve for overlapping terms of 3 years each; one third of the members first appointed [,as nearly as may be practicable,] shall be appointed for one-, two-, and three-year terms respectively. Members shall have professional, research, or personal interest in alcoholism problems. The council shall meet at least once every [3] months and report on its activities and make recommendations to the director at least once a year.

(b) The council shall advise the director on broad policies, goals, and operation of the alcoholism program and on other matters the director refers to it, and shall encourage public understanding and support of the alcoholism program.

(c) Members of the council shall serve without compensation but shall receive reimbursement for travel and other necessary expenses actually incurred in the performance of their duties.

Comment

The qualifications of the members are defined broadly. It is expected that the Governor would appoint to the council individuals representing a broad range of background and experience, including representatives of citizens groups, voluntary organizations, professional groups, and recovered alcoholics.

SECTION 8. [*Comprehensive Program for Treatment; Regional Facilities*]

(a) The division shall establish a comprehensive and coordinated program for the treatment of alcoholics and intoxicated persons. [Subject to the approval of the commissioner, the director shall divide the State into appropriate regions for the conduct of the program and establish standards for the development of the program on the regional level. In establishing the regions, consideration shall be given to city, town, and county lines and population concentrations.]

(b) The program of the division shall include:

(1) emergency treatment provided by a facility affiliated with or part of the medical service of a general hospital;

(2) inpatient treatment;

(3) intermediate treatment; and

(4) outpatient and followup treatment.

(c) The division shall provide for adequate and appropriate treatment for alcoholics and intoxicated persons admitted under sections 11 to 14. Treatment may not be provided at a correctional institution except for inmates.

(d) The division shall maintain, supervise, and control all facilities operated by it subject to policies of the department. The administrator of each facility shall make an annual report of its activities to the director in the form and manner the director specifies.

(e) All appropriate public and private resources shall be coordinated with and utilized in the program if possible.

(f) The director shall prepare, publish, and distribute annually a list of all approved public and private treatment facilities.

(g) The division may contract for the use of any facility as an approved public treatment facility if the director, subject to the policies of the department, considers this to be an effective and economical course to follow.

Comment

Whether or not the director divides the State into regional units for purposes of administration, it is desirable that all treatment services be community based. Alcoholics and other ill persons are treated more effectively through treatment services in their own communities, located conveniently to population centers so as to be quickly and easily accessible to patients and their families, rather than in large institutional settings.

The Act uses the concept of emergency treatment rather than the more popular phrase "detoxification center" as the latter concept tends to stigmatize alcoholics and set them apart from people with other illnesses or problems. These emergency services should be available 24 hours a day and readily accessible to those who need this assistance. In addition to medical services, emergency social services and appropriate diagnostic and referral services should be included.

"Inpatient treatment" refers to full-time residential treatment in an institution. Although alcoholics and intoxicated persons ordinarily do not require full-time inpatient treatment services, such care must be available for those who do need it. Since long-term inpatient services are inappropriate for alcoholics, inpatient treatment should be designed to facilitate the patient's return to his family and the community or to other appropriate care services as rapidly as possible.

"Intermediate treatment" refers to residential treatment that is less than full time and that can be provided in a variety of community facilities, such as halfway houses, day or night hospitals, or foster homes.

"Outpatient and followup treatment" includes the same wide range of treatment services and modalities offered in inpatient or intermediate service settings, but in outpatient treatment, the client is not a full or part-time resident of the treatment facility. Such services may be offered in a wide variety of settings in the community, such as clinics and social centers and even in the patient's own home.

Section 8(a) requires that all existing appropriate private and public resources be coordinated with and used whenever possible. For example, general hospitals may be used for emergency care services, and community mental health centers may be utilized for a variety of kinds of services for alcoholics. The creation of a new and separate network of treatment facilities for alcoholics would not be desirable, practical, or effective.

Section 8(c) requires the department to provide adequate and appropriate treatment for all alcoholics and intoxicated persons, including both the vast majority of persons who will come to these facilities voluntarily and the small minority who may be involuntarily committed, in accordance with the provisions of sections 13 and 14 of the Act.

SECTION 9. [*Standards for Public and Private Treatment Facilities; Enforcement Procedures; Penalties.*]

(a) The division shall establish standards for approved treatment facilities that must be met for a treatment facility to be approved as a public or private treatment facility, and fix the fees to be charged by the division for the required inspections. The standards may concern only the health standards to be met and standards of treatment to be afforded patients.

(b) The division periodically shall inspect approved public and private treatment facilities at reasonable times and in a reasonable manner.

(c) The division shall maintain a list of approved public and private treatment facilities.

(d) Each approved public and private treatment facility shall file with the division on request, data, statistics, schedules, and information the division reasonably requires. An approved public or private treatment facility that without good cause fails to furnish any data, statistics, schedules, or information as requested, or files fraudulent returns thereof, shall be removed from the list of approved treatment facilities.

(e) The division, after holding a hearing, may suspend, revoke, limit, or restrict an approval, or refuse to grant an approval, for failure to meet its standards.

(f) The [district] court may restrain any violation of this section, review any denial, restriction, or revocation of approval, and grant other relief required to enforce its provisions.

(g) Upon petition of the division and after a hearing held upon reasonable notice to the facility, the [district] court may issue a warrant to an officer or employee of the division authorizing him to enter and inspect at reasonable times, and examine the books and accounts of, any approved public or private treatment facility refusing to consent to inspection or examination by the division or which the division has reasonable cause to believe is operating in violation of this Act.

SECTION 10. [*Acceptance for Treatment;Rules.*] The director shall adopt and may amend or repeal rules for acceptance of persons into the treatment program, considering available treatment resources and facilities, for the purpose of early and effective treatment of alcoholics and intoxicated persons. In establishing the rules the director shall be guided by the following standards:

(1) If possible a patient shall be treated on a voluntary rather than an involuntary basis.

(2) A patient shall be initially assigned or transferred to outpatient or intermediate treatment, unless he is found to require inpatient treatment.

(3) A person shall not be denied treatment solely because he has withdrawn from treatment against medical advice on a prior occasion or because he has relapsed after earlier treatment.

(4) An individualized treatment plan shall be prepared and maintained on a current basis for each patient.

(5) Provision shall be made for a continuum of coordinated treatment services, so that a person who leaves a facility or a form of treatment will have available and utilize other appropriate treatment.

Comment

Section 10(1) expresses the Act's clear preference for voluntary over involuntary treatment. Voluntary treatment is more desirable from both a medical and legal point of view. Experience has shown that the vast majority of alcoholics are quite willing to accept adequate and appropriate treatment. Section 14 of the Act makes it clear that involuntary treatment is permitted only in exceptional and very clearly prescribed circumstances.

Section 10(2) is based on the fact that most alcoholics do not need long term inpatient care, but can be more successfully treated in outpatient or intermediate care settings (such as halfway houses). This section covers both voluntary and involuntary treatment, for section 14(h) allows the division to transfer a committed patient from a more restrictive to a less restrictive treatment modality whenever such transfer is "medically advisable."

Section 10(3) recognizes that alcoholics, like persons with other chronic illnesses, may relapse. Such relapses are to be expected as part of the illness and the individual should not be penalized. Prior treatment and withdrawal from treatment, even if repeated, should not bar a person from subsequent participation in a treatment program. It was deemed desirable to include this specific provision in the Act in view of the more punitive provisions against readmission in many older laws.

Section 10(4) provides that an individualized treatment plan must be prepared and maintained for each patient on a current basis. Such an individualized plan would include the factual record of all treatment provided and must be specifically tailored to meet the needs of each patient. A "boiler plate" treatment form for all patients would *not* meet the requirements of this section. This provision will ensure that patients are receiving treatment in accordance with their specific needs, and is crucial in the case of civilly committed patients in order to guard against the possibility of commitment without appropriate treatment.

Section 10(5) reinforces the Act's strong emphasis on the need for a continuum of coordinated treatment services (see also section 1 and section 8(a)) and requires the division to ensure that when a person leaves a form of treatment, other appropriate treatment services will be available to him.

SECTION 11. [*Voluntary Treatment of Alcoholics.*]

(a) An alcoholic may apply for voluntary treatment directly to an approved public treatment facility. If the proposed patient is a minor or an incompetent person, he, a parent, a legal guardian, or other legal representative may make the application.

(b) Subject to rules adopted by the director, the administrator in charge of an approved public treatment facility may determine who shall be admitted for treatment. If a person is refused admission to an approved public treatment facility, the administrator, subject to rules adopted by the director, shall refer the patient to another approved public treatment facility for treatment if possible and appropriate.

(c) If a patient receiving inpatient care leaves an approved public treatment facility, he shall be encouraged to consent to appropriate outpatient or intermediate treatment. If it appears to the administrator in charge of the treatment facility that the patient is an alcoholic who requires help, the division shall arrange for assistance in obtaining supportive services and residential facilities.

(d) If a patient leaves an approved public treatment facility, with or against the advice of the administrator in charge of the facility, the division shall make reasonable provisions for his transportation to another facility or to his home. If he has no home he shall be assisted in obtaining shelter. If he is a minor or an incompetent person the request for discharge from an inpatient facility shall be made by a parent, legal guardian, or other legal representative or by the minor or incompetent if he was the original applicant.

Comment

Most patients treated under this Act will voluntarily seek treatment. The provisions of this section allow the patient to seek treatment in the same manner as he would for any other health problem or illness. The Act encourages voluntary treatment by not requiring the patient to agree to voluntarily commit himself for a specified length of time or to accept any of the other restrictions that apply to involuntarily committed patients. Section 11 does not require either a predetermined minimum voluntary stay or a specific number of days of notice prior to seeking discharge. Such provisions would discourage treatment and would subject patients to restrictions that do not apply to patients with other medical problems.

Section 11 also requires the division to provide coordinated services (see also sections 1, 8(a), and 10(e)) and to assist the patient in getting from one service to another, including the arranging of transportation if necessary. Section 11(d) expressly provides that the division must make such provision even if the patient leaves the treatment facility against medical advice.

SECTION 12. [*Treatment and Services for Intoxicated Persons and Persons Incapacitated by Alcohol.*]

(a) An intoxicated person may come voluntarily to an approved public treatment facility for emergency treatment. A person who appears to be intoxicated in a public place and to be in need of help, if he consents to the proffered help, may be assisted to his home, an approved public treatment facility, an approved private treatment facility, or other health facility by the police or the emergency service patrol.

(b) A person who appears to be incapacitated by alcohol shall be taken into protective custody by the police or the emergency service patrol and forthwith brought to an approved public treatment facility for emergency treatment. [If no approved public treatment facility is readily available he shall be taken to an emergency medical service customarily used for incapacitated persons.] The police or the emergency service patrol, in detaining the person and in taking him to an approved public treatment facility, is taking him into protective custody and shall make every reasonable effort to protect his health and safety. In taking the person into protective custody, the detaining officer may take reasonable steps to protect himself. A taking into protective custody under this section is not an arrest. No entry or other record shall be made to indicate that the person has been arrested or charged with a crime.

220

(c) A person who comes voluntarily or is brought to an approved public treatment facility shall be examined by a licensed physician as soon as possible. He may then be admitted as a patient or referred to another health facility. The referring approved public treatment facility shall arrange for his transportation.

(d) A person who by medical examination is found to be incapacitated by alcohol at the time of his admission or to have become incapacitated at any time after his admission, may not be detained at the facility (1) once he is no longer incapacitated by alcohol, or (2) if he remains incapacitated by alcohol for more than 48 hours after admission as a patient, unless he is committed under section 13. A person may consent to remain in the facility as long as the physician in charge believes appropriate.

(e) A person who is not admitted to an approved public treatment facility, is not referred to another health facility, and has no funds, may be taken to his home, if any. If he has no home, the approved public treatment facility shall assist him in obtaining shelter.

(f) If a patient is admitted to an approved public treatment facility, his family or next of kin shall be notified as promptly as possible. If an adult patient who is not incapacitated requests that there be no notification, his request shall be respected.

(g) The police or members of the emergency service patrol who act in compliance with this section are acting in the course of their official duty and are not criminally or civilly liable therefor.

(h) If the physician in charge of the approved public treatment facility determines it is for the patient's benefit, the patient shall be encouraged to agree to further diagnosis and voluntary appropriate treatment.

Comment

A small minority of intoxicated persons are incapacitated in that they are unconscious or incoherent or similarly so impaired in judgment that they cannot make a rational decision with regard to their need for treatment. Section 12(b) authorizes the police or emergency service patrol to take such individuals into protective custody and to a public treatment facility for emergency care. This is intended to assure that those most seriously in need of care will get it.

Protective custody under (b) is similar to the way in which the police provide emergency assistance to other ill people, such as those in accidents or those who have sudden heart attacks. It is a civil procedure, and no arrest record or record which implies a criminal charge is to be made. Since the police officer may sometimes have to decide whether a man who refuses help appears to be incapacitated by alcohol or because of some other reason, section 12(g) protects the policeman should his conclusion, made in good faith, be incorrect. It provides that he cannot be held criminally or civilly liable for false arrest or imprisonment as long as he is acting in compliance with this section. Willful malice or abuse, however, would not be considered to be in compliance with this section of the Act.

Section 12(d) provides that an incapacitated person can be held at a treatment facility without consent or further civil procedures for not longer than 48 hours. By the end of 48 hours, most persons who have been incapacitated by alcohol will be sufficiently detoxified to be able to make a rational decision about their need for further treatment. To provide for those very few individuals who may still be incapacitated (perhaps even unconscious) at the end of 48 hours, section 13 provides for an emergency commitment procedure based on a written application and a certificate from a physician who is not employed by the division.

Other provisions of section 12 provide that the individual in a public treatment facility must be examined by a licensed physician as soon as possible. This is to ensure, in accordance with section 8(b), that these facilities will provide the necessary medical services.

SECTION 13. [*Emergency Commitment.*]

(a) An intoxicated person who (1) has threatened, attempted, or inflicted physical harm on another and is likely to inflict physical harm on another unless committed, or (2) is incapacitated by alcohol, may be committed to an approved public treatment facility for emergency treatment. A refusal to undergo treatment does not constitute evidence of lack of judgment as to the need for treatment.

(b) The certifying physician, spouse, guardian, or relative of the person to be committed, or any other responsible person, may make a written application for commitment under this section, directed to the administrator of the approved public treatment facility. The application shall state facts to support the need for emergency treatment and be accompanied by a physician's certificate stating that he has examined the person sought to be committed within 2 days before the certificate's date and facts supporting the need for emergency treatment. A physician employed by the admitting facility or the division is not eligible to be the certifying physician.

(c) Upon approval of the application by the administrator in charge of the approved public treatment facility, the person shall be brought to the facility by a peace officer, health officer, emergency service patrol, the applicant for commitment, the patient's spouse, the patient's guardian, or any other interested person. The person shall be retained at the facility to which he was admitted, or transferred to another appropriate public or private treatment facility, until discharged under subsection (e).

(d) The administrator in charge of an approved public treatment facility shall refuse an application if in his opinion the application and certificate fail to sustain the grounds for commitment.

(e) When on the advice of the medical staff the administrator determines that the grounds for commitment no longer exist, he shall discharge a person committed under this section. No person committed under this section may be detained in any treatment facility for more than [5] days. If a petition for involuntary commitment under section 14 has been filed within the [5] days and the administrator in charge of an approved public treatment facility finds that grounds for emergency commitment still exist, he may detain the person until the petition has been heard and determined, but no longer than 10 days after filing the petition.

(f) A copy of the written application for commitment and of the physician's certificate, and a written explanation of the person's right to counsel, shall be given to the person within 24 hours after commitment by the administrator, who shall provide a reasonable opportunity for the person to consult counsel.

Comment

The test contained in the definition of "incapacitated by alcohol" is whether the person's judgment is so impaired that he is incapable of realizing and making a rational decision with respect to his need for treatment. Section 13(a)(2) may, therefore, cover the alcoholic who threatens suicide. If he falls within the definition, he would be subject to commitment for emergency treatment.

It is anticipated that the need to resort to short term commitment for emergency medical care under this section will arise most infrequently, but the procedure does provide a means of dealing with situations not covered by other parts of the Act. It is meant to be utilized only in true emergency situations where immediate action to cope with the crisis is essential and where the delay of court proceedings would be dangerous. For example, it might be necessary to use this emergency commitment procedure for an alcoholic who becomes intoxicated at home and whose behavior becomes assaultive, or for an incapacitated alcoholic already detained involuntarily in a treatment facility for the 48-hour maximum who continues to be so severely incapacitated, perhaps because of brain damage, that he cannot make a rational decision about his continuing need for care.

SECTION 14. [*Involuntary Commitment of Alcoholics.*]

(a) A person may be committed to the custody of the division by the [district] court upon the petition of his spouse or guardian, a relative, the certifying physician, or the administrator in charge of any approved public treatment facility. The petition shall allege that the person is an alcoholic who habitually lacks self-control as to the use of alcoholic beverages and that he (1) has threatened, attempted, or inflicted physical harm on another and that unless committed is likely to inflict physical harm on another; or (2) is incapacitated by alcohol. A refusal to undergo treatment does not constitute evidence of lack of judgment as to the need for treatment. The petition shall be accompanied by a certificate of a licensed physician who has examined the person within [2] days before submission of the petition, unless the person whose commitment is sought has refused to submit to a medical examination, in which case the fact of refusal shall be alleged in the petition. A physician employed by the admitting facility or the division is not eligible to be the certifying physician.

(b) Upon filing the petition, the court shall fix a date for a hearing no later than 10 days after the date the petition was filed. A copy of the petition and of the notice of the hearing, including the date fixed by the court, shall be served on the petitioner, the person whose commitment is sought, his next of kin other than the petitioner, a parent or his legal guardian if he is a minor, the administrator in charge of the approved public treatment facility to which he has been committed for emergency care, and any other person the court believes advisable. A copy of the petition and certificate shall be delivered to each person notified.

(c) At the hearing the court shall hear all relevant testimony, including, if possible, the testimony of at least one licensed physician who has examined the person whose commitment is sought. The person shall be present unless the court believes that his presence is likely to be injurious to him; in this event the court shall appoint a guardian *ad litem* to represent him throughout the proceeding. The court shall examine the person in open court, or if advisable, shall examine the person out of court. If the person has refused to be examined by a licensed physician, he shall be given an opportunity to be examined by a court-appointed licensed physician. If he refuses and there is sufficient evidence to believe that the allegations of the petition are true, or if the court believes that more medical evidence is necessary, the court may make a temporary order committing him to the division for a period of not more than [5] days for purposes of a diagnostic examination.

(d) If after hearing all relevant evidence, including the results of any diagnostic examination by the division, the court finds that grounds for involuntary commitment have been established by clear and convincing proof, it shall make an order of commitment to the division. It may not order commitment of a person unless it determines that the division is able to provide adequate and appropriate treatment for him and the treatment is likely to be beneficial.

(e) A person committed under this section shall remain in the custody of the division for treatment for a period of [30] days unless sooner discharged. At the end of the [30] day period, he shall be discharged automatically unless the division before expiration of the period obtains a court order for his recommitment upon the grounds set forth in subsection (a) for a further period of [90] days unless sooner discharged. If a person has been committed because he is an alcoholic likely to inflict physical harm on another, the division shall apply for recommitment if after examination it is determined that the likelihood still exists.

(f) A person recommitted under subsection (e) who has not been discharged by the division before the end of the [90] day period shall be discharged at the expiration of that period, unless the division, before expiration of the period, obtains a court order on the grounds set forth in subsection (a) for recommitment for a further period not to exceed [90] days. If a person has been committed because he is an alcoholic likely to inflict physical harm on another, the division shall apply for recommitment if after examination it is determined that the likelihood still exists. Only 2 recommitment orders under subsections (e) and (f) are permitted.

(g) Upon the filing of a petition for recommitment under subsections (e) or (f), the court shall fix a date for hearing no later than [10] days after the date the petition was filed. A copy of the petition and of the notice of hearing, including the date fixed by the court, shall be served on the petitioner, the person whose commitment is sought, his next of kin other than the petitioner, the original petitioner under subsection (a) if different from the petitioner for recommitment, one of his parents or his legal guardian if he is a minor, and any other person the court believes advisable. At the hearing the court shall proceed as provided in subsection (c).

(h) The division shall provide for adequate and appropriate treatment of a person committed to its custody. The division may transfer any person committed to its custody from one approved public treatment facility to another if transfer is medically advisable.

(i) A person committed to the custody of the division for treatment shall be discharged at any time before the end of the period for which he has been committed if either of the following conditions is met:

(1) In case of an alcoholic committed on the grounds of likelihood of infliction of physical harm upon another, that he is no longer an alcoholic or the likelihood no longer exists; or

(2) In case of an alcoholic committed on the grounds of the need of treatment and incapacity, that the incapacity no longer exists, further treatment will not be likely to bring about significant improvement in the person's condition, or treatment is no longer adequate or appropriate.

(j) The court shall inform the person whose commitment or recommitment is sought of his right to contest the application, be represented by counsel at every stage of any proceedings relating to his commitment and recommitment, and have counsel appointed by the court or provided by the court, if he wants the assistance of counsel and is unable to obtain counsel. If the court believes that the person needs the assistance of counsel, the court shall require, by appointment if necessary, counsel for him

226

regardless of his wishes. The person whose commitment or recommitment is sought shall be informed of his right to be examined by a licensed physician of his choice. If the person is unable to obtain a licensed physician and requests examination by a physician, the court shall employ a licensed physician.

(k) If a private treatment facility agrees with the request of a competent patient or his parent, sibling, adult child, or guardian to accept the patient for treatment, the administrator of the public treatment facility shall transfer him to the private treatment facility.

(l) A person committed under this Act may at any time seek to be discharged from commitment by writ of habeas corpus.

[(m) The venue for proceedings under this section is the place in which the person to be committed resides or is present.]

Comment

The Act specifically states that a refusal to undergo treatment does not by itself constitute evidence of lack of judgment with respect to the need for treatment. Thus, involuntary commitment would *not* be warranted merely because the person needs treatment, or has substantially inconvenienced his family, or has frequently been intoxicated in public, or because his drinking is harmful to his health. Commitment would be warranted, however, if the alcoholic exhibited cognitive deficiencies and was so debilitated that his thinking was confused not only with respect to his drinking problem but in other areas of behavior as well.

Section 14(d) prohibits mere custodial care by providing that a person may not be committed unless the division is able to provide "adequate and appropriate treatment for him and the treatment is likely to be beneficial."

The burden of proof in each recommitment is on the petitioner since each is an independent action.

If it is necessary to hold an individual beyond the maximum period, other provisions of State law must be used.

SECTION 15. [*Records of Alcoholics and Intoxicated Persons.*]

(a) The registration and other records of treatment facilities shall remain confidential and are privileged to the patient.

(b) Notwithstanding subsection (a), the director may make available information from patients' records for purposes of research into the causes and treatment of alcoholism. Information under this subsection shall not be published in a way that discloses patients' names or other identifying information.

Comment

The treatment of privileged information in the courts and disclosure with the consent of the patient are matters of general State law. This section does, however, provide for the use of treatment records for research purposes so long as patients' names and other identifying information are not disclosed.

SECTION 16. [*Visitation and Communication of Patients.*]

(a) Subject to reasonable rules regarding hours of visitation which the director may adopt, patients in any approved treatment facility shall be granted opportunities for adequate consultation with counsel, and for continuing contact with family and friends consistent with an effective treatment program.

(b) Neither mail nor other communication to or from a patient in any approved treatment facility may be intercepted, read, or censored. The director may adopt reasonable rules regarding the use of telephone by patients in approved treatment facilities.

SECTION 17. [*Emergency Service Patrol; Establishment; Rules.*]

(a) The division and [counties, cities and other municipalities] may establish emergency service patrols. A patrol consists of persons trained to give assistance in the streets and in other public places to persons who are intoxicated. Members of an emergency service patrol shall be capable of providing first aid in emergency situations and shall transport intoxicated persons to their homes and to and from public treatment facilities.

(b) The director shall adopt rules for the establishment, training, and conduct of emergency service patrols.

Comment

The experience of using civilians and plainclothes policemen, has demonstrated the effectiveness of this method. In some communities, for example, existing rescue squads that supply help and transportation in other medical emergencies might be used to assist intoxicated and incapacitated individuals. This provision does not require the establishment of an emergency service patrol, but authorizes such a patrol, should it meet the needs of a particular community.

SECTION 18. [*Payment for Treatment; Financial Ability of Patients.*]

[(a) If treatment is provided by an approved public treatment facility and the patient has not paid the charge therefor, the division is entitled to (1) any payment received by the patient or to which he may be entitled because of the services rendered, and (2) from any public or private source available to the division because of the treatment provided to the patient.]

[(b) A patient in an approved treatment facility, or the estate of the patient, or a person obligated to provide for the cost of treatment and having sufficient financial ability, is liable to the division for cost of maintenance and treatment of the patient therein in accordance with rates established.]

[(c) The director shall adopt rules governing financial ability that take into consideration the income, savings and other personal and real property of the person required to pay, and any support being furnished by him to any person he is required by law to support.]

SECTION 19. [*Criminal Laws Limitations.*]

(a) No county, municipality, or other political subdivision may adopt or enforce a local law, ordinance, resolution, or rule having the force of law that includes drinking, being a common drunkard, or being found in an intoxicated condition as one of the elements of the offense giving rise to a criminal or civil penalty or sanction.

(b) No county, municipality, or other political subdivision may interpret or apply any law of general application to circumvent the provision of subsection (a).

(c) Nothing in this Act affects any law, ordinance, resolution, or rule against drunken driving, driving under the influence of alcohol, or other similar offense involving the operation of a vehicle, aircraft, boat, machinery, or other equipment, or regarding the sale, purchase, dispensing, possessing, or use of alcoholic beverages at stated times and places or by a particular class of persons.

Comment

An important corollary to section 19 is section 37, which provides for the repeal of the State laws that are inconsistent with this Act. Under section 37, therefore, States would be expected to repeal all the relevant portions of their criminal statutes under which drunkenness is the gravamen of the offense with the exception of (c).

SECTION 20. [*Severability.*] If any provision of this Act or the application thereof to any person or circumstance is held invalid, the invalidity does not affect other provisions or applications of the Act which can be given effect without the invalid provision or application, and to this end the provisions of this Act are severable.

[SECTION 21. [*Application of Administrative Procedure Act.*] Except as otherwise provided in this Act, the State Administrative Procedure Act applies to and governs all administrative action taken by the director.]

[SECTION 22. [*Applicability and Scope.*] Sections 23 to 34 apply to the director and prescribe the procedures to be observed by him in exercising his powers under this Act.]

[SECTION 23. [*Public Information; Adoption of Rules; Availability of Rules and Orders.*]

(a) In addition to other rule-making requirements imposed by law, the director shall:

(1) adopt as a rule a description of the organization of his office, stating the general course and method of the operations of his office and methods whereby the public may obtain information or make submissions or requests;

(2) adopt rules of practice setting forth the nature and requirements of all formal and informal procedures available, including a description of all forms and instructions used by the director or his office;

(3) make available for public inspection all rules and all other written statements of policy or interpretations formulated, adopted, or used by the director in the discharge of his functions;

(4) make available for public inspection all final orders, decisions, and opinions.

(b) No rule, order, or decision of the director is effective against any person or party, nor may it be invoked by the director for any purpose, until it has been made available for public inspection as herein required. This provision is not applicable in favor of any person or party who has knowledge thereof.]

[SECTION 24. [*Procedure for Adoption of Rules.*]

(a) Prior to the adoption, amendment, or repeal of any rule, the director shall:

(1) give at least 20 days' notice of his intended action. The notice shall include a statement of either the terms or substance of the intended action or a description of the subjects and issues involved, and the time when, the place where, and the manner in which interested persons may present their views thereon. The notice shall be mailed to all persons who have made timely request of the director for advance notice of his rule-making proceedings and shall be published in [here insert the medium of publication appropriate for the adopting State] ;

(2) afford all interested persons reasonable opportunity to submit data, views, or arguments, orally or in writing. In case of substantive rules, opportunity for oral hearing must be granted if requested by 25 persons, by a governmental subdivision or agency, or by an association having not less than 25 members. The director shall consider fully all written and oral submissions respecting the proposed rule. Upon adoption of a rule the director, if requested to do so by an interested person either prior to adoption or within 30 days thereafter, shall issue a concise statement of the principal reasons for and against its adoption, incorporating therein his reasons for overruling the considerations urged against its adoption.

(b) No rule is valid unless adopted in substantial compliance with this section. A proceeding to contest any rule on the ground of noncompliance with the procedural requirements of this section must be commenced within 2 years from the effective date of the rule.]

[SECTION 25. [*Filing and Taking Effect of Rules.*]

(a) The director shall file in the office of the [Secretary of State] a certified copy of each rule adopted by him. The [Secretary of State] shall keep a permanent register of the rules open to public inspection.

(b) Each rule hereafter adopted is effective 20 days after filing, except that, if a later date is specified in the rule, the later date is the effective date.]

[SECTION 26. [*Publication of Rules.*]

(a) The [Secretary of State] shall compile, index, and publish all effective rules adopted by the director. Compilations shall be supplemented or revised as often as necessary.

(b) Compilations shall be made available upon request to [agencies and officials of this State] free of charge and to other persons at prices fixed by the [Secretary of State] to cover mailing and publication costs.]

[SECTION 27. [*Petition for Adoption of Rules.*] An interested person may petition the director requesting the adoption, amendment, or repeal of a rule. The director shall prescribe by rule the form for petitions and the procedure for their submission, consideration, and disposition. Within 30 days after submission of a petition, the director either shall deny the petition in writing (stating his reasons for the denial) or shall initiate rule-making proceedings in accordance with the provisions on procedure for adoption of rules (section 24).]

[SECTION 28. [*Declaratory Judgment on Validity or Applicability of Rules.*]

The validity or applicability of a rule may be determined in an action for declaratory judgment in the [. . . court] if it is alleged that the rule, or its threatened application, interferes with or impairs, or threatens to interfere with or impair, the legal rights or privileges of the plaintiff. The director shall be made a party to the action. A declaratory judgment may be rendered whether or not the plaintiff has requested the director to pass upon the validity or applicability of the rule in question.]

[SECTION 29. [*Declaratory Rulings by Director.*]

The director shall provide by rule for the filing and prompt disposition of petitions of declaratory rulings as to the applicability of any statutory provision or of any rule of the director. Rulings disposing of petitions have the same status as decisions or orders in contested cases.]

[SECTION 30. [*Contested Cases; Notice; Hearing; Records.*]

(a) In a contested case, all parties shall be afforded an opportunity for hearing after reasonable notice.

(b) The notice shall include:

(1) a statement of the time, place, and nature of the hearing;

(2) a statement of the legal authority and jurisdiction under which the hearing is to be held;

(3) a reference to the particular provisions of the statutes and rules involved;

(4) a short and plain statement of the matters asserted. If the director or other party is unable to state the matters in detail at the time the notice is served, the initial notice may be limited to a statement of the issues involved. Thereafter upon

application a more definite and detailed statement shall be furnished.

(c) Opportunity shall be afforded all parties to respond and present evidence and argument on all issues involved.

(d) Unless precluded by law, informal disposition may be made of any contested case by stipulation, agreed settlement, consent order, or default.

(e) The record in a contested case shall include:

(1) all pleadings, motions, intermediate rulings;

(2) evidence received or considered;

(3) a statement of matters officially noticed;

(4) questions and offers of proof, objections, and rulings thereon;

(5) proposed findings and exceptions;

(6) any decision, opinion, or report by the officer presiding at the hearing;

(7) all staff memoranda or data submitted to the hearing officer or members of the office of the administrator in connection with their consideration of the case.

(f) Oral proceedings or any part thereof shall be transcribed on request of any party [, but at his expense].

(g) Findings of fact shall be based exclusively on the evidence and on matters officially noticed.]

[SECTION 31. [*Rules of Evidence; Official Notice.*]
In contested cases:

(1) irrelevant, immaterial, or unduly repetitious evidence shall be excluded. The rules of evidence as applied in [non-jury] civil cases in the [. . . court of this State] shall be followed. When necessary to ascertain facts not reasonably susceptible of proof under those rules, evidence not admissible thereunder may be admitted (except where precluded by statute) if it is of a type commonly relied upon by reasonably prudent men in the conduct of their affairs. The director shall give effect to the rules of privilege recognized by law. Objections to evidentiary offers may be made and shall be noted in the record. Subject to these requirements, when a hearing will be expedited and the interests of the parties will not be prejudiced substantially, any part of the evidence may be received in written form;

(2) documentary evidence may be received in the form of copies or excerpts, if the original is not readily available. Upon request, parties shall be given an opportunity to compare the copy with the original;

(3) a party may conduct cross-examinations required for a full and true disclosure of the facts;

(4) notice may be taken of judicially cognizable facts. In addition, notice may be taken of generally recognized technical or scientific facts within the director's specialized knowledge. Parties shall be notified either before or during the hearing, or by reference in preliminary reports or otherwise, of the material notices, including any staff memoranda or data, and they shall be afforded an opportunity to contest the material so noticed. The director's experience, technical competence, and specialized knowledge may be utilized in the evaluation of the evidence.]

[SECTION 32. [*Decisions and Orders.*]

A final decision or order adverse to a party in a contested case shall be in writing or stated in the record. A final decision shall include findings of fact and conclusions of law, separately stated. Findings of fact, if set forth in statutory language, shall be accompanied by a concise and explicit statement of the underlying facts supporting the findings. If, in accordance with rules of the director, a party submitted proposed findings of fact, the decision shall include a ruling upon each proposed finding. Parties shall be notified either personally or by mail of any decision or order. Upon request a copy of the decision or order shall be delivered or mailed forthwith to each party and to his attorney of record.]

[SECTION 33. [*Judicial Review of Contested Cases.*]

(a) A person who has exhausted all administrative remedies available before the director and who is aggrieved by a final decision in a contested case is entitled to judicial review under this part. This section does not limit utilization of or the scope of judicial review available under other means of review, redress, relief, or trial *de novo* provided by law. A preliminary, procedural, or intermediate action or ruling of the director is immediately reviewable if review of the final decision of the director would not provide an adequate remedy.

(b) Proceedings for review are instituted by filing a petition in the [. . . court] within [30] days after [mailing notice of] the final decision of the director or, if a rehearing is requested within [30] days after the decision thereon. Copies of the petition shall be served upon the director and all parties of record.

(c) The filing of the petition does not itself stay enforcement of the decision of the director. The director may grant, or the reviewing court may order, a stay upon appropriate terms.

(d) Within [30] days after the service of the petition, or within further time allowed by the court, the director shall transmit to the reviewing court the original or a certified copy of the entire record of the proceeding under review. By stipulation of all parties to the review proceedings, the record may be shortened. A party unreasonably refusing to stipulate to limit the record may be taxed by the court for the additional costs. The court may require or permit subsequent corrections or additions to the record.

(e) If, before the date set for hearing, application is made to the court for leave to present additional evidence, and it is shown to the satisfaction of the court that the additional evidence is material and that there were good reasons for failure to present it in the proceeding before the director, the court may order that the additional evidence be taken before the director upon conditions determined by court. The director may modify his findings and decision by reason of the additional evidence and any modifications, new findings, or decisions with the reviewing court.

(f) The review shall be conducted by the court without a jury, and shall be confined to the record. In cases of alleged irregularities in procedure before the director, not shown in the record, proof thereon may be taken in the court. The court, upon request, shall hear oral argument and receive written briefs.

(g) The court shall not substitute its judgment for that of the director as to the weight of the evidence on questions of fact. The court may affirm the decision of the director or remand the case for further proceedings. The court may reverse or modify the decision if substantial rights of the appellant have been prejudiced because the administrative findings, inferences, conclusions, or decisions are:

(1) in violation of constitutional or statutory provisions;

(2) in excess of the statutory authority of the director;

(3) made upon unlawful procedure;

(4) affected by other error of law;

(5) clearly erroneous in view of the reliable, probative, and substantial evidence on the whole record; or

(6) arbitrary or capricious or characterized by abuse of discretion or clearly unwarranted exercise of discretion.]

[SECTION 34. [*Appeals.*] An aggrieved party may obtain a review of any final judgment of the [. . . court] under this part by appeal to the [. . . court] . The appeal shall be taken as in other civil cases.]

SECTION 35. [*Short Title*] This Act may be cited as the Uniform Alcoholism and Intoxication Treatment Act.

SECTION 36. [*Application and Construction.*] This Act shall be so applied and construed as to effectuate its general purpose to make uniform the law with respect to the subject of this Act among those States which enact it.

SECTION 37. [*Repeal.*] The following Acts and parts of Acts are repealed:

(1)

(2)

(3)

SECTION 38. [*Effective Date.*] This Act shall become effective [90] days after its passage.

APPENDIX B

ALCOHOLISM – TO HEAL AND NOT TO PUNISH

by John N. Mitchell,* Attorney-General of the United States

It is a privilege to be asked to participate in this banquet honoring Brinkley Smithers. I have known and admired him for many years, and I am delighted to be able to say so to this audience tonight. I'm also pleased to bring him the good wishes of the President of the United States, who is thoroughly aware and appreciative of his leadership in the movement to control alcoholism.

I believe it is fair to say that no person in the history of this movement has approached Brinkley Smithers in the generosity of his support. Through the Christopher D. Smithers Foundation, which he founded in honor of his father in 1952, he has made repeated gifts to this cause over the past two decades.

Last July he made a personal grant of $10 million to Roosevelt Hospital in New York City for treatment and rehabilitation of alcoholics. This is the largest single gift ever made in this field, and I do not except even the various grants made in recent years by the Federal Government. I must confess that when I first read about this magnificent grant I thought some typesetter might have inadvertently added a cipher or two. It is a most extraordinary example of dedication to a cause, even by the generous standards of Brinkley Smithers.

237

Nor have the contributions of our honored guest been confined to financial values. He has given just as unstintingly of his own time and energies. If you read a list of the national and New York organizations to combat alcoholism, you will almost be reading a list of the organizations that he has founded or headed.

So I must say tonight, without fear of contradiction in this assembly of experts on the subject, that among the many world leaders in the crusade against alcoholism, no one casts a longer shadow than Brinkley Smithers.

The other reason I am happy to be here is that it gives me the chance to talk about an aspect of alcoholism that I feel needs to be addressed by a law enforcement official.

Alcoholism Is an Illness

I refer to the fact, acknowledged now by all professionals in the field, that alcoholism as such is not a legal problem—it is a health problem. More especially, simple drunkenness *per se* should not be handled as an offense subject to the processes of justice. It should be handled as an illness, subject to medical treatment.

Now, this may seem fairly obvious to most of you here in this room who are thoroughly informed on this subject. But it is not generally recognized throughout the country.

In all but a few of the States in the Union, public drunkenness is an offense punishable by a fine or jail sentence or both.

In other words, our knowledge in the field far surpasses our action. The result is that in most of the cases which come to public attention, a major disease is not being treated by doctors, therapists, or medical technicians. The disease is being treated by policemen, judges, and jailers.

This is no reproach to the latter group of professionals, many of whom know from distressing experience that this system is wrong. It is a serious misuse of their time, abilities, and resources. It is likewise a failure to use the skills of the medical practitioners who are the ones qualified for this work. And it is a desperate injustice to the victims of the disease.

I feel strongly about this situation partly because of its unnecessary drain on the resources of the criminal justice system. At least one-third of all arrests in the United States are for public drunkenness. In some cities, the proportion runs as high as three-fourths. The commitment of police on the street and for processing at the station house, the commitment of jail space and facilities, the commitment of time by judges, court administrators, and courtrooms—all this constitutes an enormous drain on a justice system that is already overtaxed by felony cases. This misuse of tax-supported resources is bad enough, and constitutes a problem crying out for solution.

Wrong Solution to Problem

But still more important is the fact that this system is absolutely ineffective as a lesson or deterrent. Those who have witnessed the arraignment of drunk arrests in the lower courts of any large city can testify that it is, indeed, a revolving door. A study in Los Angeles showed that in a given year, about one-fifth of the people arrested for drunkenness accounted for two-thirds of the total drunk arrests. In one typical case in another city, a homeless alcoholic was arrested every other day that he appeared on the street over a 4-month period.

The so-called "drying out" accomplished during such overnight jail terms has not, to anyone's knowledge, ever reformed an alcoholic. It has often, however, contributed further to any health infirmity he might have been suffering from, and has demeaned him still further with overcrowded conditions devoid of the barest human facilities.

In the process, it has also demeaned the courts and the administration of American justice. Drunk arrests in big cities are often, if not usually, brought before the judge *en masse*—10 to 20 at a time. The typical defendant is almost never represented by counsel, which means that the procedures are often perfunctory, without any real consideration of guilt or innocence.

It is not surprising that many, if not most of the policemen and judges involved, know full well that this system is a distortion of legal processes. But in most localities they also know that it is all we have for dealing with public alcoholism. They therefore tend to develop a benevolent paternalism toward their charges—taking care of them the best they can within the limits of their authority and resources. It would be the same if the police and the judges were forced by law to take care of accident victims; as compassionate human beings they would do their best, but they could not help knowing that the system was senseless.

239

Public's Right to Know

So we cannot blame the police or the courts for the system, and in many cases we must commend them for making the best of a bad situation. The blame must be faced by the public at large, which after all is the master of its own government. And if the public is unaware of this gross injustice, then it is the public that needs to be educated.

Fortunately, as many of you know, progress has been made in recent years. In 1966 the District of Columbia Circuit of the United States Court of Appeals ruled in the *Easter* case that the public drunkenness of a homeless alcoholic was involuntary. Therefore he could not be held accountable before the law. In the same year another Appellate Court made a somewhat similar ruling in the *Driver* case.

In 1967 the United States Supreme Court heard a similar case—*Powell v. Texas*. While it ruled that the defendant was accountable for being drunk in public because he did have a home to go to, a majority of the justices also expressed an opinion that coincided with that of the two Appellate decisions—that a homeless alcoholic is not accountable for his act.

The important point is that the courts have decided what the experts had been saying for years—that alcoholism in itself is involuntary and therefore is not a legal offense in the ordinary sense.

Unfortunately, these cases have not been heeded as they should be, and the constitutionality of the related laws in most States has not been challenged.

Not a Criminal Offense

However, the court rulings were taken into account by two commissions investigating the criminal justice system—the District of Columbia Crime Commission and the United States Crime Commission. They both reported in 1967 that public intoxication should be treated by public health services rather than as a criminal offense.

In turn, these recommendations influenced Congressional thinking, and new laws were forthcoming to establish this change of policy in the District of Columbia and encourage it in the States. Thoroughly associated with much of this legislation is the name of Senator Harold E. Hughes of Iowa, who of course is with us tonight. Among other things, the latest Federal legislation established an Institute on Alcohol Abuse and Alcoholism within the Department of Health, Education, and Welfare. President Nixon has shown his deep interest in this organization by asking for and receiving from Congress an additional $7 million of health initiative funds for its work.

At the same time, the court cases and the Crime Commission recommendations have been noticed by the legislatures of a few States. They have changed their laws to provide for health treatment of one kind or another, and some of them have repealed the legal sanctions against alcoholism. But the rest of the States and most of the localities have not yet responded, although some legislatures are considering the matter. Throughout most of the country, the situation remains as archaic as ever.

In fact, even in some States where the approach has been changed, new questions have arisen.

Current Factors

What is the role of a policeman?

If he can no longer make a drunk arrest, can he forcibly remove a subject to a health care center?

If the subject cannot be incarcerated, can he be committed to any kind of treatment against his will?

Fortunately, answers to some of these questions have recently been offered by several commissions that have carefully drawn up and proposed model State laws on the subject. The latest and most important is the work of the National Conference of Commissioners on Uniform State Laws, which adopted a Uniform Alcoholism and Intoxication Treatment Act last August. Among many other provisions are the following:

First, a person appearing to be incapacitated by alcohol must be taken into protective custody—not an arrest—by the police or a special emergency service patrol. He is to be taken to a public health facility for emergency treatment.

Second, if the subject has inflicted physical harm on another or may do so, he may be committed for emergency treatment for up to 5 days on the certificate of an independent physician.

Third, for a longer period up to 30 days, and with extensions for a maximum of 7 months, his commitment must be made by a court.

So as a result of developments in the past 5 years, we have made several important strides.

We have won an opinion from the courts that alcoholism in itself is involuntary and should not be subject to legal sanction.

We have secured legislation by Congress and by a few States supporting this principle and establishing civil medical treatment as an alternative.

We have a carefully drawn uniform law on the subject that can serve as a model for the States. And I would note the fact that the commission drawing up this act is composed of a representative from each State, and he is obligated to see that the act is introduced in his legislature.

Finally, we have gained enough experience from the operation of forward-looking laws in the District of Columbia and some of the States to uncover some sound operating principles.

Range of Medical Services

For instance, we know that it does little good to remove alcoholism from the purview of the law if you do not substitute a full-dress medical treatment—not only a detoxification process, but a thoroughgoing program aimed at recovery from the illness of alcoholism.

Again, the program must include the closest cooperation and communication, starting at the top level between the public health officials and law enforcement officials. The police must have an understanding that their role continues—not in an arresting capacity, but in one of helping subjects to the designated health center, voluntarily if possible, involuntarily if necessary.

Finally, the program must make a strong appeal to voluntary enrollment. We know that the street alcoholic who in the past has been the subject of most drunk arrests actually represents only from 3 percent to 5 percent of the alcoholics in this country— what we might call the tip of the iceberg. We know that some of the others who may still be living in a home environment do account for many of the arrests—perhaps one-third, as the Los Angeles survey seems to indicate. It is not only to these, but to the many more who are not arrested, that the civil treatment program must appeal if we are to reach the rest of the iceberg.

With these kinds of guidelines, and with the opportunities we now see ahead, we can perhaps venture some real hope in a field that for too long has been marked by frustration. Through the

242

processes now at work, the public itself may come to realize that our task is not to punish, but to heal. And in such a climate of belief, the work of people like Brinkley Smithers will be assisted, not by a relative few, but by all.

About the Author

Louise Bailey Burgess has always had a sensitive social conscience, especially concerning children. She has strong faith that life has meaning and purpose; that a more humane and caring generation is slowly but surely evolving. As the mother of grown sons, she returned to the University of Minnesota after her husband's death, and received a B.A., cum laude, in Child Welfare and Parent Education to add to her degree in Library Science from Western Reserve University. She later did graduate work in Family Life at the University of Chicago. Mrs. Burgess received national recognition as well as the first award in the State of Minnesota for her "Creed for Happier Family Living."

For nine years Mrs. Burgess wrote a weekly newspaper column entitled, *Let's Be Better*. She has had many articles published in national magazines, and is the author of three books: The first text book on Philately, based on the first university course in this subject taught by her husband; a compilation of her columns titled, *Let's Be Better*, and an autobiographical novel, *This Side of the Stars*.

As organizer and counselor for family life groups for over forty years, Mrs. Burgess saw the waste of human potential, the tragedies and heartbreak, and the broken homes caused by the use of beverage alcohol. As she started to collect facts and statistics on the subject, the realization that alcohol was actually the most widely used addictive drug in this country led to the publication of *Alcohol and Your Health*.